Handbook of Drug Allergy

CW01502282

Richard W. Honsinger, M.D., M.A.C.P., F.A.A.A.A.I., F.A.C.A.A.I., F.C.C.P.
*Professor of Medicine
School of Medicine
University of New Mexico;
Member, Board of Directors
American Academy of Allergy, Asthma, and Immunology;
Practicing Physician
Los Alamos, New Mexico*

George R. Green, M.D., F.A.C.P., F.A.A.A.A.I., F.A.C.A.A.I.
*Chief, Division of Allergy and Immunology
Department of Medicine
Abington Memorial Hospital
Abington, Pennsylvania;
Adjunct Professor of Medicine
School of Medicine
University of Pennsylvania
Philadelphia, Pennsylvania;
Delegate to the American Academy Medical Association
representing the
American Academy of Allergy, Asthma, and Immunology*

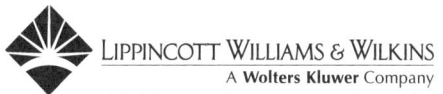

LIPPINCOTT WILLIAMS & WILKINS
A **Wolters Kluwer** Company
Philadelphia • Baltimore • New York • London
Buenos Aires • Hong Kong • Sydney • Tokyo

Acquisitions Editor: James Merritt
Developmental Editor: Stacey L. Baze
Production Editor: Jeff Somers
Manufacturing Manager: Colin Warnock
Cover Designers: Dennise and Amanda Trujillo
Compositor: TechBooks
Printer: R.R. Donnelley, Crawfordsville

© 2004 by LIPPINCOTT WILLIAMS & WILKINS
530 Walnut Street
Philadelphia, PA 19106 USA
LWW.com

Printed in the USA

Library of Congress Cataloging-in-Publication Data

Honsinger, Richard W.
 Handbook of drug allergy / editors, Richard W. Honsinger, George R. Green.
   p. ; cm.
   Includes bibliographical references and index.
   ISBN 0-7817-3934-9 (alk. paper)
   1. Drug allergy—Handbooks, manuals, etc.   2. Drug Hypersensitivity—Handbooks.   I. Honsinger, Richard W.   II. Title
   [DNLM: 1. Drug allergy—Handbooks, manuals, etc.   2. Drug Hypersensitivity—Handbooks. WD 301 H2363 2004]
   RC598. D7 H36   2004
   616.97/58 22   2003060251

Care has been taken to confirm the accuracy of the information presented and to describe generally accepted practices. However, the authors, editors and publisher are not responsible for errors or omissions or for any consequences from application of the information in this book and make no warranty, expressed or implied, with respect to the currency, completeness, or accuracy of the contents of the publication. Application of this information in a particular situation remains the professional responsibility of the practitioner.

The authors, editors and publisher have exerted every effort to ensure that drug selection and dosage set forth in this text are in accordance with current recommendations and practice at the time of publication. However, in view of ongoing research, changes in government regulations, and the constant flow of information relating to drug therapy and drug reactions, the reader is urged to check the package insert for each drug for any change in indications and dosage and for added warnings and precautions. This is particularly important when the recommended agent is a new or infrequently employed drug.

Some drugs and medical devices presented in this publication have Food and Drug Administration (FDA) clearance for limited use in restricted research settings. It is the responsibility of the health care provider to ascertain the FDA status of each drug or device planned for use in their clinical practice.

10 9 8 7 6 5 4 3 2 1

Handbook of Drug Allergy

*To Marian Honsinger and Trudy Green,
who have been supportive of our devotion to
medicine for over 40 years of marriage.*

Contents

Part 3. Special Situations and Other Issues

Contributing Authors

N. Franklin Adkinson, Jr., M. D., *Professor of Medicine, Johns Hopkins Asthma and Allergy Center, Johns Hopkins School of Medicine, Baltimore, Maryland*

Olga Bessmertny, Pharm. D., *Clinical Pharmacist, Department of Pediatric Oncology, Blood and Marrow Transplant, New York Presbyterian Hospital, New York, New York*

Leonard Bielory, M. D., *Professor, Department of Medicine, Pediatrics, and Ophthalmology, UMDNJ-New Jersey Medical School, Newark, New Jersey*

Craig F. Donatucci, M. D., *Associate Professor, Department of Surgery, Division of Urology, Duke University Medical Center, Durham, North Carolina*

Khaled M. El-Jazzar, M. D., *Senior Cardiology Fellow, Department of Cardiology, The George Washington University Medical Center, Washington, D.C.*

Adam Stuart Evans, *Medical Student, Jefferson Medical College, Philadelphia, Pennsylvania*

Mary Rachel Faris, M. D., *Rosenfeld Cancer Center, Abington Memorial Hospital, Abington, Pennsylvania*

Malcolm M. Fisher, M. D., MBChB, FJFICM, FANZCA, FRCA, *Clinical Professor, Departments of Anaesthesia and Medicine, University of Sydney, New South Wales, Australia*

Whitney S. Goldner, M. D., *Endocrinology Fellow, Department of Internal Medicine, Division of Endocrinology, University of Iowa Hospitals and Clinics, Iowa City, Iowa*

Frank M. Graziano, M. D., Ph. D., *Professor of Medicine, Department of Medicine, University of Wisconsin Hospital and Clinics, Madison, Wisconsin*

George R. Green, M. D., *Adjunct Professor of Medicine, University of Pennsylvania, Philadelphia; Chief, Allergy and Immunology Division, Abington Medical Hospital, Abington, Pennsylvania*

Paul A. Greenberger, M. D., *Professor of Medicine, Division of Allergy-Immunology, Department of Medicine, Northwestern University Feinberg School of Medicine, Chicago, Illinois*

Paul R. Gross, M. D., *Clinical Professor, Department of Dermatology, University of Pennsylvania School of Medicine, Philadelphia, Pennsylvania*

John B. Hagan, M. D., *Assistant Professor of Medicine, Division of Allergic Diseases and Internal Medicine, Mayo Clinic and Foundation, Rochester, Minnesota*

Richard Honsinger, M. D., *Clinical Professor of Medicine, University of New Mexico, Los Alamos, New Mexico*

Daniel E. Hutter, M. D., *Assistant Professor, Department of Ophthalmology and Visual Sciences, University of Wisconsin, Madison, Wisconsin*

Kimberly S. Jones, Pharm. D., *Clinical Pharmacist, Department of Pharmacy, Duke University Medical Center, Durham, North Carolina*

Renata Joffe, M. D., *Resident, Federal University of Rio de Janeiro, Rio de Janeiro, Brazil*

Kevin J. Kelly, M. D., *Professor of Pediatrics and Medicine, Department of Allergy and Immunology, Medical College of Wisconsin, Milwaukee, Wisconsin*

John M. Kelso, M. D., *Allergy Division, Naval Medical Center, San Diego, California*

Emmanuelle Lévy, M. D., F.R.C.P.(C), *Clinical Research Fellow, Department of Psychiatry, Clinical Psychopharmacology Unit, McGill University Health Centre, Montreal, Canada*

James T. Li, M. D., Ph. D., *Professor of Medicine, Divisions of Allergic Diseases and Internal Medicine, Mayo Clinic and Foundation, Rochester, Minnesota*

Richard Lockey, M. D., *Professor of Medicine, Pediatrics & Public Health, Joy McCann Culverhouse Chair in Allergy and Immunology; Director, Division of Allergy and Immunology, Department of Internal Medicine, University of South Florida College of Medicine and James A. Haley Veterans' Hospital, Tampa, Florida*

Margaret M. Lowery, M. D., *Division of Allergy-Immunology, Department of Medicine, Northwestern University Feinberg School of Medicine, Chicago, Illinois*

Omar Lupi, M. D., M. Sc., Ph. D., *Professor of Dermatology, Department of Medical Clinics (Dermatology), Federal University of Rio de Janeiro, Rio de Janeiro, Brazil*

Maria Fernanda Malaman, M. D., *Post Graduate Student, University of São Paulo Medical School; Assistant Physician, Department of Allergy and Immunology, State Public Server Hospital, São Paulo, Brazil*

Howard C. Margolese, M. D., C. M., F. R. C. P. (C), *Assistant Professor, Department of Psychiatry, Clinical Psychopharmacology Unit, McGill University Health Centre, Montreal, Canada*

David B. Nash, M. D., M. B. A., *Professor of Health Policy and Medicine, Jefferson Medical College, Philadelphia, Pennsylvania*

Bill K. Nika, M. D., *Assistant Professor of Family Medicine, Department of Family and Community Medicine, University of Illinois at Chicago College of Medicine, Rockford, Illinois*

Tony Ogburn, M. D., *Associate Professor, Department of Obstetrics and Gynecology, University of New Mexico School of Medicine, Albuquerque, New Mexico*

Jill A. Poole, M. D., *Fellow, Department of Allergy, Asthma, and Immunology, National Jewish Medical and Research Center, Denver, Colorado*

Ganesh V. Raj, M. D., Ph. D., *Chief Resident in Urology, Department of Surgery, Duke University Medical Center, Durham, North Carolina*

John Redmond, III, M. D., *Rosenfeld Cancer Center, Abington Memorial Hospital, Abington, Pennsylvania*

Lauren M. Robitaille, Pharm. D., *Clinical Pharmacist, Neonatal Intensive Care Unit, New York Presbyterian Hospital, New York, New York*

Lanny J. Rosenwasser, M. D., FAAAAI, *Professor of Medicine, Marjorie and Stephen Raphael Chair in Asthma Research, Department of Allergy, Asthma, and Immunology, National Jewish Medical and Research Center, Denver, Colorado*

Bradley B. Rowberry, M. D., *Department of Gastroenterology, Los Alamos Medical Center, Los Alamos, New Mexico*

Janet Ann Schlechte, M. D., *Professor, Department of Internal Medicine, Division of Endocrinology, University of Iowa Hospitals and Clinics, Iowa City, Iowa*

Reem A. Shalabi, Pharm. D., *Clinical Pharmacy Specialist—Bone Marrow Transplant, Clinical Center Pharmacy Department, National Institutes of Health, Bethesda, Maryland*

Gary Simpson, M.D., *Infectious Disease Bureau, State of New Mexico Health Department, Santa Fe, New Mexico*

Frederica E. Smith, M.D., *Los Alamos Medical Center, Los Alamos, New Mexico*

James H. Sussman, M.D., *Department of Pulmonology and Allergy, Los Alamos Medical Center, Los Alamos, New Mexico*

Stephen J. Tai, M.Sc., *Medical Student, Jefferson Medical College, Philadelphia, Pennsylvania*

Bruce D. Tempest, M.D., *Department of Internal Medicine, Gallup Indian Medical Center, Gallup, New Mexico*

Gisela Torres, M.D., *Clinical Research Fellow, Department of Microbiology and Immunology, Center for Clinical Studies, University of Texas Medical Branch, Houston, Texas*

Stephen K. Tyring, M.D., Ph.D., *Professor of Microbiology and Immunology, Dermatology and Internal Medicine; Director, Center for Clinical Studies, University of Texas Medical Branch-Galveston, Houston, Texas*

Andrew W. Urban, M.D., *Clinical Associate Professor, Department of Medicine, Section of Infectious Diseases, William S. Middleton VA Medical Center, Madison, Wisconsin*

Howard T. Wadstrom, M.D., *Clinical Associate Professor, Department of Obstetrics and Gynecology, University of New Mexico School of Medicine, Albuquerque, New Mexico*

Thomas J. Walsh, M.D., *Chief, Immunocompromised Host Section, Pediatric Oncology Branch, National Cancer Institute, Bethesda, Maryland*

Alan G. Wasserman, M.D., *Eugene Meyer Professor of Medicine, Chairman, Department of Medicine, The George Washington University Medical Center, Washington, D.C.*

Ralph C. Williams Jr., M.D., *Professor Emeritus, University of Florida, Gainesville, Florida*

Anthony M. Yurchak, M.D., *Clinical Assistant Professor of Medicine, Department of Medicine, SUNY at Buffalo, Buffalo, New York*

Burton Zweiman, M.D., *Professor of Medicine and Neurology, Department of Medicine, University of Pennsylvania Medical Center, Philadelphia, Pennsylvania*

Monib Zirvi, M.D., Ph.D., *Resident Physician, Department of Dermatology, University of Pennsylvania, Philadelphia, Pennsylvania*

Foreword

It is timely to write an introduction for the *Handbook of Drug Allergy* edited by my two colleagues, Richard Honsinger and George Green, because there are few books on drug allergy, and none is as complete as their review of the subject. It is fortunate to have this book available, since adverse reactions and allergic reactions are so common among our patients. There are many adverse reactions to drugs that are not truly allergic. True allergic reactions are extremely important because they are potentially the most dangerous to the patient.

Physicians of all specialties struggle with the problem of adverse reactions to drugs and drug allergy. It is among the essential aspects of medical history taking: First, to elicit an appropriate history of an adverse reaction to a drug, and second, to appropriately avoid prescribing the offending drug or a related drug. Too often, nurses and physicians incorrectly identify an adverse reaction as an allergy. Such a classification inappropriately limits a patient's access to a drug or group of drugs essential to their well being.

The utility of this book is that it is useful not only for allergists/immunologists but for all physicians. For allergists/immunologists, it is especially valuable for two reasons: The complexity and lack of knowledge about drug allergy; and the problem of diagnosis and treatment of drug allergy when a patient's life often depends on the administration of a drug to which the patient is allergic. Those of us experienced with managing drug reactions may be called for an urgent consultation because a patient is "allergic" to a medication that he or she needs. Examples abound, such as methotrexate, cyclosporin, tacrolimus, and many others. All too often, case reports are the only source of information about a rare drug allergy.

Part I of the book deals with the most commonly prescribed group that can cause allergic reactions, the antibiotics. Antituberculous, antivirals, antifungals, and antiparasitic drugs are reviewed in separate chapters.

Part II covers the major specialties concerned with drug allergy, from allergy/immunology, anesthesiology, cardiology, dermatology, gastroenterology, psychiatry, and others. There are also chapters on allergic reactions to vaccines and antivenoms and vitamins.

Part III discusses various special topics, including genetically engineered drugs, the approach to patients with multiple drug allergies, when to refer to a specialist, documentation and reporting, and the economic impact of adverse drug reactions.

All in all, this is an extraordinarily complete book written by well-known authors who are experts in their respective fields.

The book will be an outstanding addition to medical libraries and will be useful for all physicians. As for colleagues in the specialty of allergy and immunology, it will be welcomed by necessity and importance.

Richard F. Lockey, M.D.
Professor of Medicine, Pediatrics & Public Health
Joy McCann Culverhouse Chair in Allergy and Immunology
Director, Division of Allergy and Immunology
Department of Internal Medicine
University of South Florida College of Medicine and
James A. Haley Veterans' Hospital
Tampa, Florida

Introduction

The development and release of medications has increased rapidly over the last 50 years. Adverse drug reactions have paralleled this increase in drug availability and usage. The approval and surveillance of new drugs by the Food and Drug Administration does not eliminate the problem of adverse drug reactions that are often only apparent after repeated use by a large number of patients. Most physicians are only familiar with the adverse drug reaction profiles of the drugs that they commonly use.

This handbook is meant to provide a clinical perspective on the adverse drug reaction profiles of a wide range of medications. Chapters are written by practicing specialists who are familiar with the adverse drug reaction profiles of the medications used in their specialties. We do not intend to list all side effects, which may be subject to individual variation. Nor do we intend to list toxicity related to dosage or impaired metabolism or excretion.

The users of this handbook will be both generalists and specialists who need a source of information on adverse drug reactions to a wide range of medications. This will not be a laundry list of all potential adverse drug reactions, as this is already available in the *Physicians' Desk Reference* (PDR) and pharmacology texts. This handbook will focus on **allergic** (immune-related) and **idiosyncratic** (pseudoallergic) adverse drug reactions. The focus will be clinical rather than mechanistic.

The authors will indicate whether there are contraindications to the drug use, and categorize the reaction discussed as being relatively common (C) for that drug, rare (R) but characteristic for that drug, or unlikely (U) where there are few isolated reports that possibly only implicate the drug.

Table 1.

C	Relatively **Common** for drug
R	**Rare,** but characteristic for drug
U	**Unlikely** as isolated reports only implicate drug

We have classified adverse drug reactions into two categories, allergic and idiopathic:

I. Allergic (Immune-Related) Reactions
  A. Prior exposure to the drug or similar agent required for sensitization.
  B. Minute doses may cause severe reactions.
  C. Sensitization may be temporary or life-long.
  D. Several immune mechanisms are common.[*]
    1. Type I Reaction. "IgE antibody" specifically bound and excited by drug, hapten, or metabolite of a drug which often requires binding through serum proteins
      a. Prior sensitization required.

---

[*] For simplicity we have used the classical established Gel and Coombs classification, although more recent systems may be more extensive.

b. Rapid onset of action due to release of pre-formed mediators from mast cells.

c. Skin tests with wheal and flare reaction will be diagnostic if the appropriate antigen is available.

d. Most common reactions include anaphylaxis, angioneurotic edema, urticaria, and other rashes. Laryngeal edema, bronchospasm, gastrointestinal motility, uterine cramping, and hypotension may also occur.

e. Desensitization is possible by gradually increasing the dose and achieving antibody exhaustion.

f. Examples: penicillin (hapten), horse serum, egg protein, insulin. Administration causes excitation of IgE on mast cells with release of mediators and resultant immediate reaction.

2. Type II Reaction. Antigen antibody complex mediated reactions

a. Prior sensitization required.

b. Usually large amounts of immunoglobulin G or immunoglobulin M antibody present.

c. Reaction can occur rapidly.

d. Complement frequently involved.

e. Metabolic product of drug may be the relevant antigen.

f. Hematologic cells are often the target.

g. Manifestations include hemolytic anemia, leukopenia, thrombocytopenia, and drug fever.

h. Desensitization is complicated by immune complex reactions.

i. Example: Penicillin-induced hemolysis. Penicillin-specific IgG antibody reacts with membrane-fixed penicillin causing membrane damage.

3. Type III Reaction. Cytotoxic action.

a. Drug metabolite combined with a tissue protein acts as the relevant antigen.

b. Complement often involved.

c. Some forms of nephritis and vasculitis may involve this mechanism.

d. Desensitization may occasionally be possible.

e. Usually a latent phase between drug (antigen) introduction and onset of symptoms.

f. Example: A drug or drug metabolite interacts with a carrier protein to form a drug antibody complex. This attaches to a red blood cell membrane and fixes complement. The antibody is most commonly IgM, but can be IgG or IgA. This occurs with hemolysis induced by paraminosalicylic acid (PAS) or phenacetin. A similar mechanism causes platelet destruction and immune thrombocytopenia, where quinine, quinidine, chlorthiaziade, and digitoxin can be the culprits.

4. Type IV Reaction. Sensitized lymphocyte mediated.

a. Delayed reaction with frequently a 24–48 hour delay before clinical reaction occurs.

b. Lipid, heavy metals, or other chemicals are frequently the relevant allergen.

c. Dermal reactions such as contact dermatitis as well as pulmonary fibrosis and erythema may involve this mechanism.

d. Although desensitization may be possible, delayed adverse reactions can be severe such as Stevens Johnson Syndrome[#].

e. Example: Delayed Skin Rash to Para Amino Benzoic Acid (PABA) in sunscreen.

5. Reactions may involve more than one separate immune type reaction. A drug may form complexes with cell proteins. The damaged cell may release DNA that causes autosensitization and drug-induced lupus erythematosus.

II. Idiosyncratic (Pseudoallergic) Reactions

A. Unexpected reactions that occur in certain patients but are characteristic for this drug.

B. Prior exposure to drug or similar agent is not required for sensitization.

C. No antibodies or immune mechanisms can be identified.

D. Reactions are often dosage related.

E. Reactions typically recur with re-exposure.

F. Tolerance can sometimes be developed (example: aspirin).

G. A number of mechanisms have been identified.

1. Genetic

a. Reactions may be genetically controlled, and are often related to an enzyme or metabolic pathway aberration.

b. Examples: Hemolytic anemia in Glucose-6-Phosphotase Deficiency (G6PD) with dapsone.

Prolonged post-surgical paralysis from curare with abnormal cholinesterase.

2. Mediator-induced

a. Vaso-active mediator release can occur without antibody involvement.

b. Examples: Iodinated contrast material.

Angiotensin converting enzyme inhibitors.

3. Pharmacologic

a. Adverse pharmacologic effect on abnormal organ.

b. Examples: Bronchospasm from beta-blocker or sulfite.

Mediator release from aspirin causing angioedema.

4. Allergic (like)

a. Mimic allergic reactions but no immune mechanism identified.

b. Examples: Rapid infusion of gammaglobulin, which has not been stabilized. Immunoglobulin aggregates bind complement and cause mediator release.

High molecular weight iodinated radio-contrast media induces mediator release.

Aspirin-induced asthma.

c. Jarisch-Herxheimer reaction often occurs with first treatment of spirochete infections. Although mechanism is unknown it is speculated to occur due to massive release of antigen. The malaise, rigors, and high fever can be followed by severe, and rarely fatal hypotension 2–24 hours

---

[#] A bullous form of erythema multiforme which involves mucous membranes. It may involve large areas of the body and can be fatal.

after antibiotic administration. Syphilitic skin lesions and neurologic symptoms may flare.

III. Manifestations and Mechanisms of Adverse Drug Reactions

   A. The Most Characteristic and Common Adverse Drug Reactions Involve the Skin

      1. Urticaria and/or angioedema are especially common allergic reactions.

      2. Contact dermatitis is obvious from pattern of distribution and history.

      3. Other dermal reactions also occur.

        a. Acanthosis nigricans

        b. Acneform lesions

        c. Acute generalized exanthematous pustulosis

        d. Alopecia

        e. Angioedema

        f. Aphthous stomatitis

        g. Black hairy tongue

        h. Bullous eruptions

        i. Contact Urticaria

        j. Erythema multiforme and Stevens-Johnson Syndrome (SJS)

        k. Erythema nodosum

        l. Exanthems

        m. Exfoliative dermatitis

        n. Lichenoid eruptions

        o. Lupus erythematous

        p. Maculopapular eruptions

        q. Onycholysis

        r. Photoallergic reactions

          (1) Phototoxic contact dermatitis such as exposure to coal tar

          (2) Phytophotodermatitis such as furocoumarins in plants

          (3) Persistent light reactivity

          (4) Sunscreen agents can cause contact dermatitis

        s. Pigmentation

        t. Pruritus

        u. Psoriasis

        v. Purpura

        w. Raynaud's phenomenon

        x. Toxic Epidermal Necrolysis (TEN)

   B. Almost any organ can be involved as the target of an adverse drug reaction.

      1. Central nervous system

      2. Eye

      3. Ear

      4. Pulmonary

      5. Cardiac

      6. Sciatic and other nerves

      7. GI

      8. Musculoskeletal

      9. Systemic

        a. Anaphylaxis

        b. Drug fever

   c. Vasculitis
  10. Dermatologic.
C. Hepatic Metabolism and Adverse Drug Reactions
  1. Many reactions to drugs are not due to classic types I-IV mechanisms but result from reactive metabolites produced by hepatic metabolism of the drug.
  2. Acetylation, hydroxylation, or glucuronidation generally leads to nontoxic metabolites.
  3. Cytochrome P450 oxidation metabolism may result in the production of toxic reactive intermediate compounds. Cytochrome P450 systems are present in the liver and the intestinal wall. These toxic reactive intermediate compounds are usually rapidly detoxified by other enzymes.
    a. Six isoenzymes are responsible for metabolism of most drugs.

Gene Family	Sub-family	Isoenzyme
CYP 1	A	2
CYP 2	C	9
	C	19
	D	6
	E	1
CYP 3	A	4

CYP 3A4 accounts for 30% of all cytochromes in the liver.
2C9 attracts acidic drugs.
3A4 attracts lipophilic drugs
  4. Other factors may affect hepatic drug metabolism
    a. Coincident administration of other drugs metabolized by the same isoenzyme. These may induce or inhibit the enzyme resulting in decreased or increased drug levels. For example, ketoconazole inhibits CYP3A4 almost totally; erythromycin inactivates the enzyme.
    b. Acetylator status - If a patient is a slow acetylator, an increased amount of drug may be metabolized by the cytochrome system. 90% of HIV+ patients are slow acetylators versus 55% of age-matched controls.
    c. Grapefruit juice inhibits intestinal cytochrome 3A4, but not hepatic cytochrome 3A4. This may increase levels of some drugs, especially statins.
    d. St. John's Wort activates a PXR receptor, which increases production of CYP3A4, thus decreasing serum concentrations of drugs metabolized by this isoenzyme.
  5. Reactive metabolite syndromes.
    a. Idiosyncratic. Mechanisms may be different. Fever, non-urticarial rash, lymphadenopathy, hepatic and renal involvement can occur.
    b. Sometimes only one organ is involved which may hinder making a diagnosis of a drug reaction.
    c. Most patients develop symptoms 2-6 weeks after starting the drug except for cefaclor and drug-induced lupus-like reactions. See 5.e. below.
    d. Sulfamethoxazole is oxidized to a reactive metabolite, a hydroxylamine; this may be further oxidized to a nitroso derivative. These metabolites may induce symptoms by

direct toxicity. To date, there is no evidence of a specific immune reaction. In addition to slow acetylation, some HIV+ patients are deficent in glutathione which functions to enhance metabolism of the reactive metabolite. At least 90% of HIV+ patients who have developed rash and fever with sulfamethoxisole, can tolerate readministration.

e. <u>Cefaclor and cefproxil.</u> Patients develop rashes, both urticarial and maculopapular, fever, and prominent arthralgias usually occuring 1–2 weeks after starting cefaclor. In contrast to true serum sickness, vasculitis and renal problems do not occur and there is no evidence of immune complexes. The incidence is 1% in children under 14 and 0.5% overall. The usual onset is 7–12 days after starting therapy. In the few cases where the patients have been rechallenged, 60% redevelop symptoms. This has been noted with cefaclor and cefproxil, but not loracarbef (similar structure) or other cephalosporins.

f. <u>Aromatic anticonvulsants which produce arene oxide, e.g. phenytoin, carbamazine, and phenobarbitol.</u> Usually occurs within first 2 months. 90% have skin rash, 50% develop hepatitis, nephritis or blood abnormalities. There is cross-reactivity among different anticonvulsants. Affected patients appear to have an inherited deficiency of epoxide hydrolase, the enzyme that breaks down the reactive intermediate metabolic product, an epoxide; it is unclear, however, if this is the mechanism responsible for clinical symptoms.

g. <u>Antiarrythmics (procainamide, quinidine), hydralazine, chlorpromazine, isoniazid, and propylthiouracil</u> can induce lupus-like symptoms. These usually present only after at least one year of treatment. Many patients develop a positive homogeneous ANA and antihistone antibodies, but no double-stranded DNA: Most of these patients do not develop clinical symptoms. The most common symptoms are fever, musculoskeletal and cardio-pulmonary symptoms. The responsible mechanism is not known, but may involve oxidative metabolism of the drugs via myeloperoxidase in neutrophils, rather than via hepatic metabolism.

h. Rechallenge–only for sulfamethoxazole.

i. Some parents of patients who have had reactions to sulfamethoxazole, cefaclor and aromatic anticonvulsants, have altered metabolism of the same drugs.

6. Drug-induced hepatic injury

a. Can mimic all hepatobiliary diseases.

b. Drugs cause less than 5% of cases of hepatitis, but they are an important cause of severe life-threatening hepatic injury.

7. Genetic predisposition to hepatic injury. For example, halothane hepatitis.

8. <u>Allergic hepatitis.</u>

a. Immune reaction to hepatocytes.

(1) Drug-protein conjugate may stimulate drug-specific antibody and T cells. Possible future diagnosis by documenting activated T cells via flow cytometry, lymphocyte transformation tests, or lymphocyte toxicity assays.

(2) Idiosyncratic hepatitis. Results from unusual metabolism of the drug and is usually not dose-dependent, e.g. valproate, NSAIDs, aspirin, isoniazid, minocycline.

9. Dose-dependent hepatic injury, e.g. acetaminophen-induced acute hepatotoxicity, methotrexate-induced hepatic fibrosis.

IV. Diagnosis

A. History is the most important diagnostic tool. The timing of drug administration and the onset of the reaction is the most important clue. A history of previous reactions to similar drugs can often be elicited. A drug that has been administered for years without cessation is less likely to produce an allergic reaction. A simple molecule or a substance that is found in the body does not often cause an immunologic response. Hormones rarely cause reactions. An allergic response to vitamins and minerals is very unlikely.

B. Skin Testing for specific drug allergy. Before any intradermal tests are applied an epicutaneous test should first be used ("allergists always scratch first"). There are several commercial devices available that prick the epidermis. As an alternative, a drop of the solution to be tested may be placed on the skin and the skin may be pricked through the drop with a needle. The needle needs to be inserted no more than 1 mm, pricking the epidermis by pulling up on the needle point. Testing on the back is more sensitive. However, the arm can be used if the patient is suspected of having a high degree of sensitivity; as a tourniquet can be placed above the skin test if a general reaction should ensue. The test site is observed for 20 minutes. A systemic reaction to an epicutaneous test is exceedingly rare.

An intradermal test can be applied only if the epicutaneous test is negative. A small needle is inserted into the skin at an angle that is only slightly greater than parallel. The needle bevel should be down. The smallest amount can be used to make a small wheal and is injected (less than 0.05 ml). The test site is observed for 20 minutes.

When nonstandardized antigens are used, tests should also be applied to a control subject (often the investigator). Neither subject nor control should have received an antihistamine within the previous 72 hours. A positive skin test with a standard antigen and with a negative control can be helpful. A positive skin test with a nonstandard antigen can be helpful when a control subject is negative. However, negative skin test with a nonstandard antigen may only mean that you do not have the active epitope or that your reaction is not immunoglobulin E mediated. Even when tests are negative, it is good clinical practice to observe the patients carefully when the first dose is administered.

C. Patch Testing. Assessment of delayed sensitivity to topical medications (contact allergy) is best assessed by patch testing. Standardized commercial antigens are available in the form of the Hermal True Test Kit. If an antigen is used that has not been standardized, it should first be applied to a control subject to exclude irritant response. The antigen is placed on an absorbent paper under an occlusive tape. The patch test is left in place for 48–72 hours unless a severe reaction mandates early removal. The patch test is then read for erythema and vesiculation . If the test reaction is severe, a topical corticosteroid may be used to suppress the reaction. Patients with contact allergy should not have patch tests applied when their allergic reaction is in an active phase as the patch testing may aggravate the reaction. Avoidance is the only therapy for prevention of a contact allergy reaction. Desensitization is not possible.

Table 2.   Scoring patch tests

?	*Doubtful* reaction	Faint macular erythema only
+	*Weak* (nonvesicular) positive	Erythema, infiltration, possibly papules
++	Strong (vesicular) positive	Erythema, infiltration, papules, vesicles
+++	*Extreme* positive	Bullous reaction
–	*Negative*	
IR	*Irritant*	
NT	*Not Tested*	
		From *Fisher's Contact Dermatitis*

    D.   *In vitro* assay is only available for a few antigens. It may be useful when skin testing cannot be performed. However the *in vitro* assays (RAST or ELISA) have generally been less sensitive than skin testing.

V.   Management of Adverse Drug Reactions
    A.   Discontinue suspect drug or drugs.
    B.   Monitor vital signs as well as function of critical organs.
    C.   Monitor important vital functions.
    D.   Identify target organ.
    E.   Therapy. Urticaria is most often treated with H1 antihistamines. Occasionally an H2 antihistamine or a leukotriene receptor inhibitor can be helpful. Anaphylaxis or any systemic reaction is best treated with epinephrine. Epinephrine 1:1000 is administered at 0.3 ml intramuscular. Previous protocols of subcutaneous epinephrine are not as effective as intramuscular. Hypotension is best treated with epinephrine and intravenous volume expanders such as saline. Beta-adrenergic inhaled drugs such as albuterol may be necessary to treat bronchospasm. Patients who are receiving beta-adrenergic blocking agents are often resistant to epinephrine therapy and epinephrine may have to be repeated frequently. Patients who are epinephrine resistant may respond to intravenous glucagon bolus (1 mcg/kg; 1 ampule = 1000 mcg in 1 mil; Adult dose 0.5–1.0 cc). However, glucagon is a vasodilator and may potentiate hypotension, and commonly induces nausea and vomiting.

F. Late Phase Response. Although an acute reaction may be successfully treated, a late phase response may recur four to six hours later. This recurrence of symptoms can be prevented by the administration of corticosteroids at the time of initial treatment. Severe reactions need to be observed for this exacerbation and systemic corticosteroids should be administered.

G. Clarify the role of an adverse drug reaction versus a disease process.

  1. Serum tryptase level is a marker of mast cell activation.
  2. Repeat CBC.
  3. Repeat urinalysis.
  4. Hepatic function tests.
  5. Complement markers.
  6. Other tests as indicated. (See Diagnosis above)

H. Desensitization

  1. Therapy for drug allergy is primarily avoidance.
  2. When there is no substitute available, a desensitization protocol may be attempted. Desensitization protocols are included in many of the chapters. Patients must be carefully monitored. When the desensitization is complete and the patient is tolerant of the drug, the drug must be continued as it is likely that sensitization will again occur when the drug has been stopped.
  3. Desensitization is not possible for contact allergy reactions.

I. Future therapy. It has been proposed that administration of bioengineered compounds that bind immunoglobulin E will prevent drug allergy. At this time all such compounds bind circulating immunoglobulin E and do not bind the immunoglobulin E that is already attached to mast cells. Thus, theoretically the drug would have to be administered for 4 weeks prior to administration of an allergic antigen. Even then, it is likely that some reactivity would remain but desensitization would be easier. This induction of reduced reactivity has been shown in patients who had significant systemic reactions to the ingestion of peanuts.

VI. How to Use the Handbook in Clinical Practice

A. Research the drug you wish to use for clinical adverse reaction profile.

B. In a patient with adverse reaction, search by the drugs that the patient is taking with cross-reference by the type of reaction.

C. Alternatively search by signs and symptoms and cross-reference to the drugs being used.

D. Focus on the most recent drugs added to the regimen.

E. Fillers and other "inert" ingredients may be the cause. Latex contact has been a hidden culprit. Polyvinylpyrollidone (Povidone or PVP) and gelatin have caused anaphylaxis. Sulfite and metabisulfite may induce a severe bronchospastic response, probably by hypersensitivity to respiratory excretion of sulfur dioxide.

F. Many patients are also taking alternative or herbal therapy. These compounds may be antigenic or may have drug interactions.

G. In computer or PDA format, enter the symptoms of the

adverse drug reaction and enter a list of the drugs being used to get a list of the drugs that are most likely to cause the reaction.
H. Refer to other drugs which may be alternative therapy with a lower adverse reaction profile.
I. You may be able to use this reference to guide a patient through a desensitization protocol to be able to use a critical drug (example: penicillin in a pregnant patient with syphilis).
J. Each drug or drug class will be graded by its clinical frequency of reactions.
> **1.** Common (C)
> **2.** Rare but well established reaction (R)
> **3.** Very unlikely if ever causes this reaction (U)

K. Although it is not the purpose of this handbook to review use of drugs in Pregnancy, we have included an assignment of pregnancy categorization to medications that are unfamiliar to our readers. See Table 6.1, p. 50.

SELECTED READING

Grammer LC, Greenberger PA, eds. Patterson's Allergic Diseases, 6th ed. Philadelphia: Lippincott Williams and Wilkins, 2002.

Physician's Desk Reference 2003 (Physician's Desk Reference, 57th Edition). Medical Economics Company, 2002.

Rietschel RL, Fowler JF, eds. Fisher's Contact Dermatitis, 5th ed. Philadelphia: Lippincott Williams and Wilkins, 2001.

Special thanks to Gillian Shepherd, Professor of Medicine, Cornell University Medical College for her contribution on hepatic metabolism and mechanisms of drug allergy, and to Ernest N. Charlesworth, Clinical Associate Professor of Medicine in Allergy and Dermatology, University of Texas Medical School in Houston and Galveston, for his contribution to dermatologic reactions.

1

β-Lactams

Maria Fernanda Malaman, and N. Franklin
Adkinson, Jr.

I. β-Lactams
   A. **Immunochemistry of β-lactam antibiotics.** Penicillins
   constitute a large family of antibiotics whose common structural basis is a β-lactam ring joined to a thiazolidine ring. Con-
   nected to this common backbone structure are characteristi-
   cally different amide-bonded side chains in every member of
   this class of compounds. Since the penicillins are low molecular weight compounds 350 (350 to 356 daltons) they must
   combine covalently with tissue proteins to produce multivalent hapten–protein complexes, which are required for both
   the induction of an immune response and the later elicita-
   tion of an allergic reaction. The most common form of haptenation by penicillins is the penicilloyl configuration, which
   can form spontaneously under physiologic conditions, though
   studies suggest that haptenation can be facilitated by serum
   molecules.
      The penicilloyl determinant is the most abundant covalent
   derivative of penicillins in vivo and has been labeled the *major determinant*. It has a role in 75% of immunoglobulin E
   (IgE)–mediated allergic reactions and is the principal epitope
   in most types of hypersensitivity reactions, including delayed-
   type hypersensitivity (DTH). Penicillin can also be degraded by
   other metabolic pathways to form additional antigenic determinants, which are produced in smaller quantities and can vari-
   ably elicit specific immune responses; they are denominated
   collectively as *minor determinants*. Known precursors of minor determinants of penicillin include benzylpenicillin, its al-
   kaline hydrolysis product (benzylpenicilloate), and an acid hydrolysis product (benzylpenilloate), commonly used together in
   a *minor determinants mixture (MDM)*. Anaphylactic reactions
   to penicillin are usually mediated by IgE antibodies directed
   against minor determinants, although some anaphylactic reactions have occurred in patients with only penicilloyl-specific
   IgE antibodies.
   B. **Types of reactions**
      1. **Type I: immediate hypersensitivity**
         a. Type I reactions result from the synthesis of IgE an-
         tibodies specific for β-lactam antigens (major or minor de-
         terminants, or side chains).
         b. The interaction of these antigens with specific IgE
         antibodies that are bound to mast cells or basophils via
         $FC_\epsilon R_I$ [the high affinity mast cell receptor for Fe por-
         tion of IgE molecule] leads to the release of preformed
         (histamine, tryptase, etc.) and newly formed lipid media-
         tors (prostaglandins, leukotrienes, platelet activating fac-
         tor (PAF), etc.).

c. Reactions usually occur within 10 to 20 minutes of drug administration.

d. The clinical expression can be urticaria, laryngeal edema, bronchospasm, hypotension, and cardiovascular collapse in severe cases.

e. In the United States, penicillin is the most common cause of drug-induced anaphylaxis and is responsible for approximately 75% of fatal episodes of drug allergy each year. Penicillin causes fatal anaphylaxis in 0.002% of penicillin courses in the general population, or about 500 deaths per year in the United States among those using the drug.

f. Histories of nonfatal penicillin-induced anaphylaxis and urticaria range from 0.7% to 10% in the general population.

2. **Type II: cytotoxic reactions**

a. These reactions are serious and can be life threatening.

b. Cytotoxic reactions result when IgG or IgM β-lactam specific antibodies become attached to circulating blood cells or renal interstitial cells which have β-lactam antigens bound to their surface. The cytotoxic antibody usually activates the complement system, resulting in cell lysis or phagocytosis, but these reactions may also be complement independent.

c. Penicillin binding by peripheral blood cells is an essential preliminary step in the sensitization process and is more likely to occur in patients receiving large and prolonged doses of penicillin.

d. Positive direct and indirect Coombs' tests in immunohemolytic anemia may be the result of the presence of penicillin-specific IgG, complement or an autoantibody to an Rh determinant on the erythrocyte surface.

e. Clinical presentation: hemolytic anemia, thrombocytopenia, granulocytopenia or drug-induced nephritis.

3. **Type III: immune complex reactions**

a. β-Lactam-specific IgG or IgM antibodies may form circulating complexes with β-lactam antigens. These immune complexes can fix complement and then lodge in tissue sites, causing serum sickness–like reactions and possibly drug fever.

b. Clinical manifestations: fever, rash, urticaria, lymphadenopathy, and arthralgias typically appear 1 to 3 weeks in a long course of drug.

4. **Type IV: cell-mediated hypersensitivity**

a. These reactions are not mediated by antibodies but by T lymphocytes. These cells recognize the β-lactam antigen through an antigen-specific T-cell receptor, triggering cytokine release, recruitment of other cell types, and tissue inflammation.

b. Contact dermatitis is a clinical presentation of a type IV reaction. The high rate of penicillin-related contact dermatitis in the past led to the discontinuation of its use as a topical antibiotic.

c. Recent studies support the involvement of T-cell responses in penicillin allergy, showing that peripheral blood lymphocytes of patients allergic to penicillin proliferate in vitro in response to the appropriate β-lactam antibiotic. Antigen-specific T-cell clones isolated from these cultures may be of the CD4$^+$ or CD8$^+$ phenotype and synthesize a heterogeneous pattern of cytokines after specific stimulation. In allergic skin lesions studies, the T-cell phenotype identified was mainly CD8$^+$ that expressed cytolytic activity against epidermal keratinocytes and autologous B cells.

d. Drug-induced erythema multiforme minor and major (Stevens–Johnson syndrome) and toxic epidermal necrolysis syndromes are also likely to be cellular-mediated drug reactions as are simple maculopapular eruptions based on recent studies describing drug-specific T-cell clones derived from such cases as well as immunohistology of these dermal reactions.

C. Risk factors

1. Age. Although adults 20 to 49 years of age have the greatest risk for acute reactions to penicillin, reactions in elderly individuals tend to be more severe. The lower incidence in children may be related to lower cumulative penicillin exposure.

2. Immune responsiveness/genetics. Studies performed in animals and humans have indicated a genetic basis for the ability to respond immunologically to a variety of haptens and low molecular weight polymers; only about half of adult patients respond to penicillin administration with a detectable IgG or IgE antibody response.

3. Persistence of drug-specific IgE. After an IgE-mediated reaction, penicillin-specific serum IgE half-lives range from 10 to more than 1,000 days. The rate of decline of serum penicilloyl IgE is not related to the initial levels of antibodies, whether the patient previously sustained an allergic reaction to penicillin, or to the time since last therapeutic exposure to penicillin.

4. Atopy. Atopy has no effect on the frequency of drug-specific IgE antibody responses. On the other hand, an atopic background is found with high frequency among patients suffering severe and fatal anaphylactic reactions. Thus, an atopic constitution is associated with a substantial risk for serious acute allergic reactions once an IgE-antibody response has been mounted.

5. Route and dose of administration. Parenteral administration of penicillin has shown to produce more allergic reactions than oral. Whether this is attributable to the higher dose usually administered parenterally or to route-specific differences in processing or dissemination of penicillin antigens is not clear.

6. Previous exposure. IgE-dependent reactions to penicillin require previous exposure for the development of specific IgE antibodies. Most patients have a history of uneventful treatment with the drug, although this is not always the case. Rarely, patients become sensitized during an extended first course of penicillin. At least in the past, occult environmental exposures to penicillin occurred in dairy products and meat.

7. History of a previous penicillin reaction increases by four-to sixfold the risk of subsequent reactions to penicillin, compared to those without previous history. The reaction rate for probable IgE-mediated reactions after retreatment is significantly higher among patients with histories of penicillin-induced urticaria or anaphylaxis than in patients with other histories of penicillin allergy or negative history.

8. There is little evidence that the frequency of drug administration affects the likelihood of sensitization. However, the frequency of drug use has a marked influence on the likelihood of eliciting an allergic reaction.

D. Diagnosis

1. History

a. Careful history of previous and current β-lactam intake, and the temporal relationship between initiation of therapy and onset of symptoms.

b. Presence of general and specific host risk factors should be assessed in the medical history.

c. Consideration of plausible alternative explanations for the presenting manifestations or historical reactions.

2. Physical examination

a. Drug reactions can involve virtually any organ system, but cutaneous reactions are common.

b. Cutaneous lesion: describe appearance and distribution; distinction between maculopapular skin eruptions and urticaria (urticaria is more likely to be IgE mediated); angioedema; presence of purpura and petechiae are signs of vasculitis; erythema multiforme minor (target lesions); Stevens–Johnson syndrome (bullous lesions with mucosal involvement); toxic epidermal necrolysis.

c. Drug reactions can present with fever, lymphadenopathy, hepatosplenomegaly, joint tenderness and swelling, and kidney function impairment.

d. Acute anaphylactic reactions can involve upper and lower airways, and cardiovascular system: laryngeal edema, wheezing, tachycardia, hypotension.

3. Laboratory evaluation

a. General evaluation. Total blood count with eosinophil and platelet counts; sedimentation rate or C-reactive protein.

b. If anaphylaxis is suspected. Serum β-tryptase level, which peaks 1 to 2 hours after the reaction and remains elevated for 2 to 4 hours; and/or serum histamine, which appears earlier and declines rapidly.

c. If serum sickness–like syndrome is suspected. Total complement or complement components.

d. If kidney or liver involvement is suspected. aspartate aminotransferase, alanine aminotransferase, lactic dehydrogenas (LDH), urinalysis (proteinuria, casts, and eosinophils).

e. Both direct and indirect Coombs test results are often positive in drug-induced hemolytic anemia. This may reflect the presence of complement and/or penicillin antibodies on the red cell membrane, or an Rh determinant of autoantibodies.

E. Specific tests
   1. Skin test
      a. Penicillin skin testing should be done in all patients with a history of penicillin allergy for whom a β-lactam antibiotic is presently the indicated drug of choice.
      b. 80% of history-positive patients will be skin test negative and can safely receive penicillin after properly performed negative skin tests.
      c. The reagents are penicilloyl polylysine (Pre-Pen, Hollister-Stier) and an MDM. As the MDM is not commercially available in the United States, fresh benzylpenicillin diluted to a concentration of 10,000 U/mL as a substitute minor determinant reagent can be employed.
      d. If penicillin G is used instead of MDM reagent, there is a small risk that IgE antibodies to minor determinants not elicited by penicillin G may not be detected. This is particularly true when the patient's history involves anaphylactic or severe urticaria–angioedema reactions.
      e. Penicillin skin testing is considered a safe procedure when performed sequentially first with puncture and then intradermal testing including positive and negative controls. A trained specialist capable of managing anaphylaxis, including immediate access to necessary medications and equipment, also assures patient safety.
      f. After the puncture skin test, if there is no induration or systemic symptoms after 15 minutes, intradermal injections are placed, raising a 2- to 3-mm bleb in the forearm in duplicate. The diameter of the induration at 15 to 20 minutes is read; if 5 mm, the result is considered positive. If duplicates disagree, another set should be placed.
      g. Antihistamines, tricyclic antidepressants, and adrenergic drugs can inhibit skin tests results and should be discontinued before the testing procedure.
      h. Patients currently using β-adrenergic blocking drugs or angiotensin-converting enzyme inhibitors at the time of skin testing may not respond to emergency treatment with epinephrine if a systemic reaction occurs; the risk is small and generally considered assumable.
      i. Skin tests have no predictive value for non–IgE-mediated reactions, such as serum sickness, hemolytic anemia, drug fever, interstitial nephritis, or maculopapular exanthema.
      j. For a period of days or weeks after a severe systemic allergic reaction to penicillin, patients may be in a desensitized state and display falsely negative skin test results.
      k. Patients with negative benzylpenicillin skin test results can, with rare exceptions, safely receive any semisynthetic penicillin. Conversely, semisynthetic penicillin administration is contraindicated in patients with positive skin test reactions to penicilloyl polylysine and/or MDM or benzylpenicillin.
      l. Positivity to minor determinants of penicillin is associated more with anaphylactic shock than urticaria, which is clinically associated with positivity to the major penicilloyl determinant.

m. If skin test positive, an equally effective, non–cross-reacting antibiotic should be substituted when available.

n. Skin testing to penicillin should generally be done immediately before intended antibiotic use and repeated before each course of β-lactam therapy in patients with histories of convincing or serious IgE-mediated reactions. Resensitization to penicillin after oral or intravenous treatment with β-lactam antibiotic in hospitalized adult patients with a history of penicillin allergy and previous negative skin test result is about 16% per course of treatment. In one study, intravenous administration (i.e., higher doses) was responsible for all cases of resensitization.

o. Patients with a history of extensive exfoliative dermatitis, Stevens–Johnson syndrome, toxic epidermal necrolysis, or other reactions that constitute an absolute contraindication for penicillin readministration should not be evaluated by skin testing.

p. The rate of positive skin test results among history-positive patients is 7.1% to 18%, whereas among history-negative patients the rate varies from 1.7% to 4%.

q. Systemic reactions during skin testing occur in 0.12% to 1.2% of patients with a negative history and 2.3% to 9.4% in history-positive groups. Usually, the reactions are mild and resolve without treatment. Fatalities are rare, but there are case reports of anaphylactic episodes during penicillin skin testing, usually related to administration of higher doses initially or intradermal testing not preceded by puncture.

r. Reagents used during penicillin skin testing do not appear to resensitize the patient.

s. After penicillin administration to individuals with negative skin test results, acute allergic reactions can occur in about 0.5% of the subjects with negative history and in 2.9% of subjects with positive history. In all cases, the reactions are usually mild and self-limited.

2. **In vitro testing**

a. Radioallergosorbent test (RAST) can be used for the detection of penicilloyl-IgE antibodies in serum.

b. About 80% of patients with positive penicilloyl polylysine skin tests will have a positive penicilloyl RAST.

c. Whether skin test–positive, RAST-negative individuals are at lower risk of serious allergic reactions if treated is not known. However, some patients have positive skin test results with MDM or aqueous benzylpenicillin but negative results with penicilloyl RAST. Such patients are expected to be at high risk for serious systemic reactions if given penicillin.

d. No satisfactory RAST has yet been developed for minor-determinant–specific IgE antibodies. For this reason, penicilloyl RAST alone cannot be used for an accurate assessment of the risk of IgE-mediated reactions in penicillin-sensitive individuals.

F. **Penicillin desensitization**

1. Effective, non–cross-reacting alternative antibiotics to penicillin are usually available for patients with positive

penicillin skin test results. If alternative drugs fail, induce unacceptable side effects, or are less effective, then the administration of penicillin should be considered using a desensitization protocol.

2. Use of a desensitization protocol for penicillin skin test result–positive patients virtually eliminates the risk of anaphylaxis.

3. This procedure is not indicated in patients with a history of non–IgE-mediated reactions like serum sickness disease, maculopapular rash, etc.

4. Patients with a history of Stevens–Johnson syndrome and toxic epidermal necrolysis present an almost absolute contraindication to the readministration of any β-lactam antibiotic since an accelerated life-threatening reaction may occur.

5. Procedure

   a. This procedure should be performed in an intensive or intermediate care unit, by trained personnel, with the adequate emergency equipment available and only with clinically stable patients. Any β-blocking drugs should be stopped or tapered.

   b. Baseline evaluation: establishment of intravenous access, electrocardiogram, spirometry, blood pressure, pulse, respiratory rate, and clinical status. All these parameters should be reevaluated prior to the next dose, as well as 10 and 20 minutes after each dose. We do not recommend premedication with antihistamine or steroids. These drugs usually are not effective in preventing severe reactions and may cloud or mask early signs of reaction that would otherwise result in a modification of the protocol.

   c. Protocols have been developed for both oral and parenteral desensitization. The oral route seems to be safer, whereas the parenteral allows a closer monitoring of the dose and injection site reaction (Tables 1.1 and 1.2).

   d. During desensitization any dose that causes mild systemic reactions, such as pruritus, urticaria, rhinitis, or mild wheezing, should be repeated until the patient tolerates the dose without systemic symptoms or signs. More serious reactions, such as hypotension, laryngeal edema, or asthma, require appropriate treatment; if desensitization is continued, the dose should be decreased by at least tenfold and withheld until the patient is stable. Non–IgE-mediated complications like serum sickness and dermatitis can occur during and after desensitization in about 5% of patients.

   e. Once desensitized, the patient's treatment with penicillin should not lapse because the risk of an allergic reaction increases when restarting treatment. If the patient requires a β-lactam antibiotic in the future and his skin test result remains positive, desensitization is required again.

   f. Desensitization can be maintained with daily low dose administration of penicillin. Patients on chronic desensitization may be switched to a modified penicillin for acute therapy without going through a desensitization protocol. For example, a patient with penicillin allergy and an

Table 1.1. Oral penicillin desensitization protocol

Step	Phenoxymethyl Penicillin (U/mL)	Amount (mL)	Dose (U)	Cumulative Dose (U)
1	1,000	0.1	100	100
2	1,000	0.2	200	300
3	1,000	0.4	400	700
4	1,000	0.8	800	1,500
5	1,000	1.6	1,600	3,100
6	1,000	3.2	3,200	6,300
7	1,000	6.4	6,400	12,700
8	10,000	1.2	12,000	24,700
9	10,000	2.4	24,000	48,700
10	10,000	4.8	48,000	96,700
11	80,000	1.0	80,000	176,700
12	80,000	2.0	160,000	336,700
13	80,000	4.0	320,000	656,700
14	80,000	8.0	640,000	1,296,700
Observe patient for 30 minutes				
Change to benzylpenicillin IV				
15	500,000	0.25	125,000	
16	500,000	0.50	250,000	
17	500,000	1.0	500,000	
18	500,000	2.25	1,125,000	

Adapted from Sullivan TJ. Drug allergy. In: Middleton E, Reed C, Ellis E, et al., eds. *Allergy: principles and practice,* 4th ed. St. Louis: CV Mosby, 1993:1523–1543, with permission.

intermittent need for ticarcillin could be maintained on daily penicillin.

G. Cross-reactivity

1. Cephalosporins

a. Like penicillins, cephalosporins have a β-lactam ring, although the five-membered thiazolidine ring is substituted by the six-membered dihydrothiazine ring. The degree of cross-reactivity between cephalosporins and penicillins remains uncertain.

b. The incidence of clinically relevant cross-reactivity between cephalosporins and penicillins is probably small, but rare cases of life-threatening anaphylactic cross-reactivity have occurred.

c. The risk of administering a first-generation cephalosporin to a penicillin skin test–positive patient is lower than that of administering a penicillin antibiotic; however, it is not negligible. Antibodies to the second- and third-generation cephalosporins are often directed against the side chains rather than the ring structures, and therefore cross-reactivity with penicillins is less than with first-generation cephalosporins.

d. Patients with a positive skin test result to any penicillin reagent probably should not receive cephalosporin

Table 1.2.   Parenteral penicillin desensitization protocol

Injection no.	Benzylpenicillin Conc. (U/mL)	Volume/Route (mL)[b]
1[a]	100	0.1, ID
2	100	0.2, SC
3	100	0.4, SC
4	100	0.8, SC
5[a]	1,000	0.1, ID
6	1,000	0.3, SC
7	1,000	0.6, SC
8[a]	10,000	1.0, ID
9	10,000	0.2, SC
10	10,000	0.4, SC
11	10,000	0.8, SC
12[a]	100,000	0.1, ID
13	100,000	0.3, SC
14	100,000	0.6, SC
15[a]	1,000,000	0.1, ID
16	1,000,000	0.2, SC
17	1,000,000	0.2, IM
18	1,000,000	0.4, IM
19	Continuous IV infusion	1,000,000 U/hr

[a]Observe and record skin wheal-and-flare response to intradermal doses.
[b]Administer progressive doses at intervals of not less than 20 minutes.
ID, intradermal; SC, subcutaneous; IM, intramuscular; IV, intravenous.
Adapted from Weiss ME, Adkinson NF Jr. β-Lactam allergy. *Clin Allergy* 1988;18:515–540, with permission.

antibiotics unless alternative drugs are clearly less desirable. If cephalosporin drugs are to be used, they should be administered with adequate precautions, including gradual dose escalation.

e.   Before 1980, patients with positive penicillin skin test results who were given cephalosporin had a reaction rate of 10% to 20%. However, since that time the cross-reaction rate has decreased significantly and may now be only 2%. This phenomenon could be related to the more frequent use of first-generation cephalosporins at that time and by contamination of early cephalosporin products with penicillin contaminants. Since 1980, the contamination has not been reported.

f.   Recent data suggest that fewer than 20% of patients allergic to third-generation cephalosporins react to penicillin determinants. Previous studies by the same group showed that the incidence of cross-reactivity with penicillin determinants was much higher (+50%) in cephalosporin-allergic patients. This could be explained by the fact that in this previous study, some of the subjects had reacted to first-generation cephalosporins, which share more structural similarities with penicillin than third-generation antibiotics.

2. Monobactams

a. Monobactams are β-lactam antibiotics that contain a monocyclic β-lactam ring rather than the bicyclic structure of the penicillins and cephalosporins. This prototype of this class is aztreonam.

b. Aztreonam-specific antibodies are largely, if not exclusively, side chain specific. Ceftazidime, a third-generation cephalosporin, has the same bulky aminothiazolyl side chain as aztreonam, and there are case reports of cross-sensitivity to aztreonam in ceftazidime-sensitive patients.

c. Clinical studies of penicillin skin test–positive patients indicate that full doses of aztreonam are almost always well tolerated, suggesting that aztreonam may be safely administered to most, if not all, penicillin-allergic subjects.

3. Carbapenems

a. Carbapenens are another class of β-lactam antibiotics of which imipenem is the prototype. Like penicillin, this class of antibiotic has a bicyclic nucleus containing a β-lactam ring and an adjacent five-membered ring.

b. A study showed about 50% cross-reactivity in allergy skin testing between penicillin major and minor determinants and the analogous imipenem reagents, suggesting the need to withhold carbapenems from penicillin skin test–positive patients.

SELECTED READINGS

Adkinson NF Jr. Tests for immunological reactions to drugs and allergens. In: Rose NR, Macario EC, Folds JD, et al., eds. *Manual of clinical laboratory immunology,* 5th ed. Washington D.C.: American Society for microbiology, 1997:897.

Adkinson NF Jr. Immunogenicity and cross-allergenicity of aztreonam. *Am J Med* 1990;88:12S–15S.

Adkinson NF Jr. Natural history of IgE-dependent drug sensitivities. *J Allergy Clin Immunol* 1986;77:65–69.

Adkinson NF Jr. Risk factors drug allergy. *J Allergy Clin Immunol* 1984;74:567.

Adkinson NF Jr, Wheeler B. Risk factors for IgE-dependent reactions to penicillin. In: Kerr JW, Ganderton MA, eds. *Proceedings of the Eleventh International Congress of Allergology and Clinical Immunology.* London: Macmillan, 1983:55–59.

Di Piro JT, Adkinson NF Jr, Hamilton RG. Facilitation of penicillin haptenization to serum proteins. *Antimicrob Ag Chemother* 1993;July:1463–1467.

Disease management of drug hypersensitivity: a practice parameter. *Ann Allergy Asthma Immunol* 1999;83:672–400. (also available at aaaai.org)

Gadde J, Spence M, Wheeler B, et al. Clinical experience with penicillin skin testing in a large inner-city STD clinic. *JAMA* 1993; 270:2456–2463.

Neugut AI, Ghatak AT, Miller RL. Anaphylaxis in the United States. An investigation into its epidemiology. *Arch Intern Med* 2001;161:15–21.

Padovan E. T-cell response in penicillin allergy. *Clin Exp Allergy* 1998; 28:33–36.

Parker PJ, Parrinello JT, Condemi, JJ, et al. Penicillin resensitization among hospitalized patients. *J Allergy Clin Immunol* 1991;88:213–217.

Romano A, Mayorga C, Torres MJ, et al. Immediate allergic reactions to cephalosporins: cross-reactivity and selective response. *J Allergy Clin Immunol* 2000;106:17–83.

Romano A, Quaratino D, Aimone-Gastin I, et al. Cephalosporin allergy: characterization of unique and cross-reacting cephalosporin antigens. *Int J Immunopathol Pharmacol* 1997;10:187–191.

Saxon A, Adelman DC, Patel A, et al. Imipenem cross-reactivity with penicillin in humans. *JACI* 1988;82:213–217.

Sogn DD, Evans R, Shepherd GM, et al. Results of the National Institute of Allergy and Infectious Diseases Collaborative Clinical Trial to test the predictive value of skin testing with major and minor penicillin derivates in hospitalized adults. *Arch Intern Med* 1993;152:1025–1032.

Stark BJ, Earl HS, Gross GN, et al. Acute and chronic desensitization of penicillin-allergic patients using oral penicillin. *J Allergy Clin Immunol* 1987;79:523–532.

Sullivan TJ. Drug allergy. In: Middleton E, Reed C, Ellis E, et al., eds. *Allergy: principles and practice,* 4th ed. St. Louis: CV Mosby, 1993: 1523–1543.

Torres MJ, Mayorga C, Pamies R, et al. Immunologic response to different determinants of benzylpenicillin, amoxicillin and ampicillin. Comparison between urticaria and anaphylactic shock. *Allergy* 1999;54:936–943.

Valysevi MA, Van Dellen RG. Frequency of systemic reactions to penicillin skin test. *Ann Allergy Asthma Immunol* 2000;95:363–365.

Weiss ME, Adkinson NF Jr. β-Lactam allergy. *Clin Allergy* 1988;18: 515–540.

Wendel GD Jr, Stark BJ, Jamison RB, et al. Penicillin allergy and desensitization in serious infections during pregnancy. *N Engl J Med* 1985;312:1229–1232.

Other Antibiotics

Margaret M. Lowery and Paul A. Greenberger

I. Aminoglycosides. The aminoglycosides are indicated for polymicrobial and gram-negative bacillus infections in patients with intra-abdominal, urinary tract, genital tract, and nosocomial infections. They may also be used for empiric treatment in patients with neutropenic fevers. The most frequent side effects are nephrotoxicity and ototoxicity. Nephrotoxicity is reversible and seen with use of gentamicin > tobramycin > amikacin > streptomycin in order of decreasing frequency (1,2). Ototoxicity is irreversible and seen with amikacin > gentamicin > tobramycin in order of decreasing frequency (1,3). Also neuromuscular blockade occurs with rapid intravenous or copious peritoneal irrigation. This effect is more pronounced with the use of neuromuscular relaxant drugs or in patients with myasthenia gravis or other neuromuscular disorders.

Allergic reactions to aminoglycosides are very rare and have included eczematous rashes and urticaria, the latter even occurring after nebulization. Should a patient who has experienced acute urticaria require aminoglycoside treatment, successful desensitization has been accomplished beginning with intravenous 1 μg with doubling doses every 30 minutes. The cumulative dose is 80 mg.

  A. Gentamicin

    1. Precautions. Patients at risk for renal compromise, such as elderly persons or those with preexistent renal insufficiency, cardiovascular disease, diabetes, and so forth, should have renal function monitoring throughout treatment with these aminoglycoside antibiotics, including trough serum concentrations of the aminoglycoside. In addition, the patient should be well hydrated during treatment to prevent nephrotoxicity. These antibiotics should be used with caution in patients with neuromuscular disorders or patients receiving neuromuscular agents (such as for myasthenia gravis) or anesthetics (such as in surgery) because weakness or respiratory depression can occur secondary to their neuromuscular blockade side effect.

      a. Contraindications Patients with renal insufficiency should not receive aminoglycosides, or should receive them with greater dosing intervals to avoid toxicity from high trough concentrations, or hypersensitivity to gentamicin or other aminoglycoside because of known cross-reactivity among aminoglycosides.

      b. Drug interactions. Potentiation of neuromuscular block with succinylcholine or α-tubocurarine, increased potential for nephrotoxicity with concomitant use of cephalosporins, decreased gentamicin concentrations with concomitant use of carbenicillin in severely impaired renal patients, use of furosemide or ethacrynic acid may potentiate ototoxicity. Try to avoid use of other nephrotoxic/neurotoxic medications (cisplatin, vancomycin, polymyxin B, etc.).

2. Allergic reactions. Eczematous rash, urticaria, drug fever, laryngeal edema, hypersensitivity reactions (very rare).

   a. Pseudoallergic reactions. Photosensitivity, anaphylactoid reactions.

3. Adverse effects

   a. Idiosyncratic. Neuromuscular block; pseudotumor cerebri; hepatic damage; transient hepatomegaly/splenomegaly; elevated hepatic enzymes decreased calcium, sodium, magnesium, and potassium; anemia; leukopenia; agranulocytosis; eosinophilia; thrombocytopenia; pulmonary fibrosis; alopecia.

   b. Toxic effects 8.3% ototoxicity (1) (dizziness, vertigo, tinnitus, hearing loss), nephrotoxicity, increased blood urea nitrogen (BUN)/creatinine, peripheral neuropathy, paresthesias.

   c. Other adverse effects. Headache, seizures, lethargy, visual disturbances, acute organic brain syndrome, nausea, vomiting, stomatitis, increased salivation, respiratory depression, decreased appetite, weight loss, phlebitis.

B. Tobramycin

1. Precautions (see Gentamicin precautions)

   a. Contraindications. Patients with renal insufficiency should not receive aminoglycosides or receive them with greater dosing intervals to avoid toxicity from high trough concentrations, or from hypersensitivity to tobramycin or other aminoglycoside because of known cross-reactivity among aminoglycosides.

   b. Drug interactions. potentiation of neuromuscular block with succinylcholine, tubocurarine, increased incidence of nephrotoxicity with concomitant use of cephalosporins, avoid use of other nephrotoxic/neurotoxic medications (cisplatin, vancomycin, polymyxin B, etc.), use of furosemide or ethacrynic acid may potentiate ototoxicity.

2. Allergic reactions. Rash, drug fever, urticaria, exfoliative dermatitis, hypersensitivity reactions [(R) but have been reported with nebulized tobramycin (4)].

   a. Pseudoallergic reactions. Photosensitivity

3. Adverse effects

   a. Idiosyncratic. Neuromuscular block, hepatic damage, anemia, granulocytopenia, leukopenia, leukocytosis, eosinophilia, thrombocytopenia, elevated LFTs, decreased, calcium, magnesium, sodium, and potassium.

   b. Toxic effects. 6.1% ototoxicity (1) (dizziness, vertigo, tinnitus, hearing loss), nephrotoxicity, increased BUN/ creatinine. Nebulized tobramycin is associated with tinnitus, and a rare patient may develop acute renal failure.

   c. Other adverse effects. Headache, lethargy, confusion, phlebitis, nausea, vomiting, diarrhea.

C. Amikacin

1. Precautions (see Gentamicin precautions)

   a. Contraindications. Patients with renal insufficiency should not receive aminoglycosides or should receive them with greater dosing intervals to avoid toxicity from high trough concentrations, or hypersensitivity to tobramycin or other aminoglycoside because of known cross-reactivity among aminoglycosides.

   b. Drug interactions. Potentiation of neuromuscular block with succinylcholine and tubocurarine, increased incidence of nephrotoxicity with concomitant use of cephalosporins, decreased serum half-life of aminoglycosides with use of β-lactam antibiotics, use of furosemide or ethacrynic acid may potentiate ototoxicity. Avoid use of other nephrotoxic/neurotoxic medications (cisplatin, vancomycin, polymyxin B, etc.).

   2. Allergic reactions. Rash, drug fever, hypersensitivity reactions (R).

   a. Pseudoallergic reactions. Photosensitivity.

   3. Adverse effects

   a. Idiosyncratic Neuromuscular block, hepatic damage, anemia, eosinophilia.

   b. Toxic effects. 13.9% ototoxicity (1) (dizziness, vertigo, tinnitus, hearing loss), nephrotoxicity, elevated BUN/creatinine.

   c. Other adverse effects. Phlebitis, nausea, vomiting, headache, paresthesia, tremor, arthralgia, hypotension.

   D. Streptomycin (see Chapter 3)

II. Glycopeptide Antibiotics. Vancomycin is the only antibiotic in this drug class. It is useful in the management of serious gram-positive infections: methicillin-resistant *Staphylococcus aureus*, shunt infections, endocarditis, and intravenous catheter infections. This antibiotic is also used as prophylaxis prior to prosthetic implant surgery and for special procedures in patients at high risk for endocarditis.

The most common side effect is "red man syndrome," which is non–IgE-mediated release of histamine. Associated symptoms include skin erythema, pruritis, angioedema, and, occasionally, hypotension (5). This reaction can be prevented by decreasing the infusion rate to run over 1 to 4 hours and, if that is unsuccessful, premedication with antihistamines.

   A. Vancomycin

   1. Precautions. Use cautiously in patients with chronic renal insufficiency/failure. Administer the infusion over 1 to 4 hours to minimize red-man syndrome. Monitor white blood cell (WBC) count and renal function during treatment.

   a. Contraindications. Prior Stevens–Johnson syndrome (SJS) is an absolute contraindication; hypersensitivity to vancomycin.

   b. Drug interactions. Concomitant use with anesthetics is associated with erythema and histamine-like flushing; concurrent use of other nephrotoxic/neurotoxic agents requires careful monitoring (amphotericin B, aminoglycosides, bacitracin, polymyxin B, cisplatin, etc.).

   2. Allergic reactions. Hypersensitivity reactions, maculopapular or urticarial rashes, exfoliative dermatitis, SJS, toxic epidermal necrolysis (TEN), vasculitis (rare), drug fever (rare), anaphylaxis.

    a. Pseudoallergic reactions. red man syndrome-anaphylactoid reaction.

3. **Adverse effects**

    a. Idiosyncratic. Reversible neutropenia, reversible agranulocytosis (rare), thrombocytopenia (rare), eosinophilia.

    b. Toxic effects. Ototoxicity (hearing loss, vertigo, dizziness, tinnitus), nephrotoxicity (more common when vancomycin used in combination with aminoglycosides).

    c. Other adverse effects. Thrombophlebitis, nausea, pseudomembranous colitis, chemical peritonitis with intraperitoneal administration.

III. **Sulfonamides.** Trimethoprim–sulfamethoxazole (TMP-SMX) is indicated for management of urinary tract infections, upper respiratory infections, *Pneumocystis carinii* pneumonia (PCP), shigellosis, otitis media, traveler's diarrhea, and PCP prophylaxis in immunosuppressed patients. Hypersensitivity reactions occur in 3% to 4% of patients (6). Human immunodeficiency virus (HIV)–infected patients have a 65% incidence of adverse reactions to TMP-SMX. This increased effect may be the result of slow hepatic N-acetyltransferase activity (7).

Cross-reactivity between allergic reactions to sulfamethoxazole or other sulfonamide antibiotics and other medications containing the sulfonamide (SO_2NH_2) moiety appear to be extremely rare or nonexistent. The sulfonamide antibiotic contains a SO_2NH_2 moiety linking a benzene ring with a pyrazole (nitrogen-containing) ring. In contrast, furosemide and celecoxib contain the SO_2NH_2 moiety attached to a benzene ring removed from the rest of the molecule. These compounds are not strictly contraindicated in patients with sulfonamide allergy.

    A. **Trimethoprim–Sulfamethoxazole (TMP-SMX, Bactrim, Septra)**

    1. **Precautions.** Cautious use in patients with renal or hepatic failure, folate deficiency (elderly, malabsorption syndrome, anticonvulsant use).

      a. Contraindications. Previously documented SJS or TEN. Pregnancy, breast-feeding, folate or glucose-6-phosphate dehydrogenase deficiency. Age younger than 2 months. Known hypersensitivity to sulfonamides or TMP.

      b. Drug interactions. Potentiation of warfarin, phenytoin, and sulfonylureas; increase in methotrexate levels; hyperkalemia with angiotensin-converting enzyme inhibitors and potassium-sparing diuretics; increased incidence of thrombocytopenia and purpura with thiazide diuretic use in elderly patients (C).

    2. **Allergic reactions.** Hypersensitivity reactions: SJS, TEN; fever/rash (3% to 4%); maculopapular, urticarial, or morbilliform rash; erythema multiforme, purpura, anaphylaxis, angioedema, drug fever, serum sickness, acute interstitial nephritis, Henoch–Schönlein purpura.

      a. Pseudoallergic reactions. Aplastic anemia, agranulocytosis, fulminant hepatic necrosis, photosensitivity, hemolytic anemia, systemic lupus erythematosus (SLE).

3. Adverse effects
a. Idiosyncratic. Cholestatic jaundice, hepatitis, pancreatitis, hyperkalemia, hyponatremia, elevated BUN/creatinine, anemia, leukopenia, thrombocytopenia, aseptic meningitis, meningoencephalitis, pulmonary infiltrates.

b. Other adverse effects. Nausea, vomiting, diarrhea, anorexia, stomatitis, glossitis, abdominal pain, pseudomembranous enterocolitis, headache, delirium, psychosis, seizures, peripheral neuritis, arthralgia, myalgia, cough.

B. Sulfisoxazole (Pediazole)
1. Precautions.
Sulfasoxazole: Cautious use in patients with renal or hepatic failure, folic acid deficiency (elderly, malabsorption syndrome, anticonvulsant use). Erythromycin: Cautious use in patients with impaired hepatic function; may exacerbate weakness in patients with myasthenia gravis.

a. Contraindications. Breast-feeding, pregnancy, folic acid or glucose-6-phosphate dehydrogenase deficiency.

Known hypersensitivity to sulfonamides or erythromycin/macrolides. Contraindicated in patients taking terfenadine, astemizole, cisapride, and pimozide (can result in QT prolongation/ventricular arrhythmias).

b. Drug interactions Erythromycin: Inhibits P450; increases anticoagulant effects; increases digoxin, theophylline, cyclosporine, carbamazepine, phenytoin, alfentanil, disopyramide, lovastatin, benzodiazepines, and bromocriptine concentrations; rare ventricular arrhythmias; torsades de pointes. Sulfasoxazole: Competes with thiopental for plasma protein binding; therefore, patients require less thiopental for anesthesia. Displaces methotrexate from plasma protein binding sites, increasing methotrexate concentrations, potentiation of sulfonylureas resulting in hypoglycemia.

2. Allergic reactions (C).
Urticaria, angioedema, anaphylaxis, erythema multiforme, SJS, TEN, exfoliative dermatitis, serum sickness, scleral and conjunctivial injection, vasculitis, allergic myocarditis, SLE, and periarteritis nodosa.

a. Pseudoallergic reactions. Photosensitivity

3. Adverse effects
a. Idiosyncratic. Pancreatitis, pulmonary infiltrates, elevated LFTs, elevated BUN/creatinine, leukopenia, agranulocytosis, aplastic anemia, thrombocytopenia, hemolytic anemia, purpura, eosinophilia, prolonged QT interval/ventricular arrhythmias (rare).

b. Toxic effects. Transient hearing loss has been reported in patients with renal insufficiency receiving high doses of erythromycin.

c. Other adverse effects. Nausea, vomiting, diarrhea, abdominal pain, anorexia, glossitis, stomatitis, pseudomembranous colitis (rare), salivary gland enlargement, cough, shortness of breath, headache, dizziness, paresthesias, vertigo, psychosis, hallucinations.

IV. Trimethoprim

  A. Precautions. Cautious use in patients with renal or hepatic insufficiency or folate deficiency.

    1. Contraindications. Known hypersensitivity to TMP, patients with megaloblastic anemia secondary to folate deficiency.

    2. Drug interactions. Elevated phenytoin and digoxin concentrations, decreased renal tubular secretion of procainamide and the active metabolite N-acetylprocainamide increasing its concentration.

  B. Allergic reactions. Maculopapular, morbilliform rashes; anaphylaxis (R) [exfoliative dermatitis, erythema multiforme, SJS, TEN] (R).

    1. Pseudoallergic reactions

  C. Adverse effects

    1. Idiosyncratic. Elevated BUN/creatinine, hyponatremia, hyperkalemia, leukopenia, neutropenia, thrombocytopenia, megaloblastic anemia, methemoglobinemia, aseptic meningitis (R).

    2. Toxic effects. Phototoxic reaction.

    3. Other adverse effects. Nausea, vomiting, glossitis, cholestatic jaundice (R).

V. Macrolides. The macrolides are useful in the management of upper respiratory tract infections and skin infections. In general, the macrolides are safe with rare incidence of adverse effects. The most common side effects include nausea, vomiting, diarrhea, and abdominal pain. Hypersensitivity reactions are rare and can manifest as fever, rashes, and eosinophilia (8). Other rare side effects include cholestatic hepatitis with erythromycin estolate (9). Urticaria has been reported to both erythromycin and spiromycin (10).

A few studies using skin testing and patch testing to macrolides followed by oral challenge have yielded conflicting results. Igea et al. reported a series of five patients with urticarial and/or maculopapular rashes after oral spiromycin. One of these patients also took erythromycin. All of these patients had negative skin prick/patch tests to erythromycin and spiromycin but all had recurrence of rash on oral challenge to spiromycin (11). One of the patients also had recurrence of rash with oral challenge to erythromycin. Another study showed macrolide cross-reactivity in macrolide patch testing in a patient with a fixed drug eruption (FDE) to erythromycin (12).

Furthermore, erythromycin-specific IgE antibodies have been reported in the serum of one patient with a history of urticaria from erythromycin (13). In most cases of macrolide-induced hypersensitivity rash, the rash usually resolves without further complications.

  A. Erythromycin

    1. Precautions. Cautious use in patients with impaired hepatic function; may exacerbate weakness in patients with myasthenia gravis.

      a. Contraindications. Known hypersensitivity to erythromycin/macrolides.

Contraindicated in patients taking cisapride and pimozide (can result in QT prolongation/ventricular arrhythmias).

   b. **Drug interactions.** Erythromycin inhibits the hepatic cytochrome P450 enzyme system and can increase serum concentrations of theophylline, warfarin, digoxin, triazolam, alfentanil, cisapride, disopyramide, lovastatin, bromocriptine, phenytoin, valproate, carbamazepine, and cyclosporine (9); ergot toxicity; QT prolongation, cardiac arrhythmias with concomitant use of cisapride.

 2. **Allergic reactions.** Urticaria, anaphylaxis; erythema multiforme, SJS, TEN (R).

Hypersensitivity reactions are rare and can manifest with fever, rash, and eosinophilia, which occurs most often with the estolate preparation (8).

   a. **Pseudoallergic reactions.** Some patients develop a hypersensitivity syndrome to estolate that may mimic acute cholestasis, viral hepatitis, and acute pancreatitis (9).

 3. **Adverse effects**

   a. **Idiosyncratic.** [Ventricular tachycardia and QT prolongation with intravenous erythromycin, torsades de pointes] (R), transient hearing loss in patients with renal insufficiency (9).

   b. **Other adverse effects.** Nausea, vomiting, diarrhea, abdominal pain, anorexia, pseudomembranous colitis.

B. **Clarithromycin (Biaxin)**

 1. **Precautions.** Cautious use in patients with impaired hepatic function. Clarithromycin with ranitidine bismuth citrate is not given to patients with acute porphyria.

   a. **Contraindications.** Known hypersensitivity to clarithromycin/macrolides.

Contraindicated in patients taking terfenadine, astemizole, cisapride, and pimozide (can result in QT prolongation/ventricular arrhythmias).

   b. **Drug interactions.** Clarithromycin inhibits the hepatic cytochrome P450 enzyme system and can slow metabolism of carbamazepine, theophylline, digoxin, triazolam, ergotamine, cyclosporine, warfarin, valproate, disopyramide, midazolam, omeprazole, ranitidine, 3-hydroxy-3-methylglutaryl coenzyme A reductase inhibitors, and nicotine. This antibiotic conversely can lower zidovudine concentrations (9). Concomitant use with fluconazole or ritonavir increases clarithromycin concentrations. Torsades de pointes can occur with concomitant use of quinidine or disopyramide; ergot toxicity with use of ergotamine resulting in peripheral vasospasm and dysesthesia.

 2. **Allergic reactions.** Urticaria, anaphylaxis (R), SJS, TEN, acute interstitial nephritis (14).

   a. **Pseudoallergic reactions.** Pancreatitis, myasthenic syndrome, cholestatic hepatitis, and fulminant hepatic failure (9).

 3. **Adverse effects**

   a. **Idiosyncratic.** Hearing loss, elevated LFTs, elevated

BUN/creatinine, leukopenia, thrombocytopenia, QT prolongation, hepatocellular/cholestatic hepatitis.

   b.   Other adverse effects. Nausea, vomiting, diarrhea, abdominal pain, dyspepsia, anorexia, abnormal taste, glossitis, stomatitis, oral moniliasis, tongue discoloration, headache, dizziness, anxiety, confusion, seizures, hallucinations, insomnia, vertigo—all reversible.

   Patients with HIV have an increased incidence of adverse effects.

C.   Azithromycin (Zithromax)

   1.   Precautions. Cautious use in patients with impaired hepatic function and glomerular filtration rate less than 10 mL/min.

   a.   Contraindications. Known hypersensitivity to azithromycin/macrolides.

   Since erythromycin and clarithromycin are contraindicated in patients taking terfenadine, astemizole, cisapride, and pimozide (can result in QT prolongation/ventricular arrhythmias), these medications are relatively contraindicated with use of azithromycin.

   b.   Drug interactions. Contraindicated in patients receiving ergot alkaloids; monitor concentrations of digoxin, cyclosporine, phenytoin, carbamazepine concurrent with administration of azithromycin, increased azithromycin concentrations with concomitant use of nelfinavir.

   2.   Allergic reactions. Rash, urticaria, vesiculobullous rash, angioedema, hypersensitivity reaction (15) (R), erythema multiforme, SJS, TEN, anaphylaxis, acute interstitial nephritis.

   a.   Pseudoallergic reactions. Photosensitivity

   3.   Adverse effects

   a.   Idiosyncratic. Intrahepatic cholestasis (16), hepatic necrosis/failure, ventricular tachycardia, elevated aspartate aminotransferase/alanine aminotransferase (AST/ALT), elevated BUN/creatinine, abnormal neutrophil/leukocyte counts, anemia, thrombocytopenia, hearing loss, tinnitus, taste perversion (R).

   b.   Other adverse effects. Nausea, vomiting, diarrhea, abdominal pain, dyspepsia, oral moniliasis.

   Tongue discoloration (R), pseudomembranous colitis, hypotension, vaginitis, headache, dizziness, vertigo, fatigue, nervousness, insomnia, seizures.

VI.   Chloramphenicol. This antibiotic has broad-spectrum antimicrobial activity and can cross the blood–brain barrier. In the past it was used in the management of serious infections, especially meningitis. Reports of aplastic anemia and gray-baby syndrome (see below) have limited the use of chloramphenicol since safer alternative antimicrobials became available. The medication continues to be used in third-world countries because it remains efficacious and is inexpensive (17).

A.   Chloramphenicol

   1.   Precautions. Cautious use in patients with renal or hepatic disease, pregnant or lactating women, and newborns. Limit other medications that cause bone marrow suppression. Frequent monitoring of WBCs and chloramphenicol concentrations during treatment. Avoid repeated or prolonged courses of therapy.

    a.   Contraindications. Known hypersensitivity to chloramphenicol or toxic reaction; not to be used in the management of trivial infections.

    b.   Drug interactions. Inhibits hepatic enzymes, which increases serum concentrations of tolbutamide, chloropropamide, phenytoin, cyclophosphamide, and warfarin; chloramphenicol levels are decreased with rifampin, phenytoin, and phenobarbital (7).

  2.   Allergic reactions. Hypersensitivity reactions are uncommon, fever, macular and vesicular rashes, urticaria, angioedema, anaphylaxis, Jarish–Herxheimer–like reactions have been reported in patients with brucellosis, enteric fever, and syphilis (17) (R).

    a.   Pseudoallergic reactions

  3.   Adverse effects

    a.   Idiosyncratic. Irreversible aplastic anemia that is not dose related, reversible bone marrow suppression, thrombocytopenia, granulocytopenia.

    b.   Toxic effects. Gray-baby syndrome in the newborn (abdominal distention, progressive cyanosis, flaccidity), which is dose related; headache, delirium, optic and peripheral neuritis.

    c.   Other adverse effects. Depression, stomatitis, nausea, vomiting, diarrhea, *C. difficile* colitis (17)

VII.   Quinolones These compounds have a broad spectrum of antimicrobial activity. They are used in the management of uncomplicated or complicated urinary tract infections, upper respiratory infections, community-acquired pneumonia, bacterial prostatitis, sexually transmitted diseases, pelvic inflammatory disease, osteomyelitis, and mycobacterial infections. The absorption of quinolones can be blocked by multivalent metal ions: aluminum, magnesium, zinc, iron, and calcium (18).

The most common side effects are gastrointestinal (trovafloxacin > ciprofloxacin, levofloxacin > norfloxacin > ofloxacin) and central nervous system (CNS) disturbances (trovafloxacin > norfloxacin > ciprofloxacin > ofloxacin > levofloxacin) (19). The concurrent use of nonsteroidal anti-inflammatory drugs (NSAIDs) can potentiate CNS stimulation and seizure activity. Also QT prolongation has been seen: moxifloxacin > levofloxacin > gatifloxacin in order of decreasing frequency (20). Photosensitivity also occurs: ciprofloxacin > norfloxacin > ofloxacin > levofloxacin > trovafloxacin in order of decreasing frequency (19). Cystic fibrosis patients have approximately a 50% incidence of photosensitivity with the use of quinolones (21).

Furthermore, Diez et al. reported three cases of cross-reactivity with positive controlled oral provocations with a different quinolone than was associated with the initial reaction (22).

Tendonitis and tendon rupture have been reported in association with the use of norfloxacin, ciprofloxacin, and levofloxacin.

A. Trovafloxacin or Alatrofloxacin (Parenteral)

1. Precautions. Trovafloxacin has been associated with hepatitis, acute hepatic necrosis, and elevation of LFTs. This medication should *not* be used if a safer alternative is available. If used for longer than 2 weeks there is a higher risk of liver injury. Alkalinity of the urine should be avoided during treatment secondary to risk of crystalluria. Avoid NSAIDs during treatment with quinolones as the concomitant use of these medications may cause CNS stimulation and seizures. Quinolones may exacerbate weakness in myasthenia gravis patients. Dose adjustment is needed for patients with renal insufficiency. May cause hypo-/hyperglycemia in patients on oral hypoglycemic agents and insulin. Avoid excessive sunlight secondary to risk of photosensitivity. Rapid intravenous infusion of alatrofloxacin has caused hypotension; therefore, the medication should be infused over 60 to 90 minutes. Also, the bioavailability of quinolones is reduced with concomitant use of antacids and iron supplements.

a. Contraindications. Known hypersensitivity to trovafloxacin/other quinolones.

b. Drug interactions. decreased absorption with concomitant administration of antacids containing magnesium or aluminum, citric acid, sucralfate and iron, didanosine; intravenous morphine decreases absorption of trovafloxacin, enhances effect of warfarin.

2. Allergic reactions. Rash, anaphylaxis, SJS, TEN (23), acute interstitial nephritis (R).

a. Pseudoallergic reactions. Phototoxicity (U).

3. Adverse effects

a. Idiosyncratic. Hepatotoxicity, hepatitis, pancreatitis, increased AST/ALT, agranulocytosis, aplastic anemia, pancytopenia (R)

b. Other adverse effects. Nausea, vomiting, diarrhea (R), abdominal pain, vaginitis, pruritis, dizziness (3%), headaches (1% to 5%), light-headedness (2% to 4%).

B. Ciprofloxacin

1. Precautions. Dose adjustment is needed for patients with renal insufficiency. Alkalinity of the urine should be avoided during treatment secondary to risk of crystalluria. Avoid NSAIDs during treatment with quinolones as the concomitant use of these medications may cause CNS stimulation and seizures. Quinolones may exacerbate weakness in myasthenia gravis patients. May cause hypo-/hyperglycemia in patients on oral hypoglycemic agents and insulin. Avoid excessive sunlight secondary to risk of photosensitivity. Also the bioavailability of quinolones is reduced with concomitant use of antacids and iron supplements. Use ciprofloxacin 2 hours before or 6 hours after antacids.

a. Contraindications. Known hypersensitivity to ciprofloxacin/other quinolones.

b. Drug interactions. Decreased bioavailability with antacids; vitamins with iron, zinc, and calcium; didanosine. Inhibits cytochrome P450; interacts with warfarin to prolong prothrombin time (10), increased/decreased concentrations of phenytoin, elevated theophylline and caffeine concentrations; hypoglycemia with use of glyburide, transient elevated creatinine concentrations with use of cyclosporine, increased ciprofloxacin concentrations with use of probenecid.

   2. Allergic reactions. Hypersensitivity reaction: rash, urticaria, angioedema, anaphylaxis (R), acute interstitial nephritis (24), vasculitis (25) (R), TEN (26).

      a. Pseudoallergic reactions. Phototoxicity (R), increased incidence in cystic fibrosis patients) (19,21).

   3. Adverse effects

      a. Idiosyncratic. Tenosynovitis, Achilles tendonitis (<1%), tendon rupture; elevated liver enzymes (2%); hematologic side effects—leukopenia, elevated/decreased platelets, pancytopenia, eosinophilia (0.1% to 5.3%) (21), QT prolongation.

      b. Toxic effects. Headache, paresthesias, peripheral neuropathy, restlessness, seizures, somnolence, acute psychosis (21).

      c. Other adverse effects. Anorexia, nausea, vomiting, diarrhea (2% to 15%) (21), abdominal pain; arthralagia.

C. Gatifloxacin

   1. Precautions. Alkalinity of the urine should be avoided during treatment secondary to risk of crystalluria. Avoid NSAIDs during treatment with quinolones as the concomitant use of these medications may cause CNS stimulation and seizures. Quinolones may exacerbate weakness in myasthenia gravis patients. Dose adjustment is needed for patients with renal insufficiency. May cause hypo-/hyperglycemia in patients on oral hypoglycemic agents and insulin. Avoid excessive sunlight secondary to risk of phototoxicity. Also, the bioavailability of quinolones is reduced with concomitant use of antacids and iron supplements.

      a. Contraindications. Known hypersensitivity to gatifloxacin/other quinolones.

      b. Drug interactions. Decreased bioavailability with antacids; vitamins with iron, zinc, calcium, didanosine; increases digoxin concentrations; increases gatifloxacin concentrations with concomitant use of probenecid; no significant interactions have been observed with milk, calcium, cimetidine, theophylline, warfarin, midazolam, warfarin, and NSAIDs, but monitoring of anticoagulation is advised with concomitant use of gatifloxacin; use of NSAIDs with some quinolones may increase the risks of CNS stimulation and seizures, and patients should be cautioned to avoid NSAIDs while taking gatifloxacin

   2. Allergic reactions. Rash, maculopapular/vesiculobullous rash (R), angioedema, anaphylaxis (R).

      a. Pseudoallergic reactions. Phototoxicity is lower than with ciprofloxacin.

   3. Adverse effects

      a. Idiosyncratic. Seizures (R) (9), abnormal vision, taste perversion, tinnitus, torsades de pointes, hypoglycemia (R), hyperglycemia, neutropenia, thrombocytopenia, elevated LFTs, tendon rupture.

   b.   Other adverse effects. Nausea, vomiting, diarrhea, constipation, abdominal pain, anorexia, dyspepsia, glossitis, stomatitis, hepatitis, mouth ulcer, oral moniliasis, dyspnea, headache, dizziness, nervousness, insomnia, vertigo, somnolence, peripheral edema, hypertension, palpitation, [arthralgia, myalgia] (R), vaginitis.
D.   Levofloxacin
   1.   Precautions. Alkalinity of the urine should be avoided during treatment secondary to risk of crystalluria. Avoid NSAIDs during treatment with quinolones as the concomitant use of these medications may cause CNS stimulation and seizures. Quinolones may exacerbate weakness in myasthenia gravis patients. Dose adjustment is needed for patients with renal insufficiency. May cause hypo-/hyperglycemia in patients on oral hypoglycemic agents and insulin. Avoid excessive sunlight secondary to risk of phototoxicity.
   Rapid intravenous infusion has been associated with hypotension; therefore, this medication should be administered over 60 to 90 minutes. Rare cases of torsades de pointes have been associated with use of levofloxacin. Avoid use of class IA and class III antiarrhythmics with levofloxacin. Also, the bioavailability of quinolones is reduced with concomitant use of antacids and iron supplements (2 hours before and 6 hours after).
      a.   Contraindications. Known hypersensitivity to levofloxacin/other quinolones.
      b.   Drug interactions. No significant effect with use of theophylline, warfarin, cyclosporine, digoxin, probenecid, or cimetidine; increased risk of CNS stimulation and seizures with concomitant administration of NSAIDs.
   2.   Allergic reactions. Rash, urticaria, erythematous rash, anaphylaxis, SJS (R).
      a.   Pseudoallergic reactions. Anaphylactoid reaction.
   3.   Adverse effects
      a.   Idiosyncratic. Seizures (R) (9), QT prolongation, tendonitis (R), tendon rupture, hypoglycemia (R), decreased lymphocytes, taste perversion.
      b.   Other adverse effects. Nausea, diarrhea, vomiting, constipation, abdominal pain, dyspepsia, flatulence, pruritis, vaginitis, [genital moniliasis, genital pruritis, fungal infection] (R), headache, dizziness, insomnia, nervousness.
E.   Moxifloxacin
   1.   Precautions (see Ciprofloxacin)
      a.   Contraindications. Known hypersensitivity to moxifloxacin/other quinolones.
      b.   Drug interactions. Decreased bioavailability with antacids, vitamins with iron, zinc, and calcium, didanosine; does not inhibit cytochrome P450 isoenzymes; no observed interaction with NSAIDs, warfarin, itraconazole, theophylline, digoxin, probenecid, morphine, ranitidine, oral contraceptives, glyburide.
   2.   Allergic reactions rash (maculopapular, purpuric, pustular), anaphylaxis (R).
   3.   Adverse effects

    a. Idiosyncratic. Taste perversion, cholestatic jaundice, prolonged QT interval (9), tendon rupture, abnormal LFTs, thrombocytopenia, thrombocythemia, eosinophilia, leukopenia.

    b. Toxic effects. Tendon disorder (rare).

    c. Other adverse effects. Anorexia, stomatitis, glossitis, nausea, vomiting, diarrhea, constipation, abdominal pain, flatulence, dry mouth, dyspepsia (R), pruritis, dizziness, anxiety, confusion, seizures (R), tremor, vertigo, somnolence, paresthesia, hypertensive neuropathy, peripheral edema, tachycardia, arthralagia, myalgia, dyspnea, pruritis, sweating, vaginitis, vaginal moniliasis.

F. Norfloxacin

  1. Precautions (see Ciprofloxacin)

    a. Contraindications. Known hypersensitivity to norfloxacin/other quinolones; any associated tendonitis or tendon rupture associated with other quinolones

    b. Drug interactions. Increased theophylline and cyclosporine levels, enhanced effects of oral anticoagulants, decreased excretion of norfloxacin with use of probenecid. Nitrofurantoin may antagonize effect of norfloxacin, multivitamins, iron, zinc, and didanosine decreases absorption of norfloxacin, interferes with metabolism of caffeine.

  2. Allergic reactions. Rash, angioedema, vasculitis [urticaria] (R), dyspnea, arthralgia, myalgia, eosinophilia (27), eosinophilic necrotizing granulomatous hepatitis (28), acute interstitial nephritis (24), fixed drug eruption (FDE) (29), TEN, SJS, erythema multiforme, exfoliative dermatitis (R).

    a. Pseudoallergic reactions. Photosensitivity.

  3. Adverse effects

    a. Idiosyncratic. Tendon rupture, paresthesias of the finger, visual disturbances, seizures (19), cholestatic jaundice (30), increased AST, decreased WBCs, decreased platelet count, increased urine protein, decreased hemoglobin and hematocrit, increased eosinophils.

    b. Toxic effects. Headache, dizziness

    c. Other adverse effects. Anorexia (R), nausea, vomiting, diarrhea, constipation, flatulence, dyspepsia, abdominal cramping, anal/rectal pain, asthenia, hyperhidrosis.

G. Ofloxacin

  1. Precautions (see Ciprofloxacin)

    a. Contraindications. Known hypersensitivity to ofloxacin/other quinolones.

    b. Drug interactions. Decreased absorption with administration of antacids, sucralfate, metal cations, multivitamins, and didanosine; potential for interaction with cimetidine, cyclosporine, and probenecid (not studied), inhibition of cytochrome P450 may prolong half-life of theophylline and warfarin, increased risk of CNS stimulation and seizures with concomitant use of NSAIDs, hypo-/hyperglycemia with concomitant use of insulin/oral hypoglycemic agents.

  2. Allergic reactions. Rash [hypersensitivity vasculitis, angioedema, urticaria] (R), FDE, pneumonitis, stridor, serum sickness, erythema multiforme (31), SJS, TEN, conjunctivitis, vesiculobullous eruption, anaphylactic reactions, exfoliative dermatitis (R).

    a. Pseudoallergic reactions. Anaphylactoid reactions, phototoxicity.

  3. Adverse effects

    a. Idiosyncratic. Anemia leukopenia, leukocytosis, neutropenia, neutrophilia, increased band forms, lymphocytopenia, eosinophilia, lymphocytosis, thrombocytopenia, thrombocytosis, elevated erythrocyte sedimentation rate, elevated AST/ALT and alkaline phosphatase, hyper-/hypoglycemia, elevated BUN/creatinine, pancreatitis (R), tendonitis, tendon rupture.

    b. Toxic effects. Transient hearing loss (R).

    c. Other adverse effects. Nausea, vomiting, diarrhea, dysgeusia, pruritis, headache, dizziness, insomnia, [seizures, confusion] (R), genital pruritis in women, vaginitis.

VIII. Tetracyclines. The tetracyclines are used to manage respiratory, genital, systemic (Lyme disease, Rocky Mountain spotted fever, etc.), and local skin and soft-tissue infections. Since tetracycline can temporarily inhibit bone growth, its use is contraindicated during pregnancy, breast-feeding, and age younger than 8 years.

The absorption of tetracycline is decreased with the ingestion of milk; antacids containing calcium, magnesium, or aluminum; and with the use of iron supplements. Therefore, these products should be taken several hours before or after tetracycline medication. The most common side effects are gastrointestinal disturbances and photosensitivity (tetracycline > doxycycline > minocycline in order of decreasing frequency of photosensitivity reactions).

  A. Doxycycline

    1. Precautions. Absorption is decreased by use of antacids and iron supplements.

    a. Contraindications. Pregnancy, breast-feeding, and age younger than 8 years.

      Hypersensitivity to tetracyclines.

    b. Drug interactions. Potentiation of anticoagulant effects; interference with bactericidal action of penicillin; decreased absorption of antacids containing aluminum, calcium, magnesium, and iron preparations; decreased half-life of doxycycline with concomitant use of barbiturates, carbamazepine, and phenytoin; decreased effectiveness of oral contraceptives.

    2. Allergic reactions (C). Hypersensitivity reaction, maculopapular and erythematous rashes, urticaria, angioedema, anaphylaxis, exfoliative dermatitis, serum sickness, pericarditis.

    a. Pseudoallergic reactions. Photosensitivity (C), anaphylactoid purpura.

    3. Adverse effects

    a. Idiosyncratic. Pseudotumor cerebri (R), tetracycline-associated side effects: elevated BUN, hemolytic anemia, neutropenia, thrombocytopenia, eosinophilia, bulging fontanels in infants.

    b. Other adverse effects. Nausea, vomiting, esophageal ulceration (R), vaginal candidiasis, anorexia, glossitis, dysphagia, enterocolitis, anogenital candidiasis.

B. Minocycline

    1. Precautions. Cautious use in patients with hepatic dysfunction. Tetracycline absorption is decreased by use of antacids and iron supplements.

        a. Contraindications. Pregnancy, breast-feeding, and age younger than 8 years. Hypersensitivity to tetracyclines.

        b. Drug interactions. Potentiation of anticoagulant effects; may interfere with bactericidal action of penicillin; decreased absorption of tetracyclines with use of antacids containing aluminum, calcium, or magnesium and iron preparations; decreased effectiveness of oral contraceptives.

    2. Allergic reactions. Hypersensitivity reactions, maculopapular/erythematous rashes, urticaria, angioedema, anaphylaxis, FDE, erythema multiforme, SJS, TEN, vasculitis, exfoliative dermatitis, serum sickness, myocarditis, pericarditis, acute interstitial nephritis, pulmonary infiltrates with eosinophilia, exacerbation of SLE (R).

        a. Pseudoallergic reactions. Photosensitivity.

    3. Adverse effects

        a. Idiosyncratic. Vertigo, tinnitus, skin and mucous membrane pigmentation (10% in first year, 20% in four years), drug-induced lupus-like syndrome, pneumonitis, hepatitis; tetracycline associated side effects: alopecia, seizures, paresthesia, bulging fontanels in infants, pseudotumor cerebri (R), discoloration of teeth in children < 8 years, elevated LFTs, agranulocytosis, hemolytic anemia, thrombocytopenia, leukopenia, neutropenia, eosinophilia (32,33).

        b. Toxic effects. Tinnitus, decreased hearing.

        c. Other adverse effects. Nausea, vomiting, diarrhea, headache, dizziness, ataxia, dyspepsia, stomatitis, glossitis, dysphagia, pseudomembranous colitis, pancreatitis, esophagitis, hepatic cholestasis, cough, dyspnea, bronchospasm, arthralgia, myalgia.

C. Tetracycline

    1. Precautions. Tetracycline absorption is decreased by use of antacids and iron supplements.

        a. Contraindications. Pregnancy, breast-feeding, and children < 8 years, hypersensitivity to tetracyclines.

        b. Drug interactions. Potentiation of warfarin, phenytoin, barbiturates, and carbamazepine; cholestyramine and cholestipol bind tetracycline and decrease absorption; milk, antacids, iron supplements, calcium, magnesium, and aluminum decrease absorption of tetracycline, may interfere with bactericidal action of penicillin, decreased effectiveness of oral contraceptives.

    2. Allergic reactions (C). hypersensitivity reactions, urticaria, angioedema, anaphylaxis, pericarditis,

maculopapular and erythematous rashes, FDE, exfoliative dermatitis, serum sickness, exacerbation of SLE.
  a.   Pseudoallergic reactions. Photosensitivity (C).
  3.   Adverse effects
  a.   Idiosyncratic. Pseudotumor cerebri (R), discoloration of developing teeth, temporary inhibition of bone growth, hepatotoxicity, hemolytic anemia, neutropenia, thrombocytopenia, eosinophilia.
  b.   Toxic effects. Elevated BUN.
  c.   Other adverse effects. Nausea, vomiting, glossitis, esophagitis (R), diarrhea, fungal superinfection, photosensitivity, vaginal candidiasis.
IX.   Streptogramins. Quinupristin–dalfopristin is the first available antibiotic of this class. This antibiotic is reported to be effective for the management of vancomycin-resistant *Enterococcus* infections. The most common side effects reported are arthralgias and myalgias (34).
  A.   Quinupristin–Dalfopristin (Synercid)
  1.   Precautions. This medication should be infused over 60 minutes. After completion of the infusion, the vein should be flushed with 5% dextrose in water to prevent venous irritation. Note that saline and heparin are incompatible with quinupristin–dalfopristin. The frequency can be changed to q12h in patients who experience arthralgias/myalgias. If these symptoms persist then the medication should be discontinued.
    a.   Contraindications. Hypersensitivity to quinupristin–dalfopristin, pristinamycin, and virginiamycin.
    b.   Drug interactions. Inhibits cytochrome P450 (3A4) (see page xxi); inhibits digoxin's gut metabolism, which can elevate digoxin concentrations. Raises cyclosporine concentrations.
  2.   Allergic reactions. Rash, maculopapular rash, urticaria.
  3.   Adverse effects
    a.   Idiosyncratic. Significantly elevated bilirubin (25% of patients); elevated LFTs; decreased platelets, sodium, and hemoglobin levels; pancreatitis.
    b.   Other adverse effects. Nausea, vomiting, diarrhea, abdominal pain, dyspepsia, pseudomembranous colitis, stomatitis, gout, peripheral edema, arthralgia, myalgia, confusion, dizziness, insomnia, paresthesias, dyspnea, pleural effusion, pain at intravenous injection site, thrombophlebitis, vaginitis.
X.   Nitrofurantoins
This antibiotic is used in the management of uncomplicated urinary tract infections and for prophylaxis of recurrent urinary tract infections.
  A.   Nitrofuranton
  1.   Precautions. Nitrofurantoin (Macrodantin) should be taken with food to enhance tolerance and absorption. Avoid using antacids containing magnesium trisilicate in conjunction with nitrofurantoin.
    a.   Contraindications. This medication is contraindicated in patients with impaired renal function because

of increased risk of pulmonary fibrosis from decreased clearance. There is a risk of hemolytic anemia due to erythrocyte system immaturity (glutathione instability). Therefore, this medication is contraindicated at term in pregnancy (including labor and delivery) and in neonates younger than 1 month.

   b. Drug interactions. Reduced bacteriostatic activity of nalidixic acid, decreased phenytoin concentration, decreased nitrofurantoin absorption with use of antacids containing magnesium trisilicate; probenecid and sulfinpyrazone can inhibit renal tubular secretion of nitrofurantoin, thereby increasing its concentration (C).

2. Allergic reactions. Acute pneumonitis/pleural effusions. May occur within hours to 7–10 days manifested by nonproductive cough, dyspnea, pleuritic chest pain, and chest x-ray evidence of alveolar or interstitial infiltrates and pleural effusions (may be unilateral). This reaction is reversible upon withdrawal of nitrofurantoin and does not have associated eosinophilia. A distinct condition is nitrofurantoin-induced pulmonary infiltrate with peripheral eosinophilia.

   Chronic pneumonitis. Cough and dyspnea insidiously appear after one month or longer of treatment. Mimics idiopathic pulmonary fibrosis. May respond to prednisone.

   Angioedema, maculopapular or erythematous reactions, urticaria, anaphylaxis, drug fever, exfoliative dermatitis, erythema multiforme, SJS (35).

3. Adverse effects

   a. Idiosyncratic. Pancreatitis, pulmonary fibrosis, hepatitis, hepatocellular and cholestatic injury, transient alopecia, cyanosis secondary to methemoglobinemia (R), hemolytic anemia, leukopenia, megaloblastic anemia, thrombocytopenia, agranulocytosis, aplastic anemia (R), eosinophilia with pneumonitis, pseudotumor cerebri (R)

   b. Other adverse effects. Anorexia, nausea, vomiting, diarrhea, abdominal pain, sialadenitis, pseudomembranous colitis, gastrointestinal bleeding (R); polyneuropathy, peripheral neuropathy, vertigo, headache, dizziness, [confusion, psychotic reactions] (R), electrocardiographic changes (nonspecific ST/T wave changes, bundle-branch block), associated with pulmonary reactions.

XI. Nitroimidazoles

A. Metronidazole

This antibiotic is useful in the management of serious anaerobic/polymicrobial infections, including brain abscess and bone/joint infections. It has also been useful for more common problems including clostridium difficile infection, bacterial vaginosis, *Helicobacter pylori* gastritis, and acne rosacea (17). A disulfiram-like reaction can occur with concurrent ingestion of alcohol resulting in flushing, abdominal cramping, nausea, and vomiting.

   1. Precautions. Patients with severe hepatic disease need a lower dose of metronidazole since this medication is metabolized by the liver. Alcoholic beverages should be avoided because of a disulfiram-like reaction with continued avoidance for three days after completion of treatment with metronidazole.

    a. Contraindications. During first trimester of pregnancy, prior hypersensitivity to metronidazole.

    b. Drug interactions. Anticoagulant drug effects and increases lithium concentrations, disulfiram-like reaction with ingestion of alcohol, prolonged PT with warfarin (17), increased elimination of metronidazole with microsomal enzyme inducers (i.e., phenytoin, phenobarbital), increased concentrations with cimetidine.

2. Allergic reactions. Urticaria, erythematous rash, fever.

3. Adverse effects

    a. Idiosyncratic. Pancreatitis (R), metallic taste.

    b. Toxic effects. Reversible neutropenia and thrombocytopenia (R).

    Seizures, peripheral neuropathy, encephalopathy, cerebellar dysfunction.

    c. Other adverse effects. Anorexia, nausea, diarrhea, abdominal cramping, glossitis, stomatitis, dry mouth, thrush, vaginitis (17), headache, dizziness, vertigo, ataxia, insomnia, dysuria, polyuria, incontinence, flattening of T-wave on ECG readings, sodium retention with use of intravenous metronidazole and sodium containing intravenous fluids. In 1985, three patients were reported with breast cancer or cholangiocarcinoma after 4, 5, and 36 months of continuous use (36). Whether this observation is cause and effect remains unknown.

XII. Lincosamide. The only drug in this class is clindamycin. This antibiotic is used to manage anaerobic and gram-positive aerobic infections. Patch testing with clindamycin can be useful in the diagnosis of hypersensitivity. In a recent study of six patients with cutaneous reactions to clindamycin, four of six (66.6%) had a positive clindamycin patch test result (37). Oral desensitization with clindamycin was performed in an AIDS patient with *Toxoplasma* encephalitis. The protocol began with a dose of 20 mg three times daily, and the dose was doubled daily until a final dose of 600 mg four times daily was reached on day 7 (38).

  A. Clindamycin

    1. Precautions. Use with caution in patients with diarrhea and severe renal or liver disease.

      a. Contraindications. Hypersensitivity to clindamycin or lincomycin.

      b. Drug interactions. Enhances effects of neuromuscular blocking agents, antagonism between clindamycin and erythromycin.

    2. Allergic reactions. Hypersensitivity reactions (R) (39), maculopapular rash, morbilliform rash (C), vesiculobullous rash, drug fever, urticaria, eosinophilia, anaphylaxis; erythema multiforme, SJS (R) (17).

      a. Pseudoallergic reactions. Anaphylactoid reaction.

    3. Adverse effects

a. Idiosyncratic. Jaundice, metallic taste, transient elevated LFTs, neutropenia and thrombocytopenia (R) (17), agranulocytosis, eosinophilia.

b. Toxic effects. Cardiopulmonary arrest and hypotension after too rapid intravenous administration (R).

c. Other adverse effects. Diarrhea, *C. difficile* colitis (0.01% to 10%) (17), anorexia, nausea, vomiting, bitter taste, esophagitis, flatulence, abdominal distention, abdominal pain, pseudomembranous colitis, pruritis, vaginitis, exfoliative dermatitis, renal dysfunction (R), polyarthritis (R), thrombophlebitis after intravenous injection.

XIII. Phosphoric Acid

A. Fosfomycin. This is a member of the phosphoric acid antibiotic class. It is used as a single-dose regimen in the management of uncomplicated urinary tract infection. Overall this medication is well tolerated. Rosales and Vega reported a case of fosfomycin anaphylaxis with a positive skin prick and intradermal test to fosfomycin (40).

1. Precautions. Do not use more than one dose to manage acute cystitis because repeated doses increase the incidence of adverse events.

a. Contraindications. Hypersensitivity to fosfomycin.

b. Drug interactions. Metoclopramide lowers serum concentrations and urinary excretion of fosfomycin.

2. Allergic reactions. angioedema, maculopapular rash, erythematous/vesicular exanthems (41)

3. Adverse effects

a. Idiosyncratic. [Aplastic anemia, cholestatic jaundice, hepatic necrosis, toxic megacolon] (R), increased eosinophil count, increased/decreased WBCs, decreased hemoglobin/hematocrit, increased/decreased platelet.

b. Toxic effects

c. Other adverse effects. Nausea, vomiting, diarrhea, dyspepsia, abdominal pain, asthenia, rhinitis, pharyngitis, asthma (R), headache, dizziness, vaginitis, dysmenorrhea.

XIV. Monobactams

A. Aztreonam (see Chapter 1)

XV. Carbapenems/carbacephems

A. Ertapenem, Imipenem, Meropenem, Loracarbef (see Chapter 1)

XVI. Urinary agents bacteriostatic

A. Mandelamine. This drug is used as a bacteriostatic agent for urinary tract infections. It requires attention to agents that raise urine pH, which reduces the beneficial actions of mendelamine.

1. Precautions

a. Drug interactions. Antacids, ascorbic acid, and acetazolamide may cause alkalinization of the urine; this opposes the action of mandelamine, which requires an acidic pH. Avoid citric acid (lemonade), which raises the urine pH.

2. Allergic reactions

3. Adverse effects

a. Other adverse effects. Anorexia, nausea, vomiting, diarrhea.

B. Hippuric acid

1. **Precautions.** Hippuric acid is a component of cranberry juice which is beneficial for urinary tract infections because it acidifies the urine.
2. **Allergic reactions.** Erythematous rash (42) (R)
3. **Adverse effects**
   a. **Other adverse effects.** Nausea, vomiting, pruritis (42).

Acknowledgment

Supported by the Ernest S. Bazley Grant to Northwestern Memorial Hospital and Northwestern University.

REFERENCES

1. Kahlmeter G, Dahlager JI. Aminoglycoside toxicity: a review of clinical studies published between 1975 and 1982. *J Antimicrob Chemother* 1984;13:9–22.
2. Edson RS, Terrell CL. The aminoglycosides. *Mayo Clin Proc* 1999;74:519–528.
3. McGowan JP. Aminoglycosides, vancomycin, and quinolones. *Cancer Invest* 1998;16:528–537.
4. Spigarelli MG, Hurwitz ME, Nasr SZ. Hypersensitivity to inhaled TOBI following reaction to gentamicin. *Pediatr Pulmonol* 2002;33:311–314.
5. Wilhelm MP, Estes L. Vancomycin. *Mayo Clin Proc* 1999;74:928–935.
6. Masters PA, O'Bryan TA, Zurlo J, et al. Trimethoprim–sulfamethoxazole revisited. *Arch Intern Med* 2003;163:402–410.
7. Smilack JD. Trimethoprim–sulfamethoxazole. *Mayo Clin Proc* 1999;74:730–734.
8. Greenberger PA. Drug Allergy (Part B). Allergic reactions to individual drugs: low molecular weight. In: Grammer LC, Greenberger PA, eds. *Patterson's Allergic diseases,* 6th ed. Philadelphia: Lippincott Williams & Wilkins, 2002:335–385.
9. Alvarez-Elcor S, Enzler MJ. The macrolides: erythromycin, clarithromycin, and azithromycin. *Mayo Clin Proc* 1999;74:613–634.
10. DeMoly P, Benahmed S, Sahla H, et al. Allergy to macrolides: 21 cases. *Presse Med* 2000;29:294–298.
11. Igea JM, Quirce S, de la Hoz B, et al. Adverse cutaneous reactions due to macrolides. *Ann Allergy* 1991;66:216–218.
12. Saenz de SP, Gomez A, Quiralte J, et al. FDE to macrolides. *Allergy* 2002;57:55–56.
13. Pascual C, Crespo JF, Quiralte J, et al. In vitro detection of specific antibodies to erythromycin. *J Allergy Clin Immunol* 1995;95:668–671.
14. Baylor P, Williams K. Interstitial nephritis, thrombocytopenia, hepatitis, and elevated serum amylase levels in a patient receiving clarithromycin therapy. *Clin Infect Dis* 1999;29:1350–1351.
15. Cascaval R, Lancaster D. Hypersensitivity syndrome associated with azithromycin. *Am J Med* 2001;110:330–331.
16. Longo G, Valenti C, Gandini G, et al. Azithromycin-induced intrahepatic cholestasis. *Am J Med* 1997;102:217–218.

17. Kasten MJ. Clindamycin, metronidazole, and chloramphenicol. *Mayo Clin Proc* 1999;74:825–833.

18. Walker RC. The fluoroquinolones. *Mayo Clin Proc* 1999;74:1030–1037.

19. Owens RC, Ambrose PG. Clinical use of the fluoroquinolones. *Med Clin North Am* 2000;84:1447–1469.

20. Rubinstein E, Camm J. Cardiotoxicity of quinolones. *J Antimicrob Chemother* 2002;49:593–596.

21. Giamarellou H, Antoniadou A. Antipseudomonal antibiotics. *Med Clin North Am* 2001;85:19–42.

22. Davila I, Diez ML, Quirce S, et al. Cross-reactivity between quinolones: report of three cases. *Allergy* 1993;48:388–390.

23. Matthews MR, Caruso DM, Phillips BJ, et al. Fulminant toxic epidermal necrolysis induced by trovafloxacin. *Arch Intern Med* 1999;159:22–25.

24. Hadimeri H, Almroth G, Cederbrant K, et al. Allergic nephropathy associated with norfloxacin and ciprofloxacin therapy. *Scand J Urol Nephrol* 1997;31:481–485.

25. Reano M, Vives J, Rodriguez P, et al. Ciprofloxacin-induced vasculitis. *Allergy* 1997;52:599–600.

26. Moshfeghi M, Mandler HD. Ciprofloxacin-induced toxic epidermal necrolysis. *Ann Pharmacother* 1993;27:1467–1469.

27. Mofredj A, Boudjema J, Cadranel JF. Norfloxacin-induced eosinophilia in a cirrhotic patient. *Ann Pharmacother* 2002;36:1107–1108.

28. Bjornsson E, Olsson R, Remotti J. Norfloxacin-induced eosinophilic necrotizing granulomatous hepatitis. *Am J Gastroenterol* 2000;12:3662–3663.

29. Fernandez-Rivas M. Fixed drug eruption (FDE) caused by norfloxacin. *Allergy* 1997;52:477–478.

30. Lucena MI, Andrade RJ, Sanchez-Martinez H, et al. Norfloxacin-induced cholestatic jaundice. *Am J Gastroenterol* 1998;93:2309–2311.

31. Nettis E, Giordano D, Pierluigi T, et al. Erythema multiforme-like rash in a patient sensitive to ofloxacin. *Acta Dermatol Venereol* 2002;82:395–396.

32. Smilack JD. The tetracyclines. *Mayo Clin Proc* 1999;74:727–729.

33. Shapiro LE, Knowles SR, Shear NH. Comparative safety of tetracycline, minocycline and doxycycline. *Arch Dermatol* 1997;133:1224–1230.

34. Moellering RC, Linden PK, Reinhardt J, et al. The efficacy and safety of uinupristin/dalfopristin for the treatment of infections caused by vancomycin-resistant *Enterococcus faecium*. *J Antimicrob Chemother* 1999;44:251–261.

35. D'Arcy PF. Nitrofurantoin. *Drug Intell Clin Pharm* 1985;19:540–547.

36. Krause JR, Ayuyang HQ, Ellis LD. Occurrence of three cases of carcinoma in individuals with Crohn's disease treated with metronidazole. *Am J Gastroenterol* 1985;80:978–982.

37. Lammintausta K, Tokola R, Kalimo K. Cutaneous adverse reactions to clindamycin: results of skin test and oral exposure. *Br J Dermatol* 2002;146:643–648.

38. Marcos C, Sopena B, Luna I, et al. Clindamycin desensitization in an AIDS patient. *AIDS* 1995;9:1201–1202.

39. Mazur N, Greenberger PA, Regalado J. Clindamycin hypersensitivity appears to be rare. *Ann Allergy Asthma Immunol* 1999;82:443–445.
40. Rosales MJ, Vega F. Anaphylactic shock due to fosfomycin. *Allergy* 1998;53:905–907.
41. Mayama T, Yokota M, Shimatani I, et al. Analysis of oral fosfomycin calcium (Fosmicin) side-effects after marketing. *Int J Clin Pharmacol* 1993;31:77–82.
42. Gerstein AR, Okun R, Gonick HC, et al. The prolonged use of methenamine hippurate in the treatment of chronic urinary tract infection. *J Urol* 1968;100:767–771.

Antituberculous Drugs

Bruce D. Tempest and Gary Simpson

I.   First-line agents. Since tuberculosis drugs are combined for the management of disease and many of the drugs are hepatotoxic, rapid recognition of hepatitis and identification of the offending drug(s) is important. Hepatotoxicity of the first-line drugs is most commonly due to isoniazid followed in order by pyrazinamide, rifampin, and ethambutol.
  A.   Isoniazid
    1.   Contraindication. Acute liver damage; prior INH liver damage.
    2.   Caution. INH inhibits the metabolism of phenytoin and carbamazepine in some patients, increasing serum levels requiring dosage adjustment of anticonvulsant (Table 3.1).
    3.   Allergic reactions. Skin rash (R), lupus-like syndrome with arthralgia (R).
    4.   Adverse drug effects. Hepatitis, mild and self-limited (C) or progressive (R); nausea, vomiting, and/or epigastric distress (C); peripheral neuritis (R); seizures (R); ataxia (R); euphoria (R); agranulocytosis (R); thrombocytopenia (R); aplastic anemia (R).
  B.   Rifamycins (rifampin, rifabutin, rifapentine).
    1.   Contraindications. Known allergy to rifamycins.
    2.   Caution. Rifamycins induce cytochrome P450 liver enzymes, which may result in decreased levels of certain drugs administered concomitantly (Table 3.2); rifabutin is a less potent inducer of these enzymes.
    3.   Allergic reactions. Rash or urticaria (C); myalgia (C); arthralgia (C); erythema multiforme (R); vasculitis (R); chills and fever noted especially with intermittent drug administration (R).
    4.   Adverse drug effects. Leukopenia (C), especially with rifabutin; nausea, vomiting, and/or diarrhea (C); hepatitis usually mild and cholestatic (C) but may be progressive if preexisting liver disease or when combined with other hepatotoxic drugs (R); thrombocytopenia (R), especially with intermittent drug administration; hemolytic anemia (R).
  C.   Pyrazinamide
    1.   Contraindications. Severe liver damage; acute gout; known allergy.
    2.   Allergic reactions. Rash (R); urticaria (R); photosensitivity (R).
    3.   Adverse drug effects. Hepatitis (C); hyperuricemia (C), which may be asymptomatic but can precipitate gout; nausea and vomiting and/or epigastric distress (C); arthralgia (R); myalgia (R); thrombocytopenia (R).
  D.   Ethambutol
    1.   Contraindications. Optic neuritis; known allergy.

Table 3.1. Isoniazid drug interactions

Acetaminophen	Oral anticoagulants
Aluminum hydroxide	Phenytoin
Carbamazepine	Primidone
Corticosteroids	Procainamide
Cycloserine	Rifampin
Disulfiram	Selective serotonin reuptake inhibitors
Ethanol	Theophylline
Ethionamide	Valproic acid
Glucocorticoids	

Table 3.2. Rifampin drug interactions

Major significance

Oral anticoagulants	Methadone hydrochloride
Oral contraceptives	Midazolam or triazolam
Cyclosporine	Phenytoin
Digitoxin	Quinidine
Glucocorticoids	Theophylline
Itraconazole	Verapamil
Ketoconazole	

Other interactions

β-Adrenergic blocking agents	Losartan potassium
Buspirone hydrochloride	Metronidazole
Chloramphenicol	Nifedipine
Clarithromycin	Nortriptyline hydrochloride
Dapsone	Opiates (morphine and codeine)
Diazepam	Ofloxacin
Digoxin	Propafenone hydrochloride
Diltiazem	Selective serotonin receptor, Antagonists (5-HT$_3$)

Antagonist

Disopyramide	Sulfonylureas
Doxycycline	Tacrolimus
Fluconazole	Tamoxifen citrate or toremifene citrate
3-Hydroxy-3-methylglutaryl coenzyme A reductase inhibitors	Tocainide
Haloperidol	Zolpidem tartrate

Modified from Finch CK, Chrisman CR, Baciewicz AM, et al. Rifampin and rifabutin drug interactions. *Arch Intern Med* 2002;162:985–992.

    2. Allergic reactions. Rash (R); arthralgia (R); anaphylactoid reactions (R).

    3. Adverse drug effects. Optic neuritis with impaired visual and red–green discrimination (R); peripheral neuritis (R); nausea, vomiting, and/or epigastric distress (R).

  E. Aminoglycosides. [streptomycin (first line), amikacin and kanamycin (second line)].

    1. Contraindications. Pregnancy; known allergy.

    2. Caution. Renal impairment requires dose adjustment; ototoxicity and nephrotoxicity may be additive with other drugs having similar toxicities.

    3. Allergic reactions. Rash (R); urticaria (R); anaphylaxis or asthma (R), especially if the formulation contains sulfites.

    4. Adverse drug effects. Ototoxicity, either auditory or vestibular (C); nephrotoxicity (C); potentiation of neuromuscular blockade when used with neuromuscular blocking agents or general anesthetics (R).

II. Alternative drugs

  A. Macrolides (azithromycin, clarithromycin)

    1. Contraindications. Known macrolide allergy.

    2. Caution. Can inhibit metabolism of statins, theophylline, fluconazole, pimozide, and cisapride.

    3. Allergic reactions. Anaphylaxis (R); rash (R); photosensitivity (R).

    4. Adverse drug effects. Nausea, vomiting, dyspepsia, diarrhea (C); *Clostridium difficile* colitis (R), hepatitis (R); nephritis (R); hyperkalemia (R); neutropenia (R); thrombocytopenia (R); vertigo (R); malaise (R).

  B. Quinolones (ciprofloxacin, levofloxacin, ofloxacin, moxifloxacin, gatifloxacin)

    1. Contraindications. Pregnancy; children; known allergy.

    2. Caution. With use in presence of central nervous system (CNS) disorders; adjust dose with renal insufficiency; antacids decrease absorption; increases theophylline levels.

    3. Allergic reactions. Rash (R); anaphylaxis (R).

    4. Adverse drug effects. Nausea, vomiting, abdominal pain, and diarrhea (C); CNS effects including headache, dizziness, nightmares, insomnia, toxic psychosis, confusion, malaise (C); hepatitis (R); nephritis (R); arthralgia (R); leukopenia, thrombocytopenia, pancytopenia (R).

III. Second-line drugs

  A. Para-aminosalicylic acid

    1. Contradictions. Known allergy.

    2. Caution. Patients with renal, hepatic, and cardiac failure.

    3. Allergic reactions. Fever (R); rash (R); arthralgia (R); agranulocytosis (R); leukopenia (R); thrombocytopenia (R); hepatitis (R).

    4. Adverse drug effects. Nausea, vomiting, abdominal pain, and/or diarrhea (C); malabsorption of lipids, B_{12}, and/or folic acid (R).

B. Ethionamide

1. Contraindications. Severe liver damage; known allergy.

2. Caution. Monitor glucose for hypoglycemia and thyroid function tests for hypothyroidism; use caution when combining with isoniazid and/or cycloserine as CNS effects may be additive.

3. Allergic reactions. Rash (R), thrombocytopenia (R).

4. Adverse drug effects. Nausea, vomiting, abdominal pain, stomatitis, and/or diarrhea (C); hepatitis, mild and self-limited or progressive, especially in association with diabetes (R); hypoglycemia (R); hypothyroidism (R); depression (R); neuropathy (R).

C. Capreomycin

1. Cautions. Adjust dose with renal insufficiency.

2. Allergic reactions. Rash; photosensitivity.

3. Adverse drug effects. Renal (C); eighth cranial nerve (C); hypokalemia (C).

D. Cycloserine

1. Contraindications. Seizures; depression; known allergy.

2. Caution. Use with caution when INH and/or ethionimide being administered as CNS toxicity may be additive, monitor blood levels; monitor phenytoin levels as cycloserine inhibits phenytoin metabolism.

3. Allergic reactions. Rash (R); photosensitivity (R).

4. Adverse drug effects. CNS (C), including lethargy, depression, confusion, seizures; hepatitis (R).

SELECTED READINGS

Finch CK, Chrisman CR, Baciewicz AM, et al. Rifampin and rifabutin drug interactions. *Arch Intern Med* 2002;162:985–992.

McEvoy G, ed. *AHFS drug information.* American Society of Health-Systems Pharmacists, 2002.

Rom WN, Garay SM, eds. *Tuberculosis.* Boston: Little, Brown and Co., 1996.

Antivirals

Gisela Torres and Stephen K. Tyring

I. Anti-herpes simplex virus nucleoside analogs

A. **Adverse drug effects.** Drug fever is a rare adverse reaction to systemic administration of these medications. Other rare side effects of these antivirals (except topical penciclovir) include headache and gastrointestinal symptoms, such as nausea and diarrhea; seizures rarely occur (Table 4.1). Additional specific adverse effects for this class are listed below.

1. **Acyclovir (Zovirax)**

   a. **Precautions.** Coadministration with probenecid or zidovudine increases the occurrence of serious adverse events.

   b. **Allergic reactions.** Rash, drug fever, and contact dermatitis are rare but occur (R).

   c. **Adverse drug effects.** Additional reactions include crystalline nephropathy (C), renal failure (R), and neurotoxicity (R) with occurrence of extrapyramidal symptoms, seizures, delirium, tremor, and/or myoclonus.

2. **Valacyclovir (Valtrex)**

   a. **Allergic reactions.** (U)

   b. **Adverse drug effects.** Hemolytic uremic syndrome and thrombotic thrombocytopenic purpura have been reported in association with high doses of this medication in human immunodeficiency virus (HIV)–positive or bone marrow transplantation patients, but are very unlikely to occur (R).

3. **Famciclovir (Famvir)**

   a. **Allergic reactions.** (U)

   b. **Adverse drug effects.** Rare headache and gastrointestinal symptoms. (R)

4. **Penciclovir topical (Denavir)**

   a. **Allergic reactions.** Rarely causes localized erythema and pruritus; contact dermatitis (R).

   b. **Adverse drug effects.** Can lead to altered taste (R).

II. Anticytomegalovirus nucleoside analogs

A. **Adverse drug effects for the class.** Common side effects include fever, headache, and gastrointestinal symptoms (C). Myelosuppression (most commonly neutropenia and thrombocytopenia) and central nervous system symptoms (seizures, altered mental status, coma) are rare adverse effects (R).

1. **Ganciclovir (Cytovene)**

   a. **Precautions.** Concomitant administration with zidovudine may exacerbate myelosuppression.

   b. **Allergic reactions.** Contact dermatitis can occur from ganciclovir intraocular implants (U).

   c. **Adverse drug effects.** Additional adverse events include hepatotoxicity (R), muscular tremors (R), and retinal detachment (R).

Table 4.1.   Antiviral immune-related reactions

Contact dermatitis: acyclovir, penciclovir, cidofovir, foscarnet, imiquimod, doconasol, vidarabine, lamivudine, interferon intralesional injections

Drug fever: acyclovir, valacyclovir, famciclovir, ganciclovir, valganciclovir, foscarnet, cidofovir, interferon, palivizumab, stavudine, zidivudine, didanosine, zalcitabine, lamivudine, abacavir, tenofovir, efavirenz, nevirapine, delavirdine, saquinavir, ritonavir, indinavir, nelfinavir, amprenavir

Rash/urticaria: acyclovir, penciclovir, foscarnet, cidofovir, ganciclovir, valganciclovir, ribavirin, zanamivir, interferon, palivizumab, zidovudine, delavirdine, efavirenz, nevirapine, didanosine, zalcitabine, stavudine, saquinavir, ritonavir, indinavir, nelfinavir, tenofovir, lamivudine, abacavir, amprenavir

Erythema multiforme/Stevens–Johnsons syndrome: delavirdine, efavirenz, nevirapine, amprenavir

Bronchospasm: ribavirin, oseltamivir, zanamivir

Anaphylactoid reactions: zalcitabine, oseltamivir, zanamivir

Anaphylaxis: palivizumab, interferon, abacavir

Eosinophilia: nevirapine

Hemolytic anemia: indinavir, amprenavir, ribavirin

---

2.   **Valganciclovir (Valcyte)**
   a.   **Allergic reactions.** None reported (U).
   b.   **Adverse drug effects.** Can cause nephrotoxicity (R) and peripheral neuropathy (R).
3.   **Cidofovir (Vistide)**
   a.   **Interactions.** Iritis and uveitis have been reported in patients concomitantly receiving protease inhibitors.
   b.   **Allergic reactions.** Rash (R) and contact dermatitis (R).
   c.   **Adverse drug effects.** Other rare adverse reactions include nephrotoxicity, metabolic acidosis, neutropenia, and anemia.
4.   **Foscarnet (Foscavir)**
   a.   **Interactions.** Foscarnet can lead to dangerously low serum calcium if coadministered with pentamidine or other medications that cause hypocalcemia.
   b.   **Allergic reactions.** Rash and genital ulcerations rarely occur from contact dermatitis from local accumulation of foscarnet in the urine (R).
   c.   **Adverse drug effects.** Fever is a very common side effect of interferons. This is mostly due to an idiosyncratic reaction along with fatigue, myalgias, and flulike symptoms.
   d.   **Other side effects** include nephrotoxicity (R), hypocalcemia (C), hypercalcemia (R), hypo- or hyperphosphatemia (R), nephrogenic diabetes insipidus (U), and neurotoxicity including headache (C), altered mental status (R), encephalopathy (R), tremors (R), and seizures (R).

III.   **Anti-influenza antivirals**
   A.   **Amantidine (Symmetrel) and rimantadine (Flumadine)**

1. **Interactions can occur** with antihistamines, class I antiarrhythmics, and anticholinergic and psychotropic medications.
2. **Allergic reactions.** (U).
3. **Common side effects** are gastrointestinal symptoms. Adverse neurologic reactions include anticholinergic symptoms (R), muscle tremors (C), dizziness/vertigo (R), depression (R), anxiety (R), ataxia (R); and overdose can lead to seizures, hallucinations, and coma. Arrhythmias and cardiovascular complications rarely occur.

B. **Oseltamivir (Tamiflu) and zanamivir (Relenza)**
1. **Allergic reactions.** (U)
2. **Side effects include** bronchospasm (R), anaphylactoid reactions (R), oropharyngeal edema and skin rash (R).

IV. **Other antivirals**
A. **Doconasol topical (Abreva)**
1. **Allergic reactions.** Only related to rare topical skin reactions.
B. **Imiquimod topical (Aldara)**
1. **Allergic reactions.** (U)
2. **Adverse drug effects** include erythema, itching, and burning at the application sites (U).
C. **Interferons or peginterferon-α**
1. **Allergic reactions.** Drug fever as part of an allergic reaction is rare, and rash (C) and anaphylaxis (R) also occur. These medications have been shown to induce autoimmune disorders, such as autoimmune thyroiditis (R).
2. **Adverse drug effects.**
   a. **Idiopathic reactions.** Fever is a very common side effect of interferons. This is mostly due to an idiosyncratic reaction along with fatigue, myalgias, and flulike symptoms (C).
   b. **Other adverse effects.** Long-term use can result in fatigue (C), decreased appetite (C), weight loss (C), depression (C), anxiety (R), psychosis (R), hyper- or hypotension (R), acute renal insufficiency (R), alopecia (R), hepatotoxicity (R), myelosuppression (neutropenia and thrombocytopenia) (R), and neurotoxicity (seizures, altered mental status) (R).
D. **Palivizumab (Synagis) is not an antiviral per se, but is used as viral prophylaxis.**
1. **Allergic reactions.** Commonly causes injection site reactions and rare anaphylaxis and drug rash (C).
2. **Adverse drug effects.** Other rare adverse effects include gastrointestinal media symptoms, elevated transaminases, otitis media, and upper respiratory infection symptoms (R).
E. **Ribavirin (Rebetol, Virazole)**
1. **Precautions.** Long-term therapy in HIV-positive individuals can lead to lymphopenia (dose related) (R), and intravenous administration can cause extravascular hemolysis and myelosuppression leading to anemia (R).
2. **Allergic reactions.** Commonly causes conjunctival irritation, wheezing/bronchospasm, and rash (C).

3. Adverse drug effects. Rarely causes gastrointestinal complaints, headache, lethargy, insomnia, mood changes, and reversible increase in bilirubin, iron, and uric acid levels (R).

V. Antiretrovirals

A. Nucleoside analog reverse transcriptase inhibitors (NRTIs)
  1. Allergic reactions for this class include rare drug fever and rash (R).
  2. Adverse drug effects. Common adverse effects for this class include lactic acidosis and hepatomegaly. Hepatic steatosis is a rare but potentially life-threatening toxicity.

B. Stavudine (Zerit, D4T)
  1. Allergic reactions. Drug fever and rash (R).
  2. Adverse drug effects. Other adverse effects include dose-related peripheral neuropathy (C), elevated transaminases (C), myopathy (C), and pancreatitis (R).

C. Zidovudine (Retrovir)
  1. Precautions. Caution must be taken when given with other myelosuppressive drugs and to patients on methadone.
  2. Allergic reactions. Drug fever and rash (R). Rare immune-related reactions include urticaria, pruritus, and nonspecific maculopapular rash (R).
  3. Adverse drug effects. The most commonly observed side effects are anemia and neutropenia (C). Hyper- or hypopigmented skin and discolored and slow-growing nails are also common (C). Other adverse effects include nausea (R), vomiting, hepatotoxicity (R), fatigue (R), peripheral neuropathy (R), myopathy (R), myositis (R), headache, insomnia (R), and ventricular arrhythmias (U).

D. Didanosine (ddI, Videx, Videx EC)
  1. Precautions. Medications that require an acidic environment for absorption, such as ketoconazole, dapsone, indinavir, delavirdine, and quinolones, should not be given simultaneously. Medications that affect peripheral nerves, such as zalcitabine and isoniazid, should be avoided as synergistic neurotoxicity is observed.
  2. Allergic reactions. Drug fever and rash (R).
  3. Common side effects are nausea, vomiting, diarrhea, peripheral neuropathy, pancreatitis, hepatitis, dry mouth, hyperuricemia, hypertriglyceridemia, optic neuritis, and rash (C). Rarely, pancytopenia and heart block occur (R).

E. Zalcitabine (Hivid, ddC)
  1. Interactions. Drug interactions have been reported with probenecid, cimetidine, metoclopramide, and aluminum and magnesium hydroxide preparations.
  2. Allergic reactions. Drug fever and rash (R). Additional allergic reactions for this drug are urticaria (R) and anaphylactoid reactions (U).
  3. Adverse drug effects. Other side effects are gastrointestinal, including pancreatitis (C), aphthous ulcers (C), esophageal ulcers (R), and hepatomegaly with steatosis (R), peripheral neuropathy (C), and neutropenia (R).

F. Lamivudine (Epivir, 3TC)
  1. Allergic reactions. Drug fever and rash (R).

2. Adverse drug effects. Side effects include nausea (C), vomiting (C), anorexia (C), peripheral neuropathy (C), headache (C), psychosis (R), malaise (C), fatigue (C), pancreatitis (R), hyperglycemia (R), neutropenia (R), alopecia (R), rhabdomyolysis (R), and mania (R).

G. **Abacavir (Ziagen)**
   1. **Allergic reactions.** A hypersensitivity syndrome occurs in approximately 5% of treated patients and includes a centripetal macular and papular rash, evolving to urticaria (C). Fever, malaise, arthralgias, and myalgias may precede the rash. Rechallenge is contraindicated because anaphylaxis (R), hypotension (R), or death (U) could occur.
   2. **Adverse drug effects.** Other side effects include nausea (C), vomiting (C), fatigue (C), diarrhea (C), anorexia (C), malaise (C), flulike symptoms (C), headache (R), myalgias (R), hepatitis (R), and hyperbilirubinemia (R).

H. **Tenofovir (Viread)**
   1. **Allergy reactions.** Drug fever and rash (R).
   2. **Adverse drug effects.** Common toxicities include increases in creatine phosphokinase and transaminases.

I. **Nonnucleoside reverse transcriptase inhibitors (NNRTIs)**
   1. **Precautions for the class.** NNRTIs are metabolized by the cytochrome P450 system and thus may interact with other medications metabolized by this system; special care should be taken when administered with protease inhibitors as synergistic liver toxicity may occur.
   2. **Allergic reactions** for this class include rash (R) and drug fever (R).
   3. **Adverse drug effects** for the class: Increases in transaminase levels are seen (R).

J. **Nevirapine (Viramune)**
   1. **Interactions.** Significant interactions with methadone and cisapride can occur.
   2. **Allergic reactions** include rash and fever (C), Stevens–Johnson syndrome (C), and eosinophilia (R).
   3. **Adverse drug effects.** Other side effects include headache (C), hepatitis (C), liver toxicity (R), interstitial nephritis (C), interstitial nephritis(R), and myocarditis (R).

K. **Delavirdine (Rescriptor)**
   1. **Allergic reactions.** Allergic side effects include rash and Stevens– Johnson syndrome (C).
   2. **Adverse drug effects.** Other adverse effects include hepatitis (C) and headache (R).

L. **Efavirenz (Sustiva)**
   1. **Allergic reaction** commonly involves a maculopapular rash (C); erythema multiforme and Stevens–Johnson syndrome are unlikely (R).
   2. **Adverse drug effects.** Dizziness, insomnia, nightmares, delusions, hallucinations, amnesia, confusion, impaired concentration, somnolence, agitation, euphoria, depersonalization, and depression are common side effects (C). Other rare side effects include flulike symptoms, headache, dizziness, and myocarditis (R).

M. Protease inhibitors
   1. Precautions. Significant interactions with other drugs metabolized by the cytochrome P450 system can occur. Hemophiliacs on protease inhibitors have increased occurrence of spontaneous bleeding into joints, soft tissues, brain, and gastrointestinal system.
   2. Allergic reactions to the class. Drug fever and rash are rare allergic reactions to the class (R).
   3. Adverse drug effects for the class. Gastrointestinal side effects (diarrhea, nausea, vomiting, abdominal pain), lipodystrophy, and lipid abnormalities are common.
N. Saquinavir (Epivir)
   1. Allergic reactions. Drug fever and rash are rare allergic reactions to the class (R).
   2. Adverse drug effects: headache (R), hepatitis (R), diabetes mellitus (R), hyperglycemia (R), and elevated transaminases (R).
O. Ritonavir (Norvir)
   1. Allergic reactions. Drug fever and rash are rare allergic reactions to the class (R).
   2. Adverse drug effects: Headache (C), peripheral nerve and circumoral paresthesias (C), altered taste (C), hypermenorrhea (U), and elevated levels of uric acid, cholesterol, creatine phosphokinase, and transaminase occur (R).
P. Indinavir (Crixivan)
   1. Precautions. Coadministration with trimethoprim–sulfamethoxazole (Bactrim) increases risk of nephrolithiasis (C), crystalline nephropathy (R), and acute interstitial nephritis (R).
   2. Allergic reactions. Drug fever and rash are rare allergic reactions to the class (R).
   3. Adverse drug effects: Autoimmune hemolytic anemia rarely occurs (R). Dysphagia (C), headache (C), gynecomastia (C), hepatitis (R), hyperglycemia (R), diabetes mellitus (R), thrombocytopenia (R), neutropenia (R), asthenia (R), blurred vision (R), dizziness (R), metallic taste (R), and ventricular arrhythmias (U) also occur.
Q. Nelfinavir (Viracept)
   1. Precautions. Should not be given with other protease inhibitors.
   2. Allergic reactions. Drug fever and rash are rare allergic reactions to the class (R).
   3. Adverse drug effects. Common side effects include hepatitis and hyperglycemia (C).
R. Amprenavir (Agenerase)
   1. Allergic reactions. Stevens–Johnson syndrome occurs in 1% of patients (C). Drug fever and rash are rare allergic reactions to the class (R).
   2. Adverse drug effects. Other toxicities include circumoral paresthesias (C), hepatitis (R), diabetes mellitus (R), hemolytic anemia (R), and dysphagia (R).
S. Lopinavir/ritonavir (Kaletra)
   1. Allergic reactions. Drug fever and rash are rare allergic reactions to the class (R).

2. Adverse drug effects. Toxicities include exfoliative dermatitis (R), transaminase elevation (R), pancreatitis (R), hyperglycemia (C), neutropenia (R) and thrombocytopenia (R).

SELECTED READINGS

Brown TJ, Vander-Straten M, Tyring SK. Antiviral agents. *Dermatol Clin North Am* 2001:19:23–34.

Brown TJ, McCrary M, Tyring SK. Antiviral agents: nonantiviral drugs. *J Am Acad Dermatol* 2002;47:581–599.

Carrasco DA, Tyring SK. Advances in HIV treatment and treatment toxicities. *Dermatol Clin North Am* 2001;19:757–772.

Cunha BA. Antibiotic side effects. *Med Clin North Am* 2001;85:149–185.

Ford MD, Delany KA, Ling LJ, et al. *Clinical toxicology.* Philadelphia: WB Saunders, 2001.

Holdiness MR. Contact dermatitis from topical antiviral drugs. *Contact Dermatitis* 2001;44:265–269.

Tyring SK, ed. *Mucocutaneous manifestations of viral diseases.* New York: Marcel Dekker, 2002.

Ward HA, Russo GG, Shrum J. Cutaneous manifestations of antiretroviral therapy. *J Am Acad Dermatol* 2002;46:284–293.

Antifungal Compounds

Reem A. Shalabi and Thomas J. Walsh

I. Azole antifungal compounds

A. Clotrimazole (Lotromin, Mycelex)

1. **Contraindications.** Hypersensitivity reactions to clotrimazole.
2. **Allergic reactions.** Contact dermatitis (R), erythema (R), pruritus (R), urticaria (R), edema (R).
3. **Adverse drug effects.** Hepatotoxicity (R), dysuria (R), visual disturbances (R), depression (U), drowsiness (U), disorientation (U).
4. **Comments.** Pregnancy Category C. See Table 6.1.

B. Fluconazole (Diflucan)

1. **Contraindications.** Hypersensitivity reactions to fluconazole.
2. **Allergic reactions.** Itching (R), rash (R), eosinophilia (R), anaphylaxis (R), Stevens–Johnson syndrome (R), toxic epidermal necrolysis (R), fixed drug eruption (R), angioedema (U), buccal ulceration (U), acute generalized exanthematous pustulosis (U).
3. **Adverse drug effects.** Hepatotoxicity (C), dizziness (R), headache (R), hypercholesterolemia (R), hypertriglyceridemia (R), hypokalemia (R), adrenal insufficiency (R), alopecia (R), leukopenia (U), thrombocytopenia (U), seizures (U), torsades de pointes (U).
4. **Comments.** Hepatotoxicity is a class effect—elevation in transaminases. Pregnancy Category C.

C. Itraconazole (Sporonox)

1. **Contraindications.** Congestive heart failure; coadministration with astemizole, cisapride, dofetilide, midazolam, pimozide, quinidine, lovastatin, simvastatin, triazolam; hypersensitivity reactions to itraconazole.
2. **Allergic reactions.** Maculopapular rash (R), pruritus (R), photosensitivity (R), purpuric drug eruption (R), acute generalized exanthematous pustulosis (U).
3. **Adverse drug effects.** Hepatotoxicity (C), nausea (C, with oral cyclodextrin solution), peripheral edema (R), pulmonary edema (R), congestive heart failure (R), hypertension (R), neuropathy (R), headache (R), dizziness (R), fatigue (R), adrenal insufficiency (R), gynecomastia (R), renal dysfunction (R), hypokalemia (R), hypomagnesemia (R), hypercholesterolemia (R), hypertriglyceridemia (R), sexual dysfunction (R), pseudomembranous colitis (U), thrombocytopenia (U).
4. **Comments.** Pregnancy Category C.

D. Ketoconazole (Nizoral)

1. **Contraindications.** Coadministration with cisapride, astemizole, terfenadine, or triazolam; hypersensitivity reactions to ketoconazole.

    2. Allergic reactions. Rash (R), contact dermatitis (R), erythema multiforme (R), erythroderma (R), photosensitivity (R), fixed drug eruption (R), alopecia (R), facial angioedema (R), urticaria (R), pruritus (R), anaphylaxis (R).

    3. Adverse drug effects. Hepatotoxicity (C), adrenal insufficiency (R), fever (R), photophobia (R), nausea (R), papilledema (R), gynecomastia (R), impotence (R), oligospermia (R), hypertriglyceridemia (R), hypothyroidism (R), hypertension (R), paresthesia (R), headache (R), dizziness (R), somnolence (R), fatigue (R), arthralgia (R), myalgia (R), tinnitus (U), interstitial pneumonitis (U), depression (U), suicidal tendencies (U), thrombocytopenia (U), leukopenia (U), hemolytic anemia (U).

    4. Comment. Pregnancy category C.

  E. Voriconazole (Vfend)

    1. Contraindications. Hypersensitivity reactions to voriconazole; coadministration with cytochrome P450 3A4 substrates (pimozide, quinidine, sirolimus, ergot alkaloids, rifampin, carbamazepine, long-acting barbiturates, or rifabutin); galactose intolerance.

    2. Allergic reactions. Rash (R), Stevens–Johnson syndrome (R), toxic epidermal necrolysis (R), erythema multiforme (R).

    3. Adverse drug effects. Visual disturbances (C), hepatotoxicity (C), nausea (R), headache (R), hallucinations (R), peripheral edema (R), renal toxicity (U).

    4. Comment. Pregnancy Category D.

  F. As the general recommendations for management of allergic reactions to an individual azole preclude administration of another azole, there is a paucity of experience on rechallenging within the same class.

II. Polyene antifungal compounds

  A. Amphotericin B deoxycholate (Fungizone) and lipid formulations of amphotericin (Amphotec, Abelcet, Ambsome)

    1. Contraindications. Hypersensitivity to amphotericin B.

    2. Allergic reactions. Fever (C), chills (C), rigors (C), flushing (C), hypotension (C), rash (R), pruritus (R), hypoxia (R), dyspnea (R), anaphylaxis (R).

    3. Adverse drug effects. Elevation in serum creatinine (C; less common with lipid formulation), hypokalemia (C), hypomagnesemia (C), edema (C), tachycardia (C), headache (C), tachypnea (R), nephrogenic diabetes insipidus (R), hepatotoxicity (R), arrhythmias (R), bradycardia (R), hypertension (R), myalgias (R), arthralgias (R), anemia (R), thrombocytopenia (R), leukopenia (R), hyperkalemia (R), hypocalcemia (R), thrombophlebitis (R), delirium (R), confusion (R), depression (R), dizziness (R), paresthesia (R), cardiomyopathy (U), congestive heart failure (U), seizures (U), hypothermia (U), blindness (U). For management of severe acute infusion-related reactions to amphotericin B deoxycholate and its lipid formulations, there are several approaches available, depending upon severity and need for the polyene:

[1] discontinue and use another antifungal agent (especially for bronchospasm); [2] discontinue and resume under premedication; [3] for premedication for prevention of recurrent severe acute infusion-related reaction, consider acetaminophen plus diphenhydramine and hydrocortisone* (0.5–1.0 mg/kg/day up to a maximum dose of 50 mg/day). [4] meperidine 0.25–0.50 mg/kg up to a total of 25 mg during the early onset of the infusion related reaction; [5] for cases unresponsive or intolerant of these measures, lorazepam 0.02 mg/kg up to 1 mg PO or IV.

    4. Comment. Pregnancy Category B.

  B. Nystatin (Mycostatin)

    1. Contraindications. Hypersensitivity reactions to nystatin.

    2. Allergic reactions. Burning (R), itching (R), rash (R), Stevens–Johnson syndrome (U), contact dermatitis (U), exanthematous pustulosis (U).

    3. Adverse drug effects. Pain on application (R).

    4. Comment. Pregnancy Category A.

III. Allylamines

  A. Naftifine (Naftin)

    1. Contraindications. Hypersensitivity reactions to naftifine.

    2. Allergic reactions. Burning/stinging (R), dryness (R), erythema (R), itching (R), local irritation (R), contact dermatitis (U).

    3. Adverse drug effects. None.

    4. Comment. Pregnancy Category B.

  B. Terbinafine (Lamisil)

    1. Contraindications. Hypersensitivity to terbinafine.

    2. Allergic reactions. Rash (R), pruritus (R), urticaria (R), contact dermatitis (R), erythema (R), erythema multiforme (R), exanthematous pustulosis (R), toxic epidermal necrolysis (R), lupus erythematosus (R), anaphylaxis (R), Stevens–Johnson syndrome (U), pityriasis rosea (U).

    3. Adverse drug effects. Hepatotoxicity (C), nephrotoxicity (R), cholestasis (R), neutropenia (R), thrombocytopenia (R), arthralgias (R), myalgias (R), headache (R), dysgeusia (R), hyperglycemia (U).

    4. Comment. Pregnancy Category B.

IV. Echinocandins

  A. Caspofungin (Cancidas)

    1. Contraindications. Hypersensitivity to caspofungin.

    2. Allergic reactions. Fever (R), rash (R), facial edema (R), facial flushing (R), pruritus (R), erythema (R), bronchospasm (R), anaphylaxis (R).

    3. Adverse drug effects. Hepatotoxicity (R), headache (R), myalgias (R), paresthesias (R), tachycardia (R), hypokalemia (R), pulmonary edema (R), acute respiratory distress syndrome (R), tachypnea (R).

    4. Comment. Pregnancy Category C.

---

* If IV hydrocortisone is administered for >3 days, adrenal function should be monitored after discontinuation to rule out adrenal insufficiency

V. Miscellaneous

A. Flucytosine (Ancobon)

1. Contraindications. Hypersensitivity reactions to flucytosine.

2. Allergic reactions. Anaphylaxis (R), rash (R), pruritus (R), urticaria (R), photosensitivity (R), toxic epidermal necrolysis (U).

3. Adverse drug effects. Thrombocytopenia (C), leukopenia (C), anemia (C), hepatotoxicity (C), headache (R), hallucinations (R), anemia (R), peripheral neuropathy (R), liver necrosis (R).

4. Comment. Pregnancy Category C.

B. Griseofulvin (Grifulvin V)

1. Contraindications. Porphyria, hepatocellular failure, hypersensitivity reactions to griseofulvin.

2. Allergic reactions. Urticaria (R), rash (R), fixed drug eruption (R), angioneurotic edema (R), erythema multiforme (R), petechiae (R), photosensitivity (R), Stevens–Johnson syndrome (R), toxic epidermal necrolysis (R), exfoliative dermatitis (R), systemic lupus erythematosus (R), impetigo (U), allergic interstitial nephritis (U).

3. Adverse drug effects. Dysgeusia (C), proteinuria (R), leukopenia (R), dizziness (R), insomnia (R), mental confusion (R), hallucinations (R), paresthesias (R), peripheral neuropathy (U), headache (U).

4. Comment. Pregnancy Category C.

SELECTED READINGS

Groll AH, Walsh TJ. Caspofungin: pharmacology, safety and therapeutic potential in superficial and invasive fungal infections. *Expert Opin Invest Drugs* 2001;10:1545–1558.

Micromedex Healthcare Series: Micromedex. Greenwood Village, Colorado (edition expired 6/2003).

Pearson MM, Rogers PD, Cleary JD, et al. Voriconazole: a new triazole antifungal agent. *Ann Pharmacother* 2003;37:420–432.

Shoham S, Walsh TJ. Strategies for use of lipid formulations of amphotericin B. *Current treatment options in infectious diseases (in press).*

Sifton DW, ed. *Physicians' desk reference,* 57th ed. Montvale, NJ: Thompson, 2003.

Willems L, van der Geest R, de Beule K. Itraconazole oral solution and intravenous formulations: a review of pharmacokinetics and pharmacodynamics. *Clin Pharm Ther* 2001;26:159–169.

Antiparasitic Drugs

Omar Lupi and Renata Joffe

I. Antimalarial drugs

A. Chloroguanide, proguanil (Paludrine), chlorproguanil (Lapudrine)

1. **Therapeutic uses.** It is used as a safe alternative to mefloquine or other regimens for the prophylaxis of falciparum malaria or mixed vivax and falciparum infections. This drug is not available in the United States.

2. **Allergic reactions.** No allergic reactions reported (U).

3. **Adverse drug effects.** Nausea (R), diarrhea (R).

   a. Large doses (1 g daily or more). Vomiting (R), abdominal pain (C), diarrhea (C), hematuria (R), transient appearance of epithelial cells and casts in the urine (R).

   b. Pregnancy. Proguanil is considered safe for use during pregnancy (FDA Pregnancy Category A). [Pregnancy category information is listed in this chapter as many of these drugs are not available in the United States and pregnancy category information may not be readily available. See Table 6.1 for a description of the Food and Drug Administration (FDA) use-in-pregnancy ratings.]

B. Primaquine (Primaquine)

1. **Therapeutic uses.** Reserved for the terminal prophylaxis and radical cure of vivax and ovale (relapsing) malarias.

2. **Contraindications.** Acutely ill patients suffering from systemic disease characterized by a tendency to granulocytopenia (e.g., active systemic lupus erythematosus and rheumatoid arthritis). Patients receiving other potentially hemolytic drugs.

3. **Allergic reactions.** Angioedema (R), exanthemas 5% (C), pruritus (R), psoriasis (R), urticaria (R).

4. **Adverse drug effects.** Epigastric and abdominal distress (C), anemia (R), cyanosis (R) (methemoglobinemia), leukocytosis (C).

   a. High doses (60 to 240 mg daily). Methemoglobinemia (R), leukopenia (R).

   b. Overdosage. Granulocytopenia (R), agranulocytosis (R). Hypertension (R), arrhythmias (R), central nervous system (CNS) symptoms (U). Acute hemolysis and hemolytic anemia in humans with glucose-6-phosphate dehydrogenase (G6PD) deficiency (R).

5. **Pregnancy and lactation.** FDA Pregnancy Category C.

C. Chloroquine (Aralen)

1. **Therapeutic uses.** Effective in terminating or suppressing acute attacks of malaria, amebiasis.

2. **Contraindications.** Epilepsy, myasthenia gravis.

3. **Precautions.** Hepatic disease; seizures; gastrointestinal, neurologic, or blood disorders. Hemolysis can occur in patients with G6PD deficiency. Concomitant use of gold or

Table 6.1.   FDA use-in-pregnancy ratings

Category	Interpretation
A	**Controlled studies show no risk.** Adequate, well-controlled studies in pregnant women have failed to demonstrate a risk to the fetus in any trimester of pregnancy.
B	**No evidence of risk in humans.** Adequate, well-controlled studies in pregnancy woman have not shown increased risk of fetal abnormalities despite adverse findings in animals, or, in the absence of adequate human studies, animal studies show no fetal risk. The chance of fetal harm is remote but remains a possibility.
C	**Risk cannot be ruled out.** Adequate, well-controlled human studies are lacking, and animal studies have shown a risk to the fetus or are lacking as well. There is a chance of fetal harm if the drug is administered during pregnancy; but the potential benefits may outweigh the potential risk.
D	**Positive evidence of risk.** Studies in humans, or investigational or postmarketing data, have demonstrated fetal risk. Nevertheless, potential benefits from the use of the drug may outweigh the potential risk. For example, the drug may be acceptable if needed in a life-threatening situation or serious disease for which safer drugs cannot be used or are ineffective.
X	**Contraindicated in pregnancy.** Studies in animals or humans, or investigational or postmarketing reports, have demonstrated positive evidence of fetal abnormalities or risk which clearly outweighs any possible benefit to the patient.

phenylbutazone with chloroquine should be avoided (tendency to produce dermatitis). Should be avoided in patients with psoriasis because it causes severe reactions. Avoid use with mefloquine because of risk of seizures. Opposes the action of anticonvulsants and increases the risk of toxicity of these agents.

4. Allergic reactions. Dermatologic: Angioedema (<1%) (R), urticaria (R), pruritus (most commonly in dark-skinned persons) (U), contact dermatitis (U), psoriasis (C), pustular eruptions (R), Stevens–Johnson syndrome (R), toxic epidermal necrolysis (<1%) (R), lichenoid eruption (R), erythema multiforme (<1%), erythroderma, exanthemas (1% to 5%), exfoliative dermatitis (R), fixed drug eruption (<1%), photosensitivity (R), polymorphous light eruption (R), vasculitis (R), and vitiligo (R).

5. Adverse drug effects

  a. Acute toxicity. Hypotension (R), vasodilatation (R), suppressed myocardial function (R), cardiac arrhythmias

(R), cardiac arrest (R), confusion (R), convulsions (R), and coma (R). Gastrointestinal upset, headache, visual disturbances (diplopia) (R).

b. Skin side effects. Erythema annulare centrifugum (R), bleaching of hair (R), pigmentation (R), alopecia (R), gingival and oral mucosal pigmentation and ulceration (R), discoloration of the nail beds (R), porphyria (R). Widening of the QRS interval (R). Hemolysis (R), blood dyscrasias (R). Neuropsychiatric disturbances (U).

c. High daily doses (>250 mg). Irreversible retinopathy and ototoxicity (R), myopathy (R), cardiopathy (R), peripheral neuropathy (R).

d. Pregnancy and lactation. FDA Pregnancy Category D (controversial). Positive evidence for risk to human fetus; however, benefits may outweigh risks of using drug.

D. Hydroxychloroquine (Plaquenil)

1. Therapeutic uses. Effective in terminating or suppressing acute attacks of malaria, amebiasis.

2. Contraindications. Hypersensitivity, retinopathy (absolute). Pregnancy and lactation, myasthenia gravis, G6PD deficiency, psychosis (relative).

3. Allergic reactions. Angioedema (R), urticaria (R), pruritus (C), contact dermatitis (R), psoriasis (C), pustular eruptions (R), Stevens–Johnson syndrome (R), toxic epidermal necrolysis (<1%) (R), lichenoid eruption (R), erythema multiforme (<1%) (R), erythroderma (R), exanthems (1% to 5%) (C), exfoliative dermatitis (R), anaphylaxis (R).

4. Adverse drug effects

a. Headache (C), nausea (C), vomiting (U), diarrhea (R), fever (R), high levels of transaminases (R), excretion of uroporphyrins (C).

b. Restlessness (C), excitement (R), confusion (R), seizures (R), myasthenia (R), toxic psychosis (R).

c. Retinopathy (U), corneal deposits (R), and neuromuscular eye toxicity (R).

d. Hemolysis (R), blood dyscrasias (R).

e. Neuropsychiatric disturbances (U).

5. Pregnancy and lactation. FDA pregnancy FDA Pregnancy Category D (controversial). Almost all reviews suggest that hydroxychloroquine is contraindicated in pregnancy and lactation.

E. Quinine (Formula-Q, Legatrin, M-KYA, Quin-260, Quinamm, Quandan, Quiphile, Q-Vel)

1. Therapeutic uses. Treatment for malaria (chloroquine-resistant malaria).

2. Contraindications. Hypersensitivity, hemolysis, tinnitus, optic neuritis, cardiac dysrhythmias.

3. Precautions. Drug should not be given subcutaneously.

4. Interactions

a. Antacids containing aluminum may delay absorption.

b. Quinine may delay the absorption of digoxin and raise the plasma levels of warfarin.

c. Enhances the effect of neuromuscular blocking agents.

d. Renal clearance of quinine is decreased by cimetidine and increased by acidification of the urine.

5. **Allergic reactions**
   a. Fever (R), gastric distress (R), dyspnea (R), ringing in the ears (R), visual impairment (R), asthma (R).
   b. Cutaneous flushing (C), pruritus (C), skin rashes (C).
   c. Angioedema of the face (<1%) (R), contact dermatitis (R), eczematous eruption (R), erythema multiforme (<1%) (R), exanthemas (1–5%) (C), exfoliative dermatitis (R), fixed drug eruption (R), hyperhidrosis (R), hyperpigmentation, lichenoid eruption (U), photoallergic reaction (U), photosensitivity (C), pigmentation (C), purpura (R), Stevens–Johnson syndrome (R), toxic epidermal necrolysis (<1%) (R), urticaria (R), vasculitis (R), photo-onycholysis (U), oral mucosal eruption (R), bullous eruption (R), livedo racemosa (R).
   d. "Blackwater fever"—massive hemolysis, hemoglobinuria, anuria, renal failure, death (R).
6. **Adverse drug effects**
   a. Functional impairment of the eighth nerve results in tinnitus (R), decreased auditory acuity (R), and vertigo (R).
   b. Blurred vision (R), disturbed color perception (R), photophobia (C), diplopia (R), night blindness (R), constricted visual fields (R), scotomata (C), mydriasis (U) and even blindness (R) are probably the result of neurotoxicity (R).
   c. Optic atrophy (R)
   d. Nausea (U), vomiting (R), abdominal pain and diarrhea (R).
   e. Prominent sweating (R), acne (R), lichen planus (U), ochronosis (R), ulceration (R), porphyria (R).
   f. Hyperinsulinemia (R) and severe hypoglycemia (R).
   g. Severe hypotension (R), cardiac dysrhythmias (R)—sinus arrest, junctional rhythms, A-V block, and ventricular tachycardia and fibrillation (R).
   h. Hemoglobinuria (R).
   i. Excessive doses. Hypoglycemia (C) and hypotension (R). Headache (U), dysphoria (R), postural hypotension (R).
7. **Pregnancy and lactation.** FDA Pregnancy Category X.
F. **Mefloquine (Lariam, Mephaquine)**
1. **Therapeutic uses.** Should be reserved for the prevention and management of malaria caused by multidrug-resistant *Plasmodium falciparum.*
2. **Contraindications and interactions**
   a. Should be avoided during pregnancy.
   b. Should not be used in children weighing less then 5 kg.
   c. Contraindicated in patients with seizures or severe neuropsychiatric disturbances.
3. **Allergic reactions.** No allergic reactions reported (U).
4. **Adverse drug effects**
   a. Nausea (C), vomiting (C), abdominal pain (R), diarrhea (R), dysphoria (R), dizziness (C).
   b. Signs of CNS toxicity occur in half of the individuals (C).
   c. Ataxia (R), headache (C), visual or auditory disturbances (U).

d. Disorientation (R), seizures (R), encephalopathy (R), neurotic and psychotic manifestations (R).

5. Pregnancy and lactation. FDA Pregnancy Category C. Lactation Safety Unknown. Should not be used during first trimester of pregnancy. No risk to human fetus after the second trimester of pregnancy.

G. Pyrimethamine (Daraprim), pyrimethamine–sulfadoxine (Fansidar)

1. Therapeutic uses. Restricted to the suppressive management of chloroquine-resistant falciparum malaria.

2. Allergic reactions.

a. Skin rashes (C), erythema multiforme (R), Stevens–Johnson syndrome (toxic epidermal necrolysis) (R) (pyrimethamine–sulfadoxine).

b. Serum-sickness type reactions (R), urticaria (U), exfoliative dermatitis (R).

c. Acute generalized exanthematous pustulosis (R), angioedema (R), bullous eruption (R), exanthemas (C), fixed drug eruption (R), photosensitivity (R), pruritus (R), purpura (R), pustular eruption (R).

3. Adverse drug effects. Depression of hematopoiesis (C), megaloblastic anemia (C), hepatitis (R), alopecia (R), dysgeusia (R), glossitis (R), pigmentation (R).

4. Pregnancy and lactation. Risk cannot be ruled out—human studies are lacking. Animal studies may or may not show risk. Potential benefits may justify risk. FDA Pregnancy Category C. Lactation Safe.

II. Antiprotozoal drugs

A. Atovaquone (Mepron)

1. Therapeutic uses. It is used with a biguanide for management of malaria to obtain optimal clinical results and avoid emergence of drug-resistant plasmodial strains.

2. Contraindications and interactions. Contraindicated in patients with severe liver disease.

3. Allergic reactions. Maculopapular rash (C).

4. Adverse drug effects.

a. Fever (U), vomiting (R), diarrhea (R), headache (C).

b. Abnormalities of serum transaminase and amylase levels (U).

c. Hyperhidrosis (R), pruritus (R), oral candidiasis (R), dysgeusia (R).

5. Pregnancy and lactation. Can be carefully used. FDA Pregnancy Category C. Lactation Safe.

B. Eflornithine (Ornidyl)

1. Therapeutic uses. Management of West African trypanosomiasis (*Trypanosoma brucei gambiense*).

2. Allergic reactions. No allergic reaction reported (U).

3. Adverse drug effects

a. Anemia (C), diarrhea (C), leukopenia (C), convulsions (U).

b. Thrombocytopenia (U), alopecia (R), vomiting (R), abdominal pain (R), dizziness (R), fever (R), anorexia (R), headache (R).

c. Hearing loss in cases of prolonged therapy (U).

    4. Pregnancy and lactation. Should be avoided. FDA Pregnancy Category X.

C. Melarsoprol (Mel B, Arsobal)

    1. Therapeutic uses. It is the only effective drug available for the management of the late meningoencephalitic stage of both West African and East African trypanosomiasis.

    2. Precautions. *Entamoeba histolytica*

      a. The patient should remain in bed and not eat for several hours after the injection is given.

      b. Administration in leprous patients may precipitate erythema nodosum.

      c. Contraindicated during epidemics of influenza.

      d. Severe hemolytic reactions have been reported in patients with deficiency of G6PD.

    3. Allergic reactions. Febrile reaction (C), anaphylaxis (R).

    4. Adverse drug effects.

      a. Encephalopathy (U).

      b. Convulsions (R), acute cerebral edema (R), coma (R), acute nonlethal mental disturbances without neurologic signs (U), peripheral neuropathy (10%) (C).

      c. Hypertension, myocardial damage (C), shock (R).

      d. Albuminuria, vomiting, abdominal pain (C).

    5. Pregnancy and lactation. No pregnancy category has been assigned. FDA Pregnancy Category C.

D. Metronidazole (Flagyl, Metizol, Metric 21, Protostat). Available outside the United States: tinidazole (Fasigyn), secnidazole (Seczol-DS), ornidazole (Tiberal), benznidazole (Rochagan).

    1. Therapeutic uses. Genital infections with *Trichomonas vaginalis,* amebiasis (*Entamoeba histolytica*), infections due to anaerobic bacteria (*Bacterioides, Clostridium, Fusobacterium, Peptococcus, Peptostreptococcus, Eubacterium,* and *Helicobacter*).

    2. Precautions

      a. Should be used with caution in patients with active disease of the CNS (neurotoxicity).

      b. Avoid concomitant alcohol use.

    3. Allergic reactions

      a. Urticaria (R), flushing (R), pruritus (1% to 5%) (C).

      b. Acute generalized exanthematous pustulosis (R), angioedema (R).

      c. Exanthemas (R), fixed drug eruption (R), flushing (R), pityriasis rosea-like eruption (R), toxic epidermal necrolysis (R).

    4. Adverse drug effects

      a. Headache (C), nausea (U), dry mouth (R), metallic taste (C).

      b. Vomiting (R), diarrhea (C), abdominal distress (C).

      c. Furry tongue (R), glossitis (R), stomatitis (R), exacerbation of moniliasis (U).

      d. Dizziness (U), vertigo (U).

      e. Encephalopathy (R), convulsions (R), incoordination (R), ataxia (R), numbness (R), paresthesias (neurotoxic effects) (R).

f. Dysuria, cystitis, sense of pelvic pressure (R).
g. Disulfiram-like effect—abdominal distress, vomiting, flushing, headache when patients drink alcoholic beverages (R).
h. Temporary neutropenia (R).
i. Acute intermittent porphyria (R), gynecomastia (R), oral mucosal eruption and ulceration (R).
5. Pregnancy and lactation. FDA Pregnancy Category B. Should be avoided during first trimester of pregnancy. Contraindicated during lactation. Breast-feeding should be postponed for 12 to 24 hours to allow excretion of the drug.
E. Nifurtimox (Lampit, Bayer 2502)
 1. Therapeutic uses. Management of American trypanosomiasis (Chagas disease, *Trypanosoma cruzi*).
 2. Allergic reactions. Dermatitis (C), fever (R), icterus (R), pulmonary infiltrates (R), anaphylaxis (R).
 3. Adverse drug effects
  a. Headache (C), psychic disturbances (R), paresthesias (R), polyneuritis (R), and CNS excitability (R).
  b. Leukopenia (R), decreased sperm counts (U).
  c. Nausea (C), vomiting (C), myalgia (C), weakness (C), peripheral neuropathy (U), gastrointestinal symptoms (C).
 4. Pregnancy and lactation. Unrated drug. No pregnancy category has been assigned. FDA Pregnancy Category C.
F. Pentamidine (Nebupent, Pentam 300). Also see the chapter on AIDS treatment for use in *Pneumocystis carinii* prophylaxis.
 1. Therapeutic uses. Management of early lymphatic African trypanosomiasis due to *T. b. gambiense,* visceral leishmaniasis (*Leishmania donovani*), cutaneous leishmaniasis (*L. tropica).*
 2. Precautions: Toxicity and side effects occur in 50% of patients.
 3. Allergic reactions. Bullous eruption (R), exanthemas (1% to 15%) (U), Jarisch–Herxheimer reaction (R), pruritus (R), purpura (R), toxic epidermal necrolysis (R), ulcerations (R), urticaria (U), vasculitis (R), xerosis (R).
 4. Adverse drug effects
  a. Breathlessness (R), tachycardia (R), dizziness or fainting (R), headache (U), and vomiting (U).
  b. Pancreatitis (R), hypoglycemia (R), hyperglycemia (R).
  c. Thrombophlebitis (R).
  d. Thrombocytopenia (R), anemia (R), neutropenia (R).
  e. Elevation of liver enzymes (R), nephrotoxicity (C), impaired renal function (24%) (C).
  f. Ageusia (R), anosmia (R), dysgeusia (R), gingivitis (R), injection site calcification or cutaneous reaction (U), xerostomia (R).
 5. Pregnancy and lactation. FDA Pregnancy Category C. The use of pentamidine during pregnancy is controversial. Not recommended during lactation.
G. Sodium stibogluconate (sodium antimony gluconate, Pentostam; meglumine antimonate, Glucantime).

1. **Therapeutic uses.** Chemotherapy of leishmaniasis.
2. **Allergic reactions.** Skin rashes.
3. **Adverse drug effects.**
   a. Pain at the injection site (C).
   b. Chemical pancreatitis (C).
   c. Elevation of serum hepatic transaminase levels (U), bone marrow suppression (R), muscle and joint pain (C), weakness (C), malaise (U).
   d. Headache (C), nausea (C), abdominal pain (U).
   e. Reversible neuropathy (U).
   f. Hemolytic anemia (R), renal damage (R), shock (R), sudden death (R).
4. **Pregnancy and lactation.** FDA Pregnancy Category C. The use of stibogluconate during pregnancy is controversial. Not recommended during lactation.

H. **Suramin (suramin sodium, Bayer 205)**
   1. **Therapeutic uses.** Management of African trypanosomiasis caused by *T. cruzi,* and early stages of East and West African trypanosomiasis.
   2. **Precautions and contraindications.** If urine casts appear, suramin should be discontinued.
   3. **Allergic reactions**
      a. Febrile episodes (U), skin rash (C).
      b. Stomatitis (U), edema (R).
      c. Anaphylaxis (R).
   4. **Adverse drug effects**
      a. Nausea (U), vomiting (U).
      b. Shock (R), loss of consciousness (R).
      c. Malaise (C), fatigue (C).
      d. Albuminuria (renal toxicity) (R).
      e. Delayed neurologic complications (R): headache, metallic taste, paresthesias, peripheral neuropathy.
      f. Severe polyradiculoneuropathy (R).
      g. Diarrhea (U), chills (R), abdominal pain (U).
      h. Leukopenia (R), agranulocytosis (R), thrombocytopenia (R), proteinuria (R), elevation of plasma creatinine, transaminases, and bilirubin (R).
      i. Adrenal insufficiency (R), vortex keratopathy (R).
      j. Palmar-plantar hyperesthesia (R).
   5. **Pregnancy and lactation.** FDA Pregnancy Category C. The use of suramin during pregnancy is controversial. Not recommended during lactation.

III. **Antihelmintic drugs**
   A. **Thiabendazole (Mintezol)**
      1. **Therapeutic uses**–Larva migrans, *Strongyloides stercoralis.*
      2. **Precautions and contraindications.** Used with caution in patients with hepatic disease.
      3. **Allergic reactions.**
         a. Fever (U), rashes (U), exanthemas (<5%), erythema multiforme (<1%), anaphylaxis (U).
         b. Angioneurotic edema (R).
         c. Contact dermatitis (R), fixed drug eruption (<1%), flushing (U), Jarisch–Herxheimer reaction (R), perianal

rash (R), pruritus (<1%), psoriasis (R), Stevens–Johnson syndrome (R), toxic epidermal necrolysis (<1%) (R), urticaria (1% to 5%) (C).

4. Adverse drug effects
a. Anorexia (R), nausea (C), vomiting (C), dizziness (C).
b. Diarrhea (C), weariness (R), drowsiness (R), giddiness (R), headache (U).
c. Hallucinations (R), sensory disturbances (C).
d. Shock (R), tinnitus (R), convulsions (R), intrahepatic cholestasis (R).
e. Crystalluria without hematuria (U), transient leukopenia.
f. Paresthesias, xerostomia (R).

5. Pregnancy and lactation. FDA Pregnancy Category C. Pending further studies, evaluate risk/benefit ratio. The drug must be discontinued during lactation.

B. Mebendazole (Vermox)
1. Therapeutic uses. Gastrointestinal nematode infections: enterobiasis, ascariasis, trichuriasis, hookworm, cystic hydatid.
2. Contraindications.
  a. Pregnant women.
  b. Children less then 2 years of age.
3. Allergic reactions. Skin rash (U).
4. Adverse drug effects.
  a. Abdominal pain (U), abdominal distention (U), diarrhea (C).
  b. Alopecia (R), reversible neutropenia (U), agranulocytosis (U), hypospermia (R).
  c. Reversible elevation of serum transaminases (C).
5. Pregnancy and lactation. Contraindicated in pregnancy. There is no reason to risk use of the drug in pregnancy. FDA Pregnancy Category X.

C. Albendazole (Albenza)
1. Therapeutic uses. Gastrointestinal infections: ascariasis, trichuriasis, hookworm, enterobiasis, stongyloidiasis, cystic hydatid disease due to *Echinococcus granulosus,* alveolar echinococcosis due to *Echinococcus multilocularis,* and neurocysticercosis due to *Taenia solium* and *Encephalitozoon intestinale.*
2. Contraindications. This drug should not be given in pregnancy.
3. Allergic reactions. There are no allergic reactions reported (U).
4. Adverse drug effects
  a. Abdominal pain (C), diarrhea (C), nausea (C), dizziness (U), severe headache (C).
  b. Increase in serum aminotransferase activity (C).
  c. Jaundice (R), chemical cholestasis (R).
  d. Gastrointestinal pain (C), fever (R), fatigue (R), alopecia (R), thrombocytopenia (R).
5. Pregnancy and lactation. FDA unrated pregnancy category. Its use in pregnant women is not recommended. Avoid use during lactation. See pregnancy category C.

D. Diethylcarbamazine

1. **Therapeutic uses.** Chemotherapy, control of filarial disease.

2. **Precautions and contraindications.** Treatment with diethylcarbamazine should be avoided in areas where onchocerciasis or loiasis is endemic.

3. **Allergic reactions**

   a. *Mazzotti reaction* (U)–itching, skin rashes, enlargement of lymph nodes, papular rash, fever, tachycardia, arthralgia, headache.

   b. Punctate keratitis (U), uveitis (R).

   c. Eosinophilia (C).

4. **Adverse drug effects**

   a. Anorexia (U), nausea (C), headache (C), vomiting (C).

   b. Retinal hemorrhages (R), severe encephalitis (*Loaloa*) (R).

   c. Ocular complications (U): Limbitis, atrophy of retinal pigment epithelium.

   d. Leukocytosis (C).

   e. Reversible proteinuria (U).

5. **Pregnancy and lactation.** Controlled studies show no fetal risk. Appears to be safe for use during pregnancy. FDA Pregnancy Category A.

E. Ivermectin (Mectizan, Stromectol, 22,23-dihydro-avermectin B1a)

1. **Therapeutic uses.** Onchocerciasis, lymphatic filariasis, infection with intestinal nematodes.

2. **Contraindications.** Conditions associated with an impaired blood–brain barrier.

3. **Allergic reactions.** Mild itching and swollen (U), Tender lymph nodes (5% to 35%) (C).

4. **Adverse drug effects.** Fever (R), tachycardia (R), hypotension (R), prostration (R), dizziness (U), headache (C), myalgia (R), arthralgia (R), diarrhea (R), edema (R).

5. **Pregnancy and lactation.** FDA pregnancy category, risk unrated. Pending further studies, ivermectin should be avoided during pregnancy. It is excreted in milk causing no identifiable problems for the infant.

F. Piperazine (Multifuge)

1. **Therapeutic uses.** Highly effective against both *Ascaris lumbricoides* and *Enterobius vermicularis.*

2. **Contraindications.** Patients with a history of epilepsy.

3. **Allergic reactions.** Urticarial reactions (R).

4. **Adverse drug effects.** Gastrointestinal upset (C), transient neurologic effects (R).

5. **Pregnancy and lactation.** Can be used safely. FDA Pregnancy Category A.

G. Praziquantel (Biltricide, Distocide)

1. **Therapeutic uses.** Schistosomiasis, liver fluke infections.

2. **Precautions.** The bioavailability of praziquantel is reduced by carbamazepine, phenobarbital, and dexamethasone.

3. **Contraindications**

   a. Ocular cysticercosis.

   b. Driving, operating machinery should be avoided.
4. Allergic reactions. Fever (U), pruritus (C), urticaria (U), skin eruptions (U), arthralgia (c), myalgia (C).
5. Adverse drug effects. Abdominal discomfort (C), nausea (C), headache (C), dizziness (C), drowsiness (C), meningismus (R), seizures (U), mental changes (R), cerebrospinal fluid pleocytosis (U).
6. Pregnancy and lactation. Risk cannot be ruled out; human studies are lacking. Animal studies in rats showed risk of abortion. Best avoided during pregnancy. FDA Pregnancy Category X.
 H. Levamisole (Ergamisol)
   1. Therapeutic uses. Intestinal nematodes.
   2. Allergic reactions. Angioedema (<1%), erythema annulare (R), erythema multiforme (R), exanthemas (5% to 10%) (C), exfoliative dermatitis (U), fixed drug eruption (U), hemorrhagic eruption (R), lichenoid eruption (R), pemphigus-like eruption (R), pruritus (U), psoriasis (R), purpura (R), urticaria (R), vasculitis (R), anaphylaxis (R), erosive lichen planus (R), oral lesions (0.3% to 10%) (C), oral ulcerations (U), stomatitis (6%) (C).
   3. Adverse drug effects
      a. Dizziness (R), headache (C), abdominal pain (U), insomnia (R), nausea (C), vomiting (C).
      b. Xerosis (R), alopecia (R).
      c. Paresthesias (R), dysgeusia (R).
   4. Pregnancy and lactation. Can be used safely. FDA Pregnancy Category C. Lactation safety questionable.

SELECTED READINGS

Allen H, Crompton D, Silva N, et al. New policies for using antihelmintics in high risk groups. *Trends Parasitol* 2002;18:391.

Giao PT, de Vries PJ. Pharmacokinetic interactions of antimalarial agents. *Clin Pharmacokinet* 2001;40:343–73.

Griffin JP. Drug Interactions with antimalarial agents. *Adverse Drug Toxicol Rev* 1999;18:25–43.

Grover JK, Vats V, Uppal G, et al. Anthelmintics: a review. *Trop Gastroenterol* 2001;22:180–189.

Lamp KC, Freeman CD, Klutman NE, et al. Pharmacokinetics and pharmacodynamics of the nitroimidazole antimicrobials. *Clin Pharmacokinet* 1999;36:353–373.

Silva N, Guyatt H, Bundy D. Anthelmintics: a comparative review of their clinical pharmacology. *Drugs* 1997;53:769–788.

Allergy–Immunology

Burton Zweiman

I. Introduction. It seems almost paradoxical that drugs used to manage allergic disorders would themselves cause allergic reactions. However, such allergic reactions to this class of drugs do occur although they are usually rare. Nonallergic adverse reactions to these agents are more common and will also be discussed here.

II. H_1-Antihistamines, systemic therapy

A. First-generation antihistamines. Diphenhydramine (Benadryl, generic); chlorpheniramine (Chlortrimeton, many generic compounds).

    1. Contraindications. Driving, piloting plane, operating dangerous equipment, alcohol, sedatives, anticholinergic agents.

    2. Allergic reactions. (R).

    3. Adverse drug effects.

        a. Sedation, decreased cognition, decreased reflex capacity in driving, other activities (C) (frequently not recognized by patient).

        b. Other CNS effects. Stimulation, dizziness—more common in children.

        c. Anticholinergic. Dry respiratory secretions (sometimes helpful), decreased bladder function, aggravate visual problems (C).

        d. Gastrointestinal. Nausea, vomiting, diarrhea (U).

        e. Increased appetite. e.g., cyproheptadine (R), more in children.

B. Second-generation antihistamines. Terfenadine (Seldane) (withdrawn), loratadine (Claritin), astemizole (withdrawn in the United States), cetirizine (Zyrtec).

    1. Contraindications. Terfenadine, astemizole—Long QT interval, concomitant treatment with imidazole antifungal agents, macrolide antibiotics.

    2. Allergic reactions. (R).

    3. Adverse drug effects.

        a. Cardiac arrhythmias. (terfenadine, astemizole) (R).

        b. Sedation (cetirizine, 14% incidence versus 2% incidence for placebo).

C. Third-generation antihistamines. Fexofenadine (Allegra), desloratadine (Clarinex), mizolastine, ebastine (oral, topical).

    1. Contraindications. None.

    2. Allergic reactions. (R).

    3. Adverse drug effects. (R).

III. Oral sympathomimetics (decongestants)

A. Pseudoephedrine [Sudafed, component in many generic and over-the-counter (OTC) agents]

1. Contraindications. Severe hypertension, arrhythmias, monoamine oxidase inhibitor therapy, hyperthyroidism, bedtime use if insomnia, urinary outlet obstruction.

2. Allergic reactions. Fixed drug eruptions, contact dermatitis (R).

3. Adverse drug effects. Palpitations, tremor, insomnia, restlessness, increased systolic blood pressure (C); psychiatric disturbances (R).

B. Phenylephrine (Neo-Synephrine, generic component in some OTC preparations), used less commonly by oral route in recent years because of inactivation in gastrointestinal tract.

1. Allergic reactions. (R).

2. Adverse drug effects. Stimulation, but less prominent than pseudoephedrine.

C. Phenylpropanolamine. Formerly in many combination products (prescription, OTC).

1. Adverse drug effects. Headache, hypertension, CNS–psychiatric (C). Discontinued use in the United States because some reactions were severe (stroke).

IV. Ketotifen [available in United States only as eye drops (Zaditor)]

A. Contraindications (oral). Driving within several hours.

B. Allergic reactions. (R).

C. Adverse drug effects.

1. Oral. Sedation, increased appetite, seizures/infantile spasms in those with baseline seizure disorder (C).

2. Eye drops. Eye irritation (C).

V. Topical medications

A. α-Adrenergic agonists (oxymetazoline, naphazoline, brimonidine) in many nasal sprays, eye drops.

1. Contraindications. Glaucoma (eye drops), long-term use.

2. Allergic reactions. Conjunctivitis from long-term use of eye drops (likely complex mechanisms).

3. Adverse drug effects. Nasal irritation/rhinitis medicamentosa with long-term use. Benzalkonium (present in many preparations as a preservative) likely has role in irritation (C).

Local eye irritation from eye drops (burning, stinging, headache, dry mouth) (C).

B. Cromolyn, nedocromil. Available in nasal sprays, eye drops, and bronchial inhalers.

1. Contraindications. None.

2. Allergic reactions. Unknown.

3. Adverse drug effects. Local irritation common in eye; bad taste (nedocromil) (C).

C. Antihistamines

1. Azelastine (Astelin nasal spray, Optivar eye drops).

a. Allergic reactions. (U).

b. Adverse drug effects. Local irritation, taste perversion (C).

2. Doxepin cream

a. Allergic reactions. (U).

    b. Adverse drug effects. Contact dermatitis with long-term use (C).

VI. Anti IgE monoclonal antibodies.

  A. Omalizumab (Zolair)

    1. Contra indications. Hypersensitivity to Omalizumab.

    2. Allergic reactions. Anaphylaxis (R).

    3. Adverse drug effects. Injection site (C), malignancy (U).

VII. Concluding remarks. As described above, proven allergic reactions appear to be quite unusual during treatment with agents directed against allergic disorders. In most reported instances (usually case reports) the exact immune mechanisms involved have not been defined.

SELECTED READINGS

Mazzotta P, Loebstein R, Koren G. Treating allergic rhinitis in pregnancy. Safety considerations. *Drug Saf* 1999;20:361–375.

Meltzer EO. Quality of life in adults and children with allergic rhinitis. *J Allergy Clin Immunol* 2001;108:S45–S53.

Milgrom H, Bender B. Adverse effects of medications for rhinitis. *Ann Allergy Asthma Immunol* 1997;78:439–444.

Yap YG, Camm AJ. Potential cardiac toxicity of H_1-antihistamines. *Clin Allergy Immunol* 2002;17:389–419.

8

Anesthetics:

General and Analgesics

Malcolm M. Fisher

Anaphylaxis during anesthesia is rare, with an incidence of 1 in 10,000 to 200,000. In large series mortality is 4% and an additional 2% of patients sustain brain damage. The presence of an epidural increases mortality. About 95% of anaphylactic incidents occur within 5 minutes of drug administration. Neuromuscular blocking drugs (NMBDs) are the most common cause of anaphylaxis during anesthesia, followed by induction agents, antibiotics, and colloid blood volume replacement solutions. In 10% to 20% of patients no cause is found.

There is a higher incidence of asthma, atopy, and allergy in patients who develop anaphylaxis than in those who undergo uneventful anesthesia.

The diagnosis of anaphylaxis may be difficult during anesthesia, especially in the 10% of patients in whom the reaction involves a single organ system. All the signs and symptoms conventionally associated with anaphylaxis may occur in anesthesia more commonly by nonallergic mechanisms than by allergic mechanisms. Cutaneous signs may be masked by surgical drapes.

The effects of direct histamine release are common during anesthesia but are usually minor. Nonpharmacologic events, such as surgical stimulation and intubation, may also produce histamine release. Cutaneous manifestations of histamine release may occur in up to 30% of patients. There is no evidence that minor reactions are harbingers of later severe reactions. Severe reactions due to histamine release may occur with large volumes of histamine-releasing drugs (such as gelatin solutions), rapid vancomycin infusion, in a small number of patients who are "superresponders" to atracurium, and in patients with mastocytosis.

The effects of direct histamine release may be blocked by H_1 and H_2 blockers.

Recent work has shown anesthetic drugs effect different mast cell populations differently. Most drugs release histamine from skin mast cells only, and the incidence of bronchospasm is low.

Minor and delayed reactions may occur during and after anesthesia. It is very difficult to show a cause-and-effect relationship with an individual drug.

There is no evidence that other members of the family of a reactor are at risk.

    I. Induction agents. The incidence of reactions to the currently available induction agents is very low. Thiopentone anaphylaxis usually occurs after six uneventful exposures. Thiopentone is a barbiturate and may cause all of the adverse reactions associated with other barbiturates, including Stevens–Johnson syndrome. It is likely that thiopentone is the cause of most delayed reactions. Its usage has fallen over the last few years.

About 30 cases of anaphylactic reaction to propofol, 2 to midazolam, and none to ketamine have been described.

A. **Thiopentone (C).**
B. **Propofol (R).**
C. **Midazolam (R).**
D. **Ketamine (U).**

II. **Neuromuscular blocking drugs (NMBD).** Anaphylaxis occurs by bridging of cell-bound immunoglobulin E (IgE) molecules by the substituted ammonium ions on the NMBD molecule. The paired substituted ammonium ions are inherent to the structure–activity relationships of NMBDs. Thus, there is cross-sensitivity to other muscle relaxants in up to 60% of patients. Reactions have been described to more than one NMBD in a number of patients. Cross-sensitivity is not predictable without skin testing. Cisatracurium and atracurium are antigenetically identical isomers.

Reactions occur in women more commonly than in men. An unusual finding is that previous exposure to the drug causing the reaction is uncommon in NMBD anaphylaxis. The mechanism of sensitization is unknown.

Succinylcholine is the most common cause throughout the world; pancuronium is the safest.

A. **Succinylcholine (C).**
B. **Atracurium (R).**
C. **Rocuronium (R).**
D. **Vecuronium (R).**
E. **Cisatracurium (R).**
F. **Pancuronium (R).**
G. **Mivacurium (R).**

III. **Colloid solutions.** The mechanism of these reactions is complex. Patients reacting to gelatins often show positive skin tests and mast cell tryptase elevation, but antigelatin antibodies have not been detected in reactors. Gelatins are potent direct histamine releasers.

IgE antibodies to dextrans and starches are not described. Complement activation may occur in severe adverse reactions to dextrans. A dextran hapten is available that reduces the incidence of reactions to dextrans but may cause anaphylaxis.

Albumin solutions may produce both allergic and nonallergic reactions, particularly hypotension in patients on captopril.

A. **Gelatins (U).**
B. **Starches (U).**
C. **Albumin (R).**
D. **Dextrans (U).**

IV. **Narcotics.** With the exception of fentanyl the narcotics are potent releasers of histamine from skin. There is no evidence to support the commonly held belief that morphine causes bronchospasm in asthmatics. Anaphylactic reactions to these drugs has been described during anesthesia. It is very rare, with fewer than 40 cases reported. IgE antibodies to narcotics have been demonstrated by radioimmunoassay (RIA). There may be cross-sensitivity between codeine and morphine.

A. **Morphine sulfate (R).**
B. **Codeine phosphate (R).**
C. **Pethidine hydrochloride (R).**
D. **Fentanyl hydrochloride (R).**
V. **Volatile anesthetics.** Volatiles are not known to cause allergic reactions. Bronchospasm in association with enfurane has been described in a single study.
A. **Halothane (U).**
B. **Enflurane (U).**
C. **Sevoflurane (U).**
D. **Methoxyflurane (U).**
E. **Isoflurane (U).**
VI. **Other drugs used in anesthesia known to cause anaphylaxis.** Protamine may produce the clinical signs of anaphylaxis by a number of mechanisms. IgE and complement-dependent IgG antibodies have been described. The heparin–protamine complex activates complement and this is not usually of clinical significance. Protamine (and albumin solutions) has been linked to a fulminating membrane pulmonary edema occurring at the end of cardiopulmonary bypass, although a cause-and-effect relationship is not proven. The literature suggests that vasectomy, exposure to protamine insulin, and fish allergy are causative factors, but the supportive data are not convincing.
A. **Protamine (C).**
VII. **Drugs described in other sections known to cause anaphylaxis during anesthesia.** Antibiotics, local anesthetics, contrast media, sedatives, latex, patent blue, ondansetron, fragmin, ergometrine, chlorhexidene, triamcinolone, platelets, plasma, blood. Chlorbutanol (additive in synthetic oxytocin), metabisulfate, atropine neostigmine, and aprotinin have all caused anaphylactic reactions during anesthesia.
VIII. **Diagnosis of anesthetic allergy**
A. **Radioimmunoassay (RIA)** for IgE-specific antibodies is still the province of specialized laboratories. RIA inhibition with choline and RIA with morphine as the antigen improve the yield of positives for NMBDs.
B. **Lymphocyte and basophil degranulation** have been successfully used in specialized laboratories.
C. **A warning bracelet** and detailed letter should be provided to the patient. We also add a safe alternative to the culprit drug on the bracelet. The information as to what is safe is more relevant to the next anesthetist than what is not!
D. When **subsequent anesthesia** is performed with skin test–negative drugs after a properly conducted skin test, anesthesia is usually uneventful but there is a 2% rate of second reactions. There is logic, but no data, supporting pretreatment with steroids and antihistamines. Anesthetic allergy persists up to 17 years. A few patients lose their sensitivity.
E. **Mast cell tryptase.** Mast cell tryptase levels are highly specific and sensitive for IgE-mediated reactions, although they are elevated in some states where IgE is unlikely to be involved, such as in reactions to contrast media, in severe direct reactions to vancomycin, and in mastocytosis. An elevated level of mast cell tryptase indicates that testing to determine the drug

responsible is both mandatory and likely to be successful. A single sample obtained one hour after the reaction commenced is sufficient.

F. Skin testing. Skin testing is performed 4 to 6 weeks after the reaction using dilutions of the standard preparation of drug for intradermal testing or undiluted drug for prick testing. The comparative studies of the techniques show little difference. Some authorities recommend that both tests be performed. Morphine, codeine, or histamine is used as a positive control and saline as a negative control. All drugs used in the anesthetic are tested, including skin preparations. Skin tests are of little value in reactions to colloids, contrast media, and blood products.

Dilutions used for intradermal tests are 1:1,000 for NMBDs; 1:100,000 for codeine, pethidine, and morphine; and 1:100 for all others.

SELECTED READINGS

Fisher MM, Baldo BA. The incidence and clinical features of anaphylactic reactions during anaesthesia in Australia. *Ann Fr Anesth Reanim* 1993;12:97–104.

Fisher MM, Baldo BA. Mast cell tryptase in anaesthetic anaphylactoid reactions. *Br J Anaesth* 1998;80:26–29.

Genovese A, Stellato C, Marsella CV, et al. Role of mast cells, basophils and their mediators in adverse reactions to general anesthetics and radiocontrast media. *Int Arch Allergy Immunol* 1996;110:13–22.

Laroche D, Vergnaud MC, Sillard B, et al. Biochemical markers of anaphylactoid reactions to drugs. Comparison of plasma histamine and tryptase. *Anesthesiology* 1991;75:945–949.

Laxenaire MC, Mertes PM, and Groupe d'Etudes des Réactions Anaphylactoïdes Peranesthésiques. Anaphylaxis during anaesthesia. Results of a two-year survey in France. *Br J Anaesth* 2001;87:549–558.

9

Local Anesthetics

Anthony M. Yurchak

I. Local anesthetics

A. **Amides: lidocaine** (Xylocaine)
1. **Mepivacaine** (Carbocaine)
2. **Prilocaine** (Citanest)
3. **Etidocaine** (Duranest)
4. **Bupivacaine** (Marcaine, Sensocaine)
5. **Levobupivacaine** (Chirocaine)
6. **Ropivacaine** (Naropin)

B. **Esters: tetracaine** (Pontocaine)
1. **Procaine** (Novocaine)
2. **Chlorprocaine** (Nesacaine)
3. **Proparacaine** (Ophthaine) (topical only)
4. **Ethyl aminobenzoate** (benzocaine, Hurricaine) (topical only)
5. **Cocaine**

C. **Miscellaneous**
1. **Diphenhydramine** (Benadryl)
2. **Ethyl alcohol**

D. **Contraindications**
1. Drugs of the amide class often cross-react with other amides but not with drugs of the ester class.
2. Anesthetics containing epinephrine should be used with caution in patients receiving ergot oxytocin-type drugs or on monoamine oxidase or tricyclic drugs because hypertensive reactions may occur.
3. Amide-type drugs are metabolized by the cytochrome P450 system, and caution is required in debilitated patients.
4. Ester-type drugs are hydrolyzed by plasma pseudocholinesterase, and patients with abnormal pseudocholinesterase activity are at risk for systemic toxicity.

E. **Allergic reactions.** Truly immediate allergic reactions are extremely rare, occurring in less than 1 in 10,000 dental injections and possibly less often in other uses.
1. Contact dermatitis (R) from members of the older ester family of local anesthetics (procaine, benzocaine, tetracaine) are well known and may occur in 5% of patients using such products, such as in sunburn, sore throat, and hemorrhoid remedies. Benzocaine (Hurricaine gel) is commonly applied topically in dentistry. Contact dermatitis can also occur as a reaction to the acrylic materials and the dyes incorporated in them.
2. Local swelling and delayed rashes (R). Some local swelling can be expected after difficult dental extractions. Occasionally delayed swellings involve the adjacent face, which may represent a delayed hypersensitivity reaction. Patch tests and 48-hour intradermal tests suggest that this is also true of both delayed urticarial and maculopapular rashes.

Switching to a chemically unrelated anesthetic may obviate future reactions.

3. Urticaria and anaphylaxis (U). Extremely rarely patients will experience anaphylaxis, immediate urticaria, angioedema, or wheezing from the newer amide anesthetics. Older anecdotal reports did not rule out immediate-type reactions to latex, to nonsteroidal anti-inflammatory drugs, or to preservatives such as parabens and sulfites (added to epinephrine), or to formaldehyde or bleach used in root canal procedures.

F. Pseudoallergic (idiosyncratic) reactions (C). Many patients receiving local anesthetics for dental procedures experience some adverse effects. Three fourths of these patients appear to have had psychogenic reactions, and one fifth may have had excess intravascular injections.

1. Psychophysiologic symptoms occur in most patients and can be extreme in patients prone to panic attacks.

   a. Anxiety, palpitations, dizziness, and difficulty taking a deep breath.

   b. Hyperventilation requires reassurance and sometimes a rebreathing bag.

   c. Vasovagal symptoms are characterized by bradycardia, hypotension, unconsciousness, and even seizures in patients prone to such. Signs suggestive of an allergic reaction, such as urticaria or wheezing, are absent.

   d. Panic attacks can be so fearsome that even skin testing with diluted drugs is precluded.

   e. Helpful preventive measures include reassurance that these feelings can be expected, distraction with music or chatter, slow-breathing techniques, and a rehearsal for an injection using a placebo. Patients with mitral valve prolapse or chronic anxiety may require premedication with β-blockers and or diazepam, which itself abolishes the rise in endogenous plasma norepinephrine.

2. Toxic reactions from direct intravascular injection, too rapid injection, or excessive doses can occur even in experienced hands. It has been shown that small amounts of anesthetic directly injected into an artery can reach the brain by retrograde flow.

   a. Symptoms may include agitation, confusion, tremors, slurred speech, tinnitus, sweating, or seizures.

   b. Bupivacaine and etidocaine when inadvertently given intravenously have been associated with sudden bradycardia or asystole and seizures.

G. Management of reactions of patients with contact dermatitis or marked delayed swelling or rashes often requires systemic corticosteroids. Mild urticarial reactions can be treated with antihistamines, but patients with severe urticaria should receive epinephrine and corticosteroids and remain under observation.

H. Testing. Currently a reliable in vitro IgE radioallergosorbent test is not available for these drugs. It may be that, as in the penicillin system, metabolic products of these drugs are responsible for clinical reactions.

Table 9.1. Incremental test dosing

Dose	Dilution	Route
One drop	1:100	Scratch (optional)
One drop	1:1 (full strength)	Scratch
0.02 mL	1:100	Intradermal
0.1 mL	1:1	Subcutaneous
1.0 mL	1:1	Subcutaneous

1. Surprisingly, test dosing of patients who have experienced an immediate-type reaction after the use of a local anesthetic indicates that such patients often tolerate "incremental test dosing" with the suspected drug; however, prudence requires cautious evaluation. A simple protocol is given in Table 9.1 for test dosing at 15-minute intervals with resuscitative drugs and equipment available. Paraben-free products should be used. Concerns about the sulfite preservatives used with epinephrine are probably unwarranted because asthmatic individuals highly sensitive to inhaled sulfites tolerate parenteral doses ten times that found in local anesthetics.

2. If a psychological reaction is suspected, saline control doses should be inserted. Patients with alarming clinical histories may react at intradermal test doses of a 1:1,000 dilution, and additional test dilutions might be added. Some authors suggest testing such patients only with possible alternate drugs (e.g., mepivacaine or prilocaine for reactions to lidocaine). If the prior reaction was delayed and severe, a 24-hour delay might be taken before the subcutaneous challenges.

I. Emergency substitutes when time does not permit testing:

1. Injectable diphenhydramine.

2. Benzyl alcohol with or without epinephrine can be substituted for traditional amide anesthetics used for local anesthesia.

3. Use of a drug of the ester-type local anesthetic in place of traditional amide local anesthetic.

SELECTED READINGS

Bartfield JM, Jandreau SW, Raccio-Robak N. Randomized trial of diphenhydramine versus benzyl alcohol with epinephrine as an alternative to lidocaine local anesthesia. *Ann Emerg Med* 1998;32:650–654.

DeShazo RD, Kemp SF. Allergic reactions to drugs and biologic agents. *JAMA* 1997;278:1895–1906.

Nettis E, Napoli G, Ferrannini A, et al. The incremental challenge test in the diagnosis of adverse reactions to local anesthetics. *Oral Surg Oral Med Pathol Oral Radiol Endod* 2001;91:402–405.

Rood JP. Adverse reaction to dental local anaesthetic injection- "Allergy" is not the cause. *Br Dent J* 2000;189:380–384.

Soto-Aguilar MC, deShazo RD, Dawson ES. Approach to the patient with suspected local anesthetic sensitivity. *Immunol Allergy Clin North Am* 1998;18:851–865.

Schatz M. Adverse reactions to local anesthetics. *Immunol Allergy Clin North Am* 1992;12:585–609.

Tetzlaff J. *Clinical pharmacology of local anesthetics.* Boston: Butterworth–Heinemann, 2000.

10

Asthma and Pulmonology

Jill A. Poole and Lanny J. Rosenwasser

Adverse drug reactions to the drugs used for the management of asthma are uncommon and thankfully fairly rare. True allergic reactions to asthma medications and pulmonary medications are very rare, and adverse drug reactions do not often limit the therapeutic options associated with the management of allergic and other forms of asthma. Adverse drug reactions to asthma medications range from intolerance to idiosyncratic through unexplained reactions as well as to true allergic reactions. This review will briefly identify potential allergic reactions and some of the literature associated with medications in the following categories: inhaled β agonists, antileukotrienes, inhaled cromolyn/nedocromil, inhaled corticosteroids, phosphodiesterase inhibitors, inhaled cyclosporine, experimental therapy in cystic fibrosis, and α_1-antitrypsin treatment. Long-term treatment of asthma patients involves the use of controller medications including inhaled steroids, long-acting β agonists, nonsteroidal drugs such as inhaled cromolyn/nedocromil, and leukotriene modifiers ranging from zileuton through montelukast and zafirlukast. Acute management of asthma may involve the use of bronchodilators such as inhaled short-acting β agonists, inhaled corticosteroid preparations, and other treatments of unproven benefits, including inhaled diuretics and parentally administered magnesium. Adverse reactions to the acute reliever medications will be considered in conjunction with the long-term controller medications in this review.

I. **Inhaled β agonists.**
   A. **Selective β_2 agonists.** Short acting.
      1. **Albuterol sulfate** (Proventil, Ventolin)
      2. **Pirbuterol** (Maxair)
      3. **Levalbuterol** (Xopenex)
   B. **β_2 Agonists.** Long acting.
      1. **Salmeterol** (Serevent)
      2. **Formoterol** (Foradil)
   C. These medications overall have been well tolerated with few side effects at routine usage.
      1. **Allergic reactions** to the actual medication, not propellant, that have been documented include rash, angioedema, hoarseness, bronchospasm, and anaphylaxis (U). Propellant agents should be considered in questions of allergic reactions.
      2. **Adverse drug effects** are nervousness, tremor, palpitations, tachycardia, headache, dry mouth, cramp, and nausea/vomiting (C). These adverse events are increased with higher dosing. Uncommon adverse effects include slight elevation of blood glucose levels, effects on fat metabolism, hypokalemia, and possibly arrhythmias (R). Theoretical decrease in systemic vascular resistance can occur with

β_2-adrenergic agents; however, only minimal changes in blood pressure have been reported (U).

II. **Antileukotrienes**
   A. **Cysteinyl leukotriene type I receptor blockers**
      1. **Montelukast** (Singulair)
      2. **Zafirlukast** (Accolate)
   B. **Enzyme inhibitor of 5-lipoxygenase**
      1. **Zileuton** (Zyflo)
   C. Overall these medications are tolerated very well with few adverse reactions.
      1. **Allergic reactions.** None reported (U).
      2. **Adverse drug effects.** The overall incidence of adverse reactions is comparable to that of placebo. Reactions include headache, pharyngitis, abdominal pain, dyspepsia, dizziness, rash, asthenia, and cough (U). A specific note about zileuton is its potential for hepatic adverse effects; therefore, hepatic function monitoring needs to be followed at regular 3-month intervals (C).
      3. **Idiopathic.** Rare reports of occurrence of Churg–Strauss syndrome (eosinophilic vasculitis) have been associated with this class of medications. The incidence is rare and may be related to the withdrawal of oral or inhaled corticosteroids and therefore unmasking the disease process. However, in case reports of patients with Churg–Strauss syndrome given montelukast, relapses of disease have been shown.

III. **Cromolyn/Nedocromil (inhaled, nasal, and ophthalmic).** Cromolyn sodium or disodium cromoglycate (Intal, Nasalcrom, Opticrom) and nedocromil (Tilade, Alocril) are nonsteroidal anti-inflammatory medications which work principally as mast cell stabilizers. This class of medication is tolerated very well with few adverse reactions.
   A. **Allergic reactions** consistent with immediate hypersensitivity reported are rash, conjunctivitis, angioedema, urticaria, bronchospasm, and anaphylaxis (R). A case report of a patient developing liver disease, peripheral eosinophilia, and vasculitis consistent with a hypersensitivity reaction has been documented (U).
   B. **Adverse drug effects.** Unpleasant taste, nausea, headache, sore throat, and cough (C). Uncommon reactions include dermatitis, myositis, and gastroenteritis (R).

IV. **Inhaled corticosteroids** (inhaled and nasal)
   A. **Beclomethasone** (Vanceril, Beclovent, Vancenase, Beconase)
   B. **Budesonide** (Pulmicort, Rhinocort)
   C. **Flunisolide** (AeroBid, Nasarel)
   D. **Fluticasone** (Flovent, Flonase)
   E. **Mometasone** (Nasonex)
   F. **Triamcinolone acetonide** (Azmacort, Nasacort)
   G. Overall these medications are tolerated well with few adverse reactions.
      1. **Allergic reactions.** One study found positive dermal responses with patch testing. Budesonide has been found to provoke allergic contact dermatitis, and it can cross-react with triamcinolone and possibly other corticosteroids (R).

2. Adverse drug effects. Common reactions reported for nasal corticosteroids are dry nose, unpleasant taste, epistaxis, and headache (C). Common reactions for inhaled corticosteroids are pharyngitis, throat irritation, hoarseness, dysphonia, oral candidiasis, thinning of skin, and easy bruising (C). The potential for inhaled and nasal corticosteroids to cause systemic adverse effects such as hypothalamic–pituitary–adrenal axis suppression, osteoporosis or changes in bone mineral density, growth retardation in children, cataracts, and glaucoma are very uncommon to nonexistent at licensed doses (U). Reactions can occur with nasal corticosteroids, consisting of nasal congestion, pruritus, worsening of rhinitis, perforation of the nasal septum, and development of eczematous lesions. Inhalation corticosteroids have been reported to cause pruritus, dryness, erythema and edema of the mouth, cough, odynophagia, eczematous and erythematous lesions of the face and body, and urticaria. These represent local adverse effects of corticosteroids.

V. Phosphodiesterase inhibitors
  A. Theophylline (Slo-bid, Theo-dur)
  B. Aminophylline (salt of theophylline, ethylenediamine)
    1. Allergic reactions to theophylline have been rarely reported. These include angioedema, urticaria, pruritus, and rash. However, an increased frequency of allergic reactions to aminophylline have been reported, including rash, urticaria, angioedema, pruritus, high fever, and exfoliative dermatitis (R). Interestingly, such reactions appear to be related to ethylenediamine rather than the xanthine component of aminophylline. Ethylenediamine is unique to aminophylline.
    2. Adverse drug effects. Reactions to these medications are related to toxic reactions associated with overdosage. Common adverse reactions are nausea, headache, insomnia, flushing, nervousness, agitation, tremor, tachycardia, and palpitations (C). Severe reactions include tachycardia, flushing, vomiting, urinary symptoms, seizures, arrhythmia, and death (R).

VI. Inhaled immunosuppressants
  A. Cyclosporin A (CsA)
  B. Tacrolimus
  C. New therapies are being investigated for treating severe asthma patients. Preparations (dilauroylphosphatidylcholine liposome aerosol and ADI628) and delivery systems, including meter-dose inhaler and nebulized forms, are in trials.
  D. Potential Reactions
    1. Allergic reactions. (U).
  E. Adverse drug effects. Preliminary data show tracheal irritation and intermittent cough. No evidence for immune suppression has been observed in small trials. Larger trials are needed.

VII. Mucolytics or expectorants
  A. Bromhexine, Sodium 2-mercaptoethanesulfonate, Guaifenesin, S-Carboxymethylcysteine
    1. Reports on these medications are sparse (U).

B.   Nacystelyn, a salt derivative of *N*-acetylcysteine and lysine, is a new mucolytic agent developed for management of cystic fibrosis.

   1.   Allergic reactions. (U).

   2.   Adverse drug effects reported in small dose finding studies were wheezing, worsening of dyspnea, cough, and throat irritation. Clearly more data are needed.

C.   Potassium iodide

   1.   Allergic reactions have been reported to include fever, rash, urticaria, eosinophilia, lymphadenopathy, arthralgia, and submucosal hemorrhage (U). Hematuria, proteinuria, asthma, fever, pulmonary edema, and iododerma have also been reported (U).

   2.   Adverse drug effects. Most common adverse reactions are secondary to iodide ingestion and include direct effects on thyroid function.

VIII. α_1-Antitrypsin deficiency replacement therapy

   A. α_1-Antitrypsin deficiency replacement therapy has been used in short-term studies as an intravenous infusion.

   1.   Allergic reactions. None known (U).

   2.   Adverse drug effects. Most commonly reported effect is fever associated with the infusion (C). Adverse reactions included headache and dyspnea (R). One patient experienced fever, hypotension, and hypoxemia with specific lots from the manufacturer that were thought to contain a pyrogen. More long-term studies are needed.

IX.   Experimental therapy in cystic fibrosis. Cystic fibrosis transmembrane conductance regulator gene replacement is an experimental approach to decreasing morbidity and mortality from cystic fibrosis. Aerosolized delivery systems are under investigation to minimize the adverse effects of alveolar exposure to the vector. More data are needed.

X.   Discussion. Adverse reactions to the drugs used for asthma management are uncommon and fairly rare. True allergic reactions to asthma medications and pulmonary medication are very rare, and adverse drug reactions do not often limit the therapeutic options associated with the management of allergic and other forms of asthma. Adverse drug reactions to asthma medications range from intolerance of medications to idiosyncratic reactions. This chapter has briefly identified potential adverse and allergic reactions and some of the literature associated with medications in the following categories; inhaled β agonists, antileukotrienes, inhaled cromolyn/nedocromil, inhaled corticosteroids, phosphodiesterase inhibitors, inhaled cyclosporine, experimental therapy in cystic fibrosis, and α_1-antitrypsin treatment. Long-term treatment of asthma involves the use of controller medications, including inhaled steroids, long-acting β agonists, nonsteroidal drugs such as inhaled cromolyn/nedocromil, and leukotriene modifiers ranging from zileuton through montelukast and zafirlukast. Acute management of asthma may involve the use of bronchodilators, such as inhaled short-acting β agonists, inhaled and parenterally administered steroid preparations, and other treatments of unproven benefits including inhaled diuretics and parenteral magnesium.

SELECTED READINGS

Barker AF, Siemsen F, Pasley D, et al. Replacement therapy for hereditary alpha1-antitrypsin deficiency. A program for long-term administration. *Chest* 1994;105:1406–1410.

Ellis EF. Theophylline toxicity. *J Allergy Clin Immunol* 1985;76:297–301.

Flotte TR, Laube BL. Gene therapy in cystic fibrosis. *Chest* 2001;120:124S–131S.

Hatton MQ, Allen MB, Mellor EJ, et al. Salmeterol rash. *Lancet* 1991;337:1169–1170.

Huang TY, Peterson GH. Pulmonary edema and iododerma induced by potassium iodide in the treatment of asthma. *Ann Allergy* 1981;46:264–266.

Ibanez MD, Laso MT, Mercedes I, et al. Anaphylaxis to disodium cromoglycate. *Ann Allergy Asthma Immunol* 1996;77:185–186.

Isaksson M, Bruze M. Allergic contact dermatitis in response to budesonide reactivated by inhalation of the allergen. *J Am Acad Dermatol* 2002;46:880–885.

Lilly CM, Churg A, Lazarovich M, et al. Asthma therapies and Churg–Strauss syndrome. *J Allergy Clin Immunol* 2002;109:S1–S20.

Prenner BM. Safety, efficacy and bronchodilator-sparing effects of nebulized cromolyn sodium solution in the treatment of asthma in children. *Ann Allergy* 1982;49:186–190.

Shurman A. Passero MA. Unusual vascular reactions to albuterol. *Arch Intern Med* 1984;144:1771–1772.

Spector SL; The Antileukotriene Working Group. Safety of antileukotriene agents in asthma management. *Ann Allergy Asthma Immunol* 2001;86(6 Suppl 1):18–23.

Cardiac Drugs and Antihypertensives

Alan G. Wasserman and Khaled M. El-Jazzar

I. **Angiotensin-converting enzyme inhibitors (ACEIs).**
A. Benazepril (Lotensin), captopril (Capoten), enalapril (Vasotec), fosinopril (Monopril), lisinopril (Prinivil, Zestril), moexipril (Univasc), perindopril (Aceon), quinapril (Accupril), ramipril (Altace), trandalopril (Mavik).
  1. **Contraindications.** ACEIs are contraindicated if there is a history of hypersensitivity to any of the above-mentioned products.
  2. **Allergic reactions.**
     a. **Anaphylactoid reactions during desensitization (U).** Report of patients undergoing desensitization to hymenoptera venom sustained life-threatening reactions that were avoided upon discontinuation of the drug.
     b. **Anaphylactoid reactions during membrane exposure (R).** Reported in patients dialyzed with high-flux membranes and in patients undergoing low-density lipoprotein apheresis with dextran sulfate.
     c. Autoimmune (C). Rash with pruritus, fever, arthralgia, and eosinophilia, and antinuclear antibody (ANA) positive.
  3. **Adverse drug effects.**
     a. **Angioedema (R).** Involving the face, lips, mucous membranes, tongue, glottis, or larynx.
     b. **Impaired kidney function (C).** Twenty percent of patients develop stable elevations in blood urea nitrogen (BUN) and creatinine greater than 20% above baseline level. Less than 5% require discontinuation of treatment.
     c. **Hyperkalemia (C).**
     d. **Cough (C).**
     e. **Proteinuria (R).** More common in patients with pre-existing renal disease.
     f. **Agranulocytosis/neutropenia (R).** Neutropenia with myeloid metaplasia has resulted from use of *captopril*. It was also described with the use of other ACEIs; however, studies were insufficient to establish a cause–effect relationship. It is usually detected in the first 3 months of initiation of treatment with a 13% case fatality rate. The neutrophil count returns to normal within 2 weeks of discontinuation of treatment. Patients with renal impairment and/or congestive heart failure (CHF) are at higher risk.
     g. **Dysgeusia (C).** Reversible and self-limited diminution or loss of taste.
     h. **Dermatologic (C).** Rash, pruritus.

i. GI (U). Pancreatitis, glossitis, dyspepsia, jaundice, hepatitis.

j. Others (U). Myalgia, myasthenia, hyponatremia, blurred vision, impotence.

II. Angiotensin receptor blockers (ARBs).

A. Candesartan (Atacand), eprosartan (Teveten), irbesartan (Avapro), losartan (Cozaar), telmisartan (Micardis), valsartan (Diovan).

1. Contraindications. ARBs are contraindicated if there is a history of hypersensitivity to any of the above-mentioned products.

2. Allergic reactions (U).

3. Adverse drug effects

a. Central nervous system (C). Headache, dizziness, insomnia.

b. Renal (C). Worsening renal function in susceptible patients. Patients with known renal impairment, severe CHF, dehydration, renal artery stenosis are most at risk. In most of the cases, these effects were reversible upon discontinuation of the drug.

c. Hyperkalemia (C).

d. Hematologic (R). Anemia, neutropenia.

e. GI (R). Abdominal pain, diarrhea, dyspepsia, hepatitis, elevated liver function test (LFT) result.

f. Others (R). Upper respiratory symptoms, fatigue, myalgia, back pain, cough.

III. Antidysrhythmic

A. Adenosine (Adenocard)

1. Contraindications. Adenosine is contraindicated if there is a history of hypersensitivity to this medication. Adenosine is also contraindicated in patients with second- and third-degree A-V block and patients with sinus node disease.

2. Allergic reactions (U).

3. Adverse drug effects

a. Cardiovascular (C). Flushing, headache, sweating, palpitations, chest pain, hypotension. A variety of new rhythms, including premature atrial contractions, premature ventricular contractions (PVCs), bradycardia, and A-V block, are very common following adenosine injection.

b. Respiratory (C). Shortness of breath, chest pressure.

c. Central nervous system (C). Light-headedness, dizziness, body pain.

d. GI (C). Nausea, vomiting, metallic taste.

4. Warning. Adenosine has been reported to cause bronchoconstriction in asthmatic patients and its use should be avoided in these patients and in patients with obstructive lung disease and hyperactive airways.

B. Amiodarone (Cordarone, Pacerone)

1. Contraindications. Amiodarone is contraindicated in patients with known hypersensitivity to this medication. It is also contraindicated in severe sinus node disease, second- and third-degree A-V block, bradycardia-induced syncope.

2. Allergic reactions (U). Cases of angioedema, vasculitis, thrombocytopenia, serositis, toxic epidermal necrolysis, and organizing pneumonia have been reported.

3. Adverse drug effects

a. Pulmonary toxicity (C). Cough, dyspnea, chest x-ray changes, hypersensitivity pneumonitis, interstitial/alveolar pneumonitis. These reactions can be fatal in up to 10% of patients. It is usually reversible within 2 months of discontinuation of treatment. A baseline chest x-ray should be taken and another obtained upon the appearance of any new respiratory symptoms. The presence of baseline lung disease does not affect the incidence of these reactions. A rechallenge at a lower dose can de done with caution. Some patients with hypersensitivity pneumonitis may need a short course of steroids.

b. Cardiovascular (C). Various types of ventricular arrhythmias have been reported.

c. Thyroid abnormalities (C). Hypo- and hyperthyroidism. A baseline thyroid function tests should be obtained and followed regularly. Patients who present with new arrhythmias should be investigated for possible hyperthyroid-induced arrhythmias.

d. CNS (C). Malaise, fatigue, dizziness, tremor, poor coordination, peripheral neuropathy.

e. Dermatologic (C). Solar dermatitis, photosensitivity, skin discoloration.

f. GI (C). Nausea and vomiting, elevated LFT. Rare cases of hepatitis cholestatic hepatitis, cirrhosis, and pancreatitis are reported.

g. Ophthalmic (R). Cases of optic neuritis with progression to permanent blindness, papilledema, corneal degeneration, and macular degeneration have been reported. Asymptomatic corneal deposit is virtually present in all patients receiving amiodarone for more than 6 months.

4. Warning. Amiodarone should be used with extreme caution when combined with other antiarrhythmics (increase in arrhythmia and QT), *digitalis* (increased level), *cyclosporine* (elevated LFT), and *warfarin* (dose of *warfarin* should be reduced by one-third to one-half, and prothrombin time should be monitored closely).

C. Atropine

1. Contraindications. Glaucoma, obstructive uropathy, paralytic ileus, severe ulcerative colitis, myasthenia gravis.

2. Allergic reactions (U)

3. Adverse drug effects

a. Anticholinergic (C). Xerostomia, urinary hesitancy, blurred vision, mydriasis, increase ocular tension, loss of taste.

b. CNS (C). Headache, nervousness, excitement, drowsiness.

c. GI (C). Nausea, vomiting, constipation.

D. Azimilide

1. Contraindications. Azimilide is contraindicated in patients with known hypersensitivity to the drug. It is also contraindicated in patients with prolonged QT, unstable angina,

bradycardia (less than 50 beats per minute), decompensated CHF.
2. **Allergic reactions (U).**
3. **Adverse drug effects**
 a. **Cardiovascular (R).** QT prolongation, ventricular arrhythmia, torsade de pointes (TDP).
 b. **GI (C).** Nausea, vomiting, diarrhea.
 c. **CNS (C).** Headache, dizziness
4. **Warning.** No data pertaining to azimilide on anterograde conduction in patients with Wolff–Parkinson–White syndrome are available, so azimilide should be avoided in this group of patients.
E. **Bretylium** (Bretylol, Bretylate)
 1. **Contraindications.** Bretylium is contraindicated in patients with known hypersensitivity to the drug.
 2. **Allergic reactions (U).**
 3. **Adverse drug effects**
 a. **Cardiovascular (C).** Hypotension, bradycardia, PVCs, angina, initial increase in arrhythmias.
 b. **GI (C).** Nausea, vomiting, abdominal pain.
 c. **Dermatologic (R).** Flushing, erythematous macular rash, mild conjunctivitis.
 4. **Warning.** Bretylium should be used with caution in patients with severe aortic stenosis (AS) or pulmonary hypertension because of excessive hypotension. Moreover, norepinephrine release from the administration of bretylium can exacerbate digitalis toxicity.
F. **Digitalis** (Lanoxin, Lanoxicaps, Digitek)
 1. **Contraindications.** Known hypersensitivity to this medication. It is also contraindicated in patients with recent ventricular fibrillation.
 2. **Allergic reactions (U).**
 3. **Adverse drug effects**
 a. **Cardiovascular (R).** First-, second-, and third-degree A-V block, accelerated junctional rhythm, ventricular ectopia (C).
 b. **GI (C).** Nausea, vomiting, diarrhea.
 c. **CNS (R).** Headache, weakness, dizziness, visual disturbance.
 d. **Other.** Gynecomastia (R), thrombocytopenia (R), rash (R).
G. **Digoxin-immune Fab** (Digibind)
 1. **Contraindications.** No known contraindications.
 2. **Allergic reaction** (R). Most common in patients with antibiotic allergies.
 3. **Adverse drug effects**
 a. **Cardiovascular (C).** Rapid ventricular response in patients with atrial fibrillations (a-fib) or flutter (a-flut), exacerbation of heart failure.
 b. **Hypokalemia** (C).
H. **Dofetilide** (Tikosyn)
 1. **Contraindication.** Known hypersensitivity to this medication. It is also contraindicated in patients with long QT interval, severe kidney disease, concomitant use of verapamil, cimetidine, terfenadine, ketoconazole.

2. **Allergic reactions (U).**
3. **Adverse drug effects**
    a. **Cardiovascular (R-C).** Ventricular arrhythmia mostly TDP. Patients with hypomagnesemia are more susceptible, and prompt correction of magnesium is warranted. Chest pain with no evidence of ischemia is also commonly reported.
    b. **Miscellaneous.** Headache, dizziness, dyspnea, flulike syndrome (C). Diarrhea, abdominal pain, rash (R).
4. **Warning.** Dofetilide should not be combined with other antiarrhythmics that can prolong the QT interval. Dofetilide should be started in a hospital where electrocardiographic activity is continuously monitored.

I. **Epinephrine**
    1. **Contraindications.** None.
    2. **Allergic reactions (U).**
    3. **Adverse drug effects**
        a. **Cardiovascular (C).** Tachycardia, palpitations, sweating, hypertension, chest pain. Rare cases of myocardial ischemia/infarction.
        b. **CNS (C).** Dizziness, tremor, headache, anxiety, pallor.
        c. **GI (C).** Nausea, vomiting, diarrhea.
    4. **Warning.** Epinephrine should be used with care in patients with coronary artery disease (CAD) and history of arrhythmias.

J. **Ibutilide** (Corvert)
    1. **Contraindication.** Known hypersensitivity to this medication.
    2. **Allergic reactions (U).**
    3. **Adverse drug effects**
        a. **Cardiovascular (C).** Ventricular arrhythmias including sustained and nonsustained ventricular tachycardias, TDP, A-V block, PVCs, bundle-branch block, bradycardia, tachycardia/supraventricular tachycardia, hypotension, QT prolongation.
        b. **Other (C).** Nausea, headache.

K. **Procainamide** (Procanbid, Pronestyl)
    1. **Contraindication.** Known hypersensitivity to this medication. It is also contraindicated in patients with previous severe allergic reaction to procaine or ester-type local anesthetics, patients with systemic lupus erythematosus (SLE), complete heart block, TDP.
    2. **Allergic reaction.** Two types of reactions (R).
        a. Lupus like reaction with arthralgia, serositis, arthritis, fever, chills, positive ANA.
        b. Angioneurotic edema, urticaria, pruritus, flushing, maculopapular rash.
    3. **Adverse drug effects**
        a. **Cardiovascular (R).** Hypotension, dizziness, arrhythmia, second degree A-V block.
        b. **GI (C).** Nausea, vomiting, diarrhea, elevated LFT.
        c. **CNS (R).** Psychosis, hallucinations.
        d. **Hematologic (R).** Neutropenia, thrombocytopenia, hemolytic anemia.

  e. Idiosyncratic reactions (R). Pancytopenia, neutropenia, aplastic anemia.
 4. Warning
  a. Patients with a-fib or a-flut should be cardioverted or digitalized prior to use of *procainamide* because it can enhance A-V conduction.
  b. Procainamide should be avoided in patients with CHF because of its myocardial depressive effect.
  c. Procainamide should be used with caution in patients with renal insufficiency.
  d. Procainamide may worsen symptoms of myasthenia gravis.
L. Quinidine (Quinidex, Quinore)
 1. Contraindications. Known hypersensitivity to this medication or history of thrombotic thrombocytopenic purpura (TTP) or history of quinidine-induced TTP. It is also contraindicated in patients with junctional or idioventricular pacemaker.
 2. Allergic reaction (R). TTP, urticaria, fever, rash, exfoliative dermatitis, psoriasiform rash, lymphadenopathy, vasculitis, uveitis, sicca syndrome, SLE, pneumonitis, and ataxia.
 3. Adverse drug effects
  a. Cardiovascular (C). Arrhythmia, TDP, QT prolongation. Rarely it can enhance A-V conduction in patients with atrial fibrillation precipitating rapid ventricular response.
  b. GI (C). Diarrhea, nausea, vomiting, abdominal pain.
  c. CNS (C). Headache and dizziness.
  d. Fever and rash (C).
  e. Cinchonism (R). Consists of nausea, vomiting, tinnitus, hearing loss, vertigo, blurred vision, diplopia, photophobia, headache, confusion, delirium.
M. Sotalol (Betapace, Sotacar, Rytosol)
 1. Contraindications. Known hypersensitivity to this medication. It is also contraindicated in patients with bronchial asthma, bradycardia, second- and third-degree A-V block, long QT, cardiogenic shock, uncontrolled CHF.
 2. Allergic reactions (U).
 3. Adverse drug effects
  a. Cardiovascular (C). Ventricular arrhythmias including TDP, bradycardia, hypotension, worsening CHF.
  b. CNS (C). Fatigue, dizziness, asthenia, dyspnea, visual problems.
  c. GI (C). Nausea, vomiting, abdominal pain, elevated LFT.
  d. Metabolic (R). Worsening hyperglycemia with need of adjustment of diabetic medications.
N. Vascor (Bepridil)
 1. Contraindication. Known hypersensitivity to this medication. It is also contraindicated in patients with history of serious ventricular arrhythmias, sick sinus syndrome, second- or third-degree A-V block, prolonged QT, hypotension, decompensated CHF. Moreover, in clinical trials,

patients who had a myocardial infarction within the past 3 months were excluded.

2. Allergic reactions (U).

3. Adverse drug effects

  a. Cardiovascular (R). Worsening of arrhythmia, TDP, CHF.

  b. GI (C). Nausea, dyspepsia, abdominal pain, diarrhea. Elevated LFT (R).

  c. CNS (C). Dizziness, asthenia, nervousness.

  d. Dermatologic (R). Rash, sweating, skin irritation.

  e. Other (U). Neutropenia, pulmonary infiltrates.

IV. Antihyperlipidemic

  A. Bile acid sequestrants. Cholestyramine (Questran, Questran Light, Prevatile, LoCholest, LoCholest Light).

    1. Contraindications. Cholestyramine is contraindicated in patients with known hypersensitivity to the drug. Cholestyramine is also contraindicated in patients with complete biliary obstruction. Questran light contains phenylalanine; therefore, patients with phenylketonuria should avoid it.

    2. Allergic reactions (U).

    3. Adverse drug effects

      a. GI (C). Constipation, abdominal pain, flatulence, nausea, vomiting, steatorrhea, hemorrhoidal bleed, fat-soluble vitamin deficiency (R), elevated LFT (R).

      b. Dermatologic (R). Rash, irritation of the skin, tongue, and perianal area.

  B. Colsevelam (Welchol)

    1. Contraindications. Welchol is contraindicated in patients with bowel obstruction and in individuals with a history of hypersensitivity to any of its components.

    2. Allergic reactions (U).

    3. Adverse drug effects

      a. GI (C). Flatulence, constipation, diarrhea, nausea, dyspepsia.

      b. Upper respiratory. (C) Sinus congestion, increased cough, rhinitis.

      c. Vitamin K deficiency (C) and other fat-soluble vitamin deficiencies. Common in susceptible individuals with malabsorption syndromes or patients on warfarin.

      d. Others (R). Myalgia, back pain, headache, asthenia.

  C. Colestipol (Colestid, Colestid flavored)

    1. Contraindications. Colestid is contraindicated in patients with bowel obstruction and in individuals with a history of hypersensitivity to any of its components.

    2. Allergic Reactions (R). Rash has been infrequently reported with rare reports of severe anaphylactic reactions.

    3. Adverse drug effects

      a. GI (C). Constipation, abdominal pain, indigestion, heart burn, diarrhea, nausea, vomiting, hemorrhoids. Elevated LFT (R).

      b. GI (U). Peptic ulceration, cholelithiasis, cholecystitis, difficulty swallowing, transient esophageal obstruction.

      c. Neurologic (R). Headache, dizziness.

  D. 3-Hydroxy-3-methylglutaryl coenzyme A reductase

inhibitors (statins) Atorvastatin (Lipitor), cerivastatin (Baycol), fluvastatin (Lescol), lovastatin (Mevacor), pravastatin (Pravachol), simvastatin (Zocor). The following contraindications, adverse reactions, and allergic reactions are common to all statins except as otherwise noted.

    1. Contraindications. Statins are contraindicated if there is a history of hypersensitivity to any of the above-mentioned products. Statins are also contraindicated in patients with severe liver disease, unexplained elevation in LFT, or known myopathy. Cerivastatin is contraindicated in patients taking gemfibrozil.

    2. Allergic reactions (U).

    3. Adverse drug effects

        a. Elevated LFT (C). Dose dependent and reversible upon discontinuation or reduction of dose. Patients should have a baseline LFT and 12 weeks after following initiation or change in the dosage of the drug. Rare cases of persistent elevation in LFT have been reported even after the drug is stopped.

        b. Skeletal muscle (C). Myalgia is common; however, cases of myopathy with tenfold elevation in creatine phosphokinase (CK) are well reported. Rarely cases with rhabdomyolysis with renal failure resulting from myoglobinuria have been reported.

        c. GI (R). Constipation, nausea, diarrhea.

        d. CNS (U). Animal data showed hemorrhage and edema in multiple areas of the brain as well as cataract acceleration. These effects were observed at drug levels 12 to 50 times higher than mean human therapeutic drug levels.

    4. Warning. The risk of myopathy increases with the concurrent administration of the following medications: cyclosporine, fibric acid derivatives, niacin, erythromycin, and azole antifungals.

E. Fibric acid derivatives (FADs) Fenofbrate (Tricor), gemfibrizol (Lopid), clofibrate (Atromid)

    1. Contraindications. FADs are contraindicated if there is a history of hypersensitivity to any of the above-mentioned products. FADs are also contraindicated in patients with severe hepatic and kidney impairment and in patients with preexisting gallbladder disease. Cerivastatin is contraindicated in patients taking gemfibrozol.

    2. Allergic Reactions (U): Cases of anaphylaxis, laryngeal edema, and lupus-like reactions have been reported with no clear relationship to the drug.

    3. Adverse drug effects

        a. GI (C). Elevated LFT, cholelithiasis, dyspepsia, abdominal pain, diarrhea. Pancreatitis (R).

        b. Myositis and myopathy (R).

        c. CNS (R). Headache, vertigo, fatigue.

        d. Hematologic (R). Mild hemoglobin, hematocrit, and white blood cell count reductions have been observed with no clinical consequences.

        e. Dermatologic (R). Rash, urticaria.

    4. Warning. Combined use of FADs and statins and cyclosporine should be done with caution because of increased risk of myopathy and liver disease. Warfarin dose should be reduced and close monitoring of prothrombin time should be done in patients receiving FADs.

F. Niacin (nicotinic acid, vitamin B$_3$, Niacor, Niacor, Niaspan)

   1. Contraindications. Niacin is contraindicated if there is a history of hypersensitivity to this drug and in patients with severe liver impairment.

   2. Allergic reactions (U).

   3. Adverse drug effects

   a. Elevated LFT (R). Dose dependent and reversible.

   b. Rhabdomyolysis (R).

   c. Thrombocytopenia (R).

   d. Hypophosphatemia and glucose intolerance (R).

   e. Flushing, dizziness, tachycardia, and palpitations (C). This is more common upon initiation of the treatment and gradual increase in dose is recommended. Patients who live in a more temperate climate are more susceptible. Some of these effects can be reduced by pretreatment with *aspirin* 30 minutes prior to administration of the drug.

G. Ezetimibe (Zetia)

   1. Contraindications. History of hypersensitivity to this drug.

   2. Allergic reactions (U).

   3. Adverse drug effects Few adverse reactions, including upper respiratory symptoms (C), headache (C), back pain (C), and elevated LFT (R).

V. Antihypertensives

A. Clonidine (Catapress), transdermal patch (Catapress-TTS)

   1. Contraindications: Clonidine is contraindicated if there is a history of hypersensitivity to this drug.

   2. Allergic reactions (U).

   3. Adverse drug effects

   a. Dry mouth, drowsiness, dizziness, and constipation (C). In rare cases localized or generalized rash, hives and urticaria. Transdermal patch is commonly associated with erythema, vesiculation, hyperpigmentation, and edema.

   4. Warning. Severe rebound hypertension commonly occurs upon abrupt discontinuation of the medication. Patient should be advised that discontinuation of the medication should be done under medical supervision. Withdrawal symptoms that can be encountered include nervousness, agitation, headache, and tremor.

B. Hydralazine (Apresoline)

   1. Contraindications. Hydralazine is contraindicated in patients with known hypersensitivity to the drug.

   2. Allergic reactions (R). Rash, urticaria, pruritus, lupuslike reaction including fever, chills, arthralgia, chills, arthralgia, eosinophilia, glomerulonephritis, and hepatitis.

   3. Adverse drug effects

   a. CNS (C). Headache, dizziness.

   b. GI (C). Anorexia, vomiting, diarrhea. Peripheral neuritis (R) occasionally responsive to pyridoxine; tremor (R).

 c. Cardiovascular (C). Palpitations, tachycardia, angina.
 d. Hematologic (R). Blood dyscrasia, lymphadenopathy, splenomegaly.
4. Warning. Patients receiving hydralazine should be monitored for signs of lupus-like reaction. Patients with CAD can have angina pectoris upon initiation of the medication and *hydralazine* should be avoided in these patients.

C. Minoxidil (Loniten)
 1. Contraindications. Minoxidil is contraindicated in patients with known hypersensitivity to the drug. Minoxidil is also contraindicated in patients with pheochromocytoma because it may stimulate secretion of catecholamine from the tumor through its antihypertensive action.
 2. Allergic reactions (R). Rash, including rare reports of bullous eruptions, and Stevens–Johnson syndrome.
 3. Adverse drug effects
  a. Cardiovascular (C). Salt and water retention and CHF. Patients on this medication should be on a diuretic to prevent fluid overload. Rarely refractory fluid retention may require discontinuation of this medication. Tachycardia and exacerbation of angina is common, and it is advisable that patients with CAD should be on a BB. Pericarditis, pericardial effusion, and tamponade (R), more common in patients with reduced renal function. Changes in direction and magnitude of T-waves are also reported very commonly with no clinical implication and reversal upon discontinuation of the drug.
  b. Hematologic (R). Thrombocytopenia, leukopenia, anemia.
  c. GI (C). Nausea, vomiting, elevated LFT.
  d. Dermatologic (C). Hypertrichosis with elongation, thickening, and enhanced pigmentation of fine hair first on the temples, between eyebrows, side burns, and later extending to other sites of the body.
 4. Warning. Minoxidil can produce serious adverse effects and should be reserved for patients who do not respond to other antihypertensive agents. In experimental animals, it caused several kinds of myocardial lesions of unknown clinical significance in humans.

D. Nitroprusside
 1. Contraindications. Nitroprusside is contraindicated in patients with known hypersensitivity to the drug. Nitroprusside is also contraindicated in patients with compensatory hypertension such as aortic coarctation or arteriovenous shunting. Patients with congenital (Leber) optic atrophy or with tobacco amblyopia have high cyanide/thiocyanate ratios, and in such patients nitroprusside should be avoided.
 2. Allergic reactions (U).
 3. Adverse drug effects
  a. Cardiovascular. Excessive hypotension can result from transient excessive use of nitroprusside. This is usually self-limited within 10 minutes of discontinuation of the infusion.

b. Cyanide toxicity and methemoglobinemia. Rarely occur when the maximum recommended dose at 10 μg/kg per minute is exceeded. This manifests with lactic acidosis, air hunger, confusion, and death. Hypertensive patients on other antihypertensive medications are more sensitive to this effect than normal subjects.

c. Miscellaneous (R). Flushing, increased intracranial pressure, hypothyroidism.

4. Warning. Nitroprusside should be used with care in patients with hepatic insufficiency.

VI. Antiplatelets

A. 2b3a Inhibitors (2b3a): abciximab (Reopro), eptifibatide (Integrelin), tirofiban (Aggrastat). The following contraindications, adverse reactions, and precautions are common to all 2b3a unless otherwise noted.

1. Contraindications. 2b3a are contraindicated if there is a known hypersensitivity to any of the above-mentioned drugs. 2b3a are also contraindicated in the following situations:

a. Active internal bleeding

b. Recent (<6 weeks) GI or genitourinary (GU) bleeding or major surgery or trauma.

c. History of cerebral cardiovascular accident (CVA) within 2 years or CVA with significant residual deficit.

d. Bleeding diathesis.

e. Patient on oral anticoagulant unless partial thromboplastin time (PTT) is less than 2.

f. Thrombocytopenia less than 100,000.

2. Allergic reactions (U).

3. Adverse drug effects

a. Hematologic. Bleeding [major (R), minor (C)], thrombocytopenia [mild (C), severe (R)].

b. GI (C). Dyspepsia, diarrhea, nausea, vomiting.

c. Others. Hypotension and bradycardia (C), back and chest pain (C), dizziness, headache, and anxiety (C), peripheral edema (C).

4. Warning. Tirofiban is partially renally excreted, and dose adjustment is needed if creatinine is greater than 2.

B. Acetyl salicylic acid (aspirin)

1. Contraindications. Aspirin is contraindicated if there is a known hypersensitivity to the drug or any other nonsteroidal anti-inflammatory medication. Aspirin is also contraindicated in children or teenagers with viral infection due to the possibility of Reye syndrome.

2. Allergic reactions (R). Acute anaphylaxis, angioedema, urticaria, rash.

3. Adverse drug effects

a. GI. Stomach pain, heart pain, nausea, and vomiting (C), GI bleed (R), elevated LFT and hepatitis (R), Reye syndrome (R), hypoglycemia (R).

b. CNS (R). Hearing loss, tinnitus, confusion.

c. Hematologic (R). Thrombocytopenia.

C. Clopidogrel (Plavix)

1. Contraindications. Clopidogrel is contraindicated if there is a known hypersensitivity to the drug and if there is a known pathologic bleeding such as peptic ulcer disease or intracranial hemorrhage.

 2. Adverse drug effects

  a. Hematologic. Bleeding [minor (C), major (R)], thrombocytopenia (R), neutropenia (R), TTP (U), rash (R).

  b. GI (C). Abdominal pain, gastritis.

D. Ticlopidine (Ticlid)

 1. Contraindications. Ticlopidine is contraindicated if there is a known hypersensitivity to the drug. Ticlopidine is also contraindicated in patients with:

  a. History of hematopoietic disorder.

  b. History of ticlopidine-induced hematopoietic abnormalities.

  c. GI bleeding or liver impairment.

 2. Allergic reactions (R). Rash, urticaria, exfoliative dermatitis, Stevens–Johnson syndrome, erythema multiforme.

 3. Adverse drug effects

  a. Hematologic. Neutropenia (C), thrombocytopenia (R), TTP (R), aplastic anemia (R).

  b. GI (C). Diarrhea, nausea, vomiting, abdominal pain, increased cholesterol.

VII. β-Blockers (β-B)

A. Acebutolol (Sectral, Monitan)*, atenolol (Tenormin)*, betaxolol (Kerlone)*, bisoprolol (Zebeta)*, carvedilol (Coreg), esmolol (Breviblock)*, labetolol (Trandate, Normodyne), metoprolol (Lopressor, Toprol XL, Betaloc)*, nadolol (Corgard), pindolol (Visken), propranolol (Inderal), timolol (Blocarden) [*β_1 selective]. The following contraindications, adverse reactions, and allergic reactions are common to all βBs except as otherwise noted.

 1. Contraindications. βBs are contraindicated if there is a history of hypersensitivity to any of the above-mentioned products. βBs are also contraindicated in patients with the following conditions:

  a. Persistently severe bradycardia.

  b. Second- and third-degree A-V block.

  c. Cardiogenic shock.

  d. β_1 selective agents are contraindicated in patients with pheochromocytoma.

  e. Carvedilol is contraindicated in patients with asthma and liver impairment.

 2. Allergic reactions. Patients on βBs commonly develop ANA-positive serology. In rare cases, however, severe allergic reactions have been reported, including SLE-like reaction, rash of various types, Peyronie disease, and reversible vascular disease.

 3. Adverse drug effects

  a. Cardiovascular (R). Exacerbation of heart failure in patients with New York Heart Association (NYHA) III and IV disease, bradycardia, hypotension, hypertensive crisis in patients with pheochromocytoma (more likely with β_1 selective agents).

  b. Respiratory (R). Bronchospasm in patients with history of bronchospastic disease. The risk is higher with nonselective βBs.

    c. **CNS (C).** Depression, fatigue, impotence (R).

    d. **Elevated LFT (R).** Severe hepatocellular injury may occur rarely with case reports of hepatic necrosis and death.

    e. **Muscular (R).** Exacerbation of muscle weakness in patients with myopathy or myasthenia gravis.

  4. **Warning.** βBs should be used with caution in the following patients:

    a. Patients with history of severe anaphylactic reactions to environmental and synthetic agents.

    b. Patients with thyrotoxicosis.

    c. Patients prone to hypoglycemia.

    d. Patients on haloperidol because hypotension and cardiac arrest have been reported in patients taking the combination.

    e. Intravenous labetolol and halothane are synergistic, so that care should be used in managing hypertension during anesthesia with intravenous labetolol.

VIII. **Calcium channel blockers (CCBs)**

A. **Dihydropyridine CCBs (DHPCCBs), Amlodipine (Norvasc), felodipine (Plendil, Renedil), isradipine (DynaCirc, DynaCirc CR), nicardipine (Cardene), nifedipine (Procardia, Procardia XL, Adalat XL).** The following contraindications, adverse reactions, and allergic reactions are common to all DHPCCBs except as otherwise noted.

  1. **Contraindications.** DHPCCBs are contraindicated if there is a history of hypersensitivity to any of the above-mentioned products. Nifedipine is contraindicated in the management of hypertension and within the first 2 weeks of myocardial infarction or acute coronary syndrome.

  2. **Allergic reactions (R).** Procardia and Procardia XL are rarely associated with severe allergic reaction, including arthritis with ANA-positive serology and exfoliative dermatitis.

  3. **Adverse drug effects**

    a. CNS (C): Headache, flushing, dizziness.

    b. GI (C): Abdominal pain, constipation, elevated LFT.

    c. Peripheral edema (C) and gynecomastia (R).

B. **Nondihydropyridine CCBs (NDHPCCBs),** Diltiazem (Cardizem, Diltia XL, Tiazac, Dilacor, Tiamate), verapamil (Isoptin, Calan, Cover H-S, Veralan PM, Chronovera). The following contraindications, adverse reactions, and allergic reactions are common to all NDHPCCBs except as otherwise noted.

  1. **Contraindications.** NDHPCCBs are contraindicated if there is a history of hypersensitivity to any of the above-mentioned products. NDHPCCBs are also contraindicated in patients with the following conditions:

    a. Sick sinus syndrome or second- and third-degree A-V block.

    b. A-fib with Wolf–Parkinson–White syndrome.

    c. Hypotension or cardiogenic shock.

    d. Severe left ventricular dysfunction.

  2. **Allergic reactions (R).** Angioedema (facial and periorbital), alopecia, erythema multiforme, exfoliative dermatitis are rarely reported with diltiazem

3. **Adverse drug effects**
   a. CNS (C): Headache, dizziness, flushing.
   b. GI: Constipation (C), elevated LFT.
   c. Peripheral edema (C), rash (R).
4. **Warning.** NDHPCCBs should be used with caution in patients with severe liver or kidney impairment. Verapamil may reduce neuromuscular junction in patients with Duchenne muscular dystrophy.

IX. **Diuretics**
  A. **Loop diuretics**
   1. **Bumetanide (Bumex)**
      a. **Contraindications.** Bumetanide is contraindicated in patients with known hypersensitivity to the drug. Bumetanide is also contraindicated in patients with anuria or in those in hepatic coma. Patients who are allergic to sulfonamides may show hypersensitivity to the drug.
      b. **Allergic reactions (U).**
      c. **Adverse drug effects**
         (1) CNS (C): Dizziness, hypotension (volume depletion and electrolyte disturbance), weakness.
         (2) Metabolic (C): Electrolyte disturbance, hyperglycemia, hyperuricemia.
         (3) Other: Thrombocytopenia, drop in hemoglobin and white blood cell count (R).
      d. **Warning.** In the presence of impaired kidney function, combined use of *bumetanide* and other ototoxic medications, such as aminoglycosides, should be avoided.
   2. **Ethacrynic acid (Edecrin)**
      a. **Contraindications.** Ethacrynic acid is contraindicated if there is a known hypersensitivity to the drug. Ethacrynic acid is also contraindicated in patients with anuria or a history of severe diarrhea induced by ethacrynic acid.
      b. **Allergic reactions.** Fever, chills, and arthralgia (R), Henoch–Schönlein purpura (U).
      c. **Adverse drug effects**
         (1) GI: Anorexia, malaise, abdominal pain, nausea, and vomiting (C), sudden-onset severe diarrhea (R): upon occurrence of severe diarrhea, *ethacrynic acid* should be stopped immediately and should never be administered to that patient again; pancreatitis (R), elevated LFT (R).
         (2) Hematologic (R): Neutropenia, thrombocytopenia.
         (3) CNS (R): Headache, deafness, tinnitus, vertigo, fatigue, blurred vision, confusion.
         (4) Acute gout (R).
   3. **Furosemide (Lasix)**
      a. **Contraindications.** Furosemide is contraindicated if there is a known hypersensitivity to the drug. Furosemide is also contraindicated in patients with anuria.
      b. **Allergic reactions (R).** Erythema multiforme, exfoliative dermatitis, urticaria, rash, purpura, photosensitivity, necrotizing angiitis, systemic vasculitis.
      c. **Adverse drug effects**
         (1) GI: Anorexia, cramping, diarrhea, nausea, and vomiting (C); pancreatitis and jaundice (R).

(2)   CNS (C): Tinnitus, headache, dizziness, vertigo, blurred vision, paresthesias.

(3)   Hematologic (R): Aplastic anemia, thrombocytopenia, hemolytic anemia, neutropenia, anemia.

(4)   Others (R): Hyperglycemia, hyperuricemia, weakness, fever, urinary bladder spasm, muscle spasm.

d.   Warning. Cases of tinnitus and reversible or irreversible hearing loss have been reported. These cases were mostly associated with the use of other ototoxic medications and high doses of furosemide.

4.   Torsemide (Demadex)

a.   Contraindications. Torsemide is contraindicated if there is a known hypersensitivity to the drug. Torsemide is also contraindicated in patients with anuria and in those with a known hypersensitivity to sulfonylureas.

b.   Allergic reactions (U).

c.   Adverse drug effects

(1)   CNS (C): Dizziness, headache.

(2)   GI (C): Nausea, hyperglycemia.

d.   Warning. Torsemide should be used with caution in patients with hepatic disease and cirrhosis. Cases of tinnitus and hearing loss have been rarely reported following rapid intravenous infusion.

B.   Potassium-sparing diuretics: Amiloride (Midamor), spironolactone (Aldactone) and triamterene (Dyrenium).

1.   Contraindications. Potassium-sparing diuretics are contraindicated if there is a known hypersensitivity to the drug. Potassium-sparing diuretics are also contraindicated in patients with anuria, hyperkalemia, and diabetic nephropathy.

2.   Allergic reactions (U).

3.   Adverse drug effects

a.   GI (C). Nausea, abdominal pain, flatulence. Elevated LFT (U).

b.   Others (U). Activation of peptic ulcer disease, aplastic anemia, neutropenia, rash.

C.   Thiazides: Cholorothiazide (Diuril), chlorthalidone (Hygrolon, Thalitone), hydrochlorothiazide (HCTZ), indapamide (Lozol), metalozone (Zaroxolyn, Mykrox). The following contraindications, adverse reactions, and allergic reactions are common to all thiazides except as otherwise noted.

1.   Contraindications. Thiazides are contraindicated if there is a known hypersensitivity to the drug. Thiazides are also contraindicated in patients with anuria. Hydrocholorothiazide is contraindicated in patients with hypersensitivity to sulfonamide.

2.   Allergic reactions (R)

3.   Adverse drug effects

a.   CNS (C). Headache, fatigue, nervousness, back pain, irritability. Syncope, neuropathy, vertigo, depression, and impotence (R).

b.   GI (R). Hepatitis, pancreatitis, jaundice, constipation, anorexia.

c.   Hematologic (R). Aplastic anemia, neutropenia, thrombocytopenia.

    d. Metabolic (C). Decrease serum level of Na, K, P, Mg, Cl. Increase serum level of glucose, calcium, and uric acid.

   4. Warning. Thiazides should be used with care in patients with liver impairment.

X. Nitrates

  A. Oral: isosorbide dinitrates (Isordil, Sorbitrate, Dilatrate SR), isosorbide mononitrate (ISMO, Monoket, Imdur)

   1. Nitroglycerin. Intravenous (Tridil, Nitro-Bid IV), ointment (Nitrobid, Nitrol), spray (Nitrolingual), sublingual (Nitrostat), sustained release (Nitrong, Nitrogyn), transdermal (Deponit, Minitran, Nitrodisc, Nitro-dur, Transderm-Nitro, Trinipatch)

    a. Contraindication. Nitrates are contraindicated if there is a known hypersensitivity to any of the above-mentioned drugs. Nitrates are relatively contraindicated in patients with severe anemia, increase intracranial pressure, and use of Viagra within past 12 hours.

    b. Allergic reactions (R). Rash, erythema multiforme, exfoliative dermatitis.

    c. Adverse drug effects

      (1) CNS (C). Headache, dizziness, flushing

      (2) GI (C). Nausea, vomiting.

      (3) Methemoglobinemia (U).

    d. Warning. Sildenafil can amplify the vasodilatory effect of nitrates, and nitrates should not be used if sildenafil was used within the past 12 hours.

XI. Pressors

  A. Dobutamine (Dobutrex)

   1. Contraindications. Dobutamine is contraindicated if there is a known hypersensitivity to the drug. Dobutamine is also contraindicated in patients with hypertrophic obstructive cardiomyopathy.

   2. Allergic reactions (R). Skin rash, fever, eosinophilia, bronchospasm. Sodium bisulfite can cause anaphylactic and life-threatening reaction, which is more common in patients with a history of asthma.

   3. Adverse drug effects

    a. Cardiovascular (C). Angina, hypotension, tachyarrhythmias, tachycardia, shortness of breath.

    b. Other (C). Nausea, phlebitis at injection site.

  B. Dopamine (Intropin)

   1. Contraindications. Dopamine is contraindicated in patients with known hypersensitivity to the drug. Dopamine is also contraindicated in patients with pheochromocytoma.

   2. Allergic reactions (U)

   3. Adverse drug effects. The following adverse reactions have been reported but there are not enough data to support an estimate of their frequency.

    a. Cardiovascular: Ventricular arrhythmia, ectopic beats, tachycardia, palpitations, hypertension, Raynaud phenomenon.

    b. Endocrinologic (C). Infusion of dopamine suppresses pituitary secretion of thyroid-stimulating hormone, growth hormone, and prolactin.

c. **Other.** Headache, nausea, vomiting, piloerection, gangrene of the extremity with high doses for prolonged periods.

4. **Warning.** Dopamine should be used with caution in patients with a history of occlusive vascular disease. Patients receiving monoamine oxidase inhibitors within the last 2 to 3 weeks should receive only one-tenth the usual dose. Lastly, the infusion contains sodium bisulfite, which may cause an anaphylactic reaction in patients with asthma.

C. **Midodrine (Proamatine)**

1. **Contraindications.** Midodrine is contraindicated if there is a known hypersensitivity to the drug. Midodrine is also contraindicated in patients with severe organic heart disease, acute renal disease, urinary retention, pheochromocytoma, thyrotoxicosis, and excessive supine hypertension.

2. **Allergic reactions (U)**

3. **Adverse drug effects.** Midodrine has very few adverse reactions attributed to α-adrenergic stimulation, including paresthesia, pruritus, piloerection, and urinary symptoms (C), chills (C), rash (R).

4. **Warning.** The most potentially serious reaction is marked elevation in supine blood pressure.

D. **Milrinone (Primacor)**

1. **Contraindications.** Milrinone is contraindicated if there is a known hypersensitivity to the drug. Milrinone is also contraindicated in patients with hypertrophic obstructive cardiomyopathy.

2. **Allergic reactions (U)**

3. **Adverse drug effects**

a. **Cardiovascular (C).** Ventricular and supraventricular arrhythmias, hypotension.

b. **Other.** Headache (C), hypokalemia (R), tremor (R), thrombocytopenia (R).

XII. **Thrombolytics**

A. **Reteplase (Retavase), streptokinase (Streptase, Kabikinase), tenecteplase (TNKase), tissue plasminogen activator (TPA).** The following contraindications, adverse reactions, and allergic reactions are common to all thrombolytics except as otherwise noted.

1. **Contraindications.** Thrombolytics are contraindicated if there is a known hypersensitivity to any of the above-mentioned drugs. They are also contraindicated or relatively contraindicated in the following group of patients:

a. History of CVA

b. Recent (<6 months) GI or GU bleeding or serious trauma.

c. Uncontrolled hypertension (systolic blood pressure >180, or diastolic blood pressure >110).

d. High likelihood of left heart thrombus.

e. Hemostatic defect, oral warfarin.

f. Diabetic hemorrhagic retinopathy or other hemorrhagic ophthalmic condition.

g. Recent puncture from a noncompressible arterial site.

    h. Pregnancy, advanced age (>75).
    i. Subacute bacterial endocarditis.
2. Allergic reactions (R). Anaphylactoid reactions with laryngeal edema, rash, and urticaria. Hypotension not secondary to bleeding or anaphylaxis has been described during intravenous streptokinase infusion. Cases of noncardiogenic pulmonary edema polyneuropathy, Guillain–Barré syndrome were also described rarely with streptokinase.
3. Adverse drug effects
    a. Bleeding. Minor (C), major (R).
    b. Cardiovascular (U). Arrhythmias, A-V block, pericardial, effusion, pulmonary edema, pericarditis.
4. Warning. Cases of cholesterol emboli have been reported with all thrombolytics. This is in association with invasive vascular procedures. The true incidence is unknown.

SELECTED READINGS

Dujovne CA, et al. Efficacy and safety of a potent new selective cholesterol inhibitor, Ezetimibe, in patients with primary hypercholesterolemia. *Am J Cardiol* 2002;90:1092.

Kjekshus J, et al. Randomized trial of cholesterol lowering in 4444 patients with coronary heart disease. The Scandinavian Simvastatin Survival Study. *Lancet* 1994;344:1383–1389.

Lincoff AM, et al. Complementary clinical benefits of coronary stenting with use of platelet glycoprotein IIb/IIa receptors. *N Engl J Med* 1999;341:319–327.

Page RL. Antiarrhythmic effects of azimilide in paroxysmal supraventricular tachycardia. Efficacy and dose response. *Am Heart J* April 2002;143:643–649.

Physician's desk reference, 22nd ed. Oradell, NJ: Medical Economics, 2001.

Van de Werf F, et al. Safety assessment of a single bolus administration of TNK–tissue plasminogen activator in acute myocardial infarction. The ASSENT-1 trial. *Am Heart J* 1999;137:186–191.

12

Dermatology

Paul R. Gross and Monib Zirvi

12.1. DRUG ERUPTIONS

Drug eruptions are one of the most common reasons for consultation with a dermatologist. Often patients are on a number of medications that may be responsible for a drug eruption. It is important in such cases that a careful medication timeline be constructed to help narrow down the potential causative medication. In many cases such a timeline still leaves a number of potential offending agents. In these cases, sometimes the specific morphology of the eruption can point to the most likely cause. In this chapter, a list of the most common medications associated with specific morphologies of drug eruptions is presented. In addition, medications commonly associated with drug reactions are also listed. Potential drug reactions associated with commonly used classes of medications are summarized. Finally, unique eruptions that are classically associated with certain medications are presented. This information may be helpful for guiding the perplexing process of identifying the cause of a drug eruption in a patient taking numerous medications.

I. Drug eruptions
  A. **Drugs commonly associated with drug eruptions**
    1. Amoxicillin, trimethoprim–sulfamethoxazole, cephalosporins, antimalarials, gentamicin, diuretics, dapsone, heparin, sulfonamides, anticonvulsants, quinolones, tetracyclines, nonsteroidal anti-inflammatory drugs (NSAIDs), macrolides, azidothymidine (zidovudine, AZT).
  B. **Drugs frequently associated with severe drug eruptions**
    1. Allopurinol, anticonvulsants, sulfonamides, furosemide, penicillamine, thiazide, diuretics
  C. **Drugs associated with specific skin eruptions**
    1. Acne. corticosteroids, halogens (bromides/iodides), haloperidol, steroid hormones, isoniazid, lithium, phenytoin
    2. Acute generalized exanthematous pustulosis. Penicillins, cephalosporins, macrolides, allopurinol, carbamazepine, tetracyclines, calcium channel blockers, furosemide, hydroxychloroquine, imipenem, isoniazid, phenytoin, vancomycin
    3. Alopecia. Allopurinol, anticoagulants, azathioprine, bromocriptine, β-blockers, cyclophosphamide, hormones, NSAIDs, phenytoin, methotrexate (MTX), valproate
    4. Bullous pemphigoid. Penicillamine, furosemide, neuroleptics, penicillins, psoralen ultraviolet A (PUVA), sulfasalazine
    5. Erythema nodosum. Halogens, oral contraceptives, penicillin, sulfonamides, tetracyclines

6. Erythroderma. Allopurinol, anticonvulsants, barbiturates, captopril, carbamazepine, chloroquine, chlorpromazine, calcium channel blockers, lithium, sulfonamides
7. Fixed drug eruptions. Anticonvulsants, aspirin, NSAIDs, barbiturates, benzodiazepines, dapsone, metronidazole, oral contraceptives, penicillins, sulfonamides, tetracyclines
8. Hypersensitivity syndrome [fever, adenopathy, elevated liver function test (LFT) results, and drug eruptions]. Allopurinol, carbamazepine, dapsone, minocycline, NSAIDs, phenobarbital, phenytoin, sulfonamides
9. Lichenoid reactions. Antimalarials, β-blockers, angiotensin-converting enzyme (ACE) inhibitors, furosemide, gold, penicillamine, tetracyclines, thiazides
10. Linear IgA dermatosis. Captopril, diclofenac, lithium, vancomycin
11. Lupus-like eruption. Hydralazine, procainamide, minocycline, hydrochlorothiazide, calcium channel blockers, griseofulvin, terbinafine
12. Morbilliform. ACE inhibitors, allopurinol, amoxicillin, ampicillin, anticonvulsants, barbiturates, carbamazepine, isoniazid, NSAIDs, penicillin, phenytoin, quinolones, sulfonamides, thiazides
13. Pemphigus. Captopril, penicillamine, cephalosporins, penicillins, phenobarbital, piroxicam, progesterone, propranolol
14. Photosensitivity. Amiodarone, chlorpromazine, furosemide, griseofulvin, lovastatin, piroxicam, quinolones, sulfonamides, tetracyclines, thiazide
15. Pseudoporphyria. Barbiturates, sulfonamides, isoniazid, NSAIDs, oral contraceptives, androgens, tetracyclines
16. Psoriasis (exacerbation). ACE inhibitors, granulocyte-macrophage colony-stimulating factor (GM-CSF), lithium, gold, β-blockers, antimalarial agents, interferon-α (IFN-α), NSAIDs, clonidine, tetracycline, terfenadine
17. Stevens–Johnson syndrome. Allopurinol, anticonvulsants, NSAIDs, barbiturates, carbamazepine, codeine, diltiazem, furosemide, penicillins, phenytoin, sulfonamides, tetracyclines
18. Toxic epidermal necrolysis (TEN). Allopurinol, anticonvulsants, NSAIDs, isoniazid, penicillins, phenytoin, sulfonamides, tetracyclines, vancomycin, and nevirapine
19. Urticaria. ACE inhibitors, aspirin, NSAIDs, cephalosporins, opiates, penicillins, contrast dye, vaccines
20. Vasculitis. Allopurinol, barbiturates, chlorpromazine, NSAIDs, gold, hydralazine, penicillins, phenytoin, propylthiouracil, quinolones, sulfonamide, tetracyclines, thiazides
21. Vesiculobullous eruptions. NSAIDs, barbiturates, captopril, cephalosporins, furosemide, griseofulvin, penicillamine, penicillins, sulfonamides, thiazides
D. Chemotherapeutic agents associated with specific morphologic patterns
  1. Acneiform. Dactinomycin, vinblastine

2. **Alopecia.** Alkylating agents, anthracycline, bleomycin, doxorubicin, hydroxyurea, MTX, mitomycin, mitoxantrone, vinblastine, vincristine, cyclophosphamide

3. **Erythema multiforme.** Chlorambucil, cyclophosphamide, diethylstilbestrol (DES), etoposide, hydroxyurea, MTX, mitomycin C, paclitaxel

4. **Fixed drug eruptions.** Dacarbazine, hydroxyurea, paclitaxel, procarbazine

5. **Hyperpigmentation.** Busulfan, nitrogen mustard, cyclophosphamide, ifosfamide, carmustine (BCNU), fotemustine, cisplatin, thiotepa, 5-fluorouracil (5-FU), MTX, bleomycin, dactinomycin, daunorubicin, doxorubicin, mithramycin, mitoxantrone, hydroxyurea, procarbazine

6. **Lichenoid.** Hydroxyurea

7. **Systemic lupus erythematosus (SLE).** DES, hydroxyurea, leuprolide

8. **Morbilliform.** Bleomycin, carboplatin, chlorambucil, cytarabine, DES, doxorubicin, etoposide, 5-FU, hydroxyurea, MTX, mitomycin C, mitotane, mitoxantrone, paclitaxel, thiotepa

9. **TEN.** Asparaginase, bleomycin, chlorambucil, cytarabine, doxorubicin, 5-FU, MTX

10. **Urticaria.** Bleomycin, busulfan, carboplatin, chlorambucil, cisplatin, cyclophosphamide, cytarabine, daunorubicin, DES, doxorubicin, etoposide, 5-FU, mechlorethamine, melphalan, MTX, mitomycin C, mitotane, mitoxantrone, paclitaxel, pentostatin, thiotepa, vincristine

11. **Vasculitis.** Busulfan, cyclophosphamide, cytarabine, hydroxyurea, 6-mercaptopurine, MTX, mitoxantrone, tamoxifen

E. **Cutaneous reactions to cytokine therapy**

1. **Granulocyte colony-stimulating factor (G-CSF).** Sweet syndrome, leukocytoclastic vasculitis, localized pruritus, localized erythema

2. **GM-CSF.** Maculopapular eruptions, exfoliative dermatitis, urticaria, pruritus, purpura, alopecia, flushing, epidermolysis, localized erythema

3. **Tumor necrosis factor-α (TNF-α).** Erythroderma and localized erythema

4. **IFN-α.** Alopecia, pruritus, psoriasis, SLE

5. **Interleukin-1 (IL-1).** Phlebitis, mucositis

6. **IL-2.** Erythema, pruritus, desquamation, erythroderma, necrosis, urticaria, blisters, exacerbation of autoimmune skin disorders, flushing, telogen effluvium, cutaneous ulcers, erythema nodosum, TEN

F. **Nail changes associated with medications**

1. **Anonychia.** Oral retinoids

2. **Beau lines.** Chemotherapy and other cytotoxic medications

3. **Splinter hemorrhages.** Tetracyclines

4. **Longitudinal pigmented streaks.** Bleomycin, busulfan, daunorubicin, nitrogen mustard, hydroxyurea, methotrexate, cyclophosphamide, 5-FU, PUVA, zidovudine, gold, antimalarials, ketoconazole, tetracyclines, phenytoin, sulfonamides

5. Blue nails. Minocycline, bleomycin, zidovudine, antimalarials

6. Terry nails (half-and-half nail = proximal white, distal pink). Prednisone, cyclophosphamide, methotrexate, doxorubicin, vincristine

7. Onycholysis. Bleomycin, doxorubicin, 5-FU, oral retinoids

8. Photo-onycholysis. Tetracyclines, chlorpromazine, thiazides, PUVA

9. Paronychia. Oral retinoids

G. Dermatologic adverse reactions of commonly used classes of medications

1. β-Blockers. Pruritus (C), xerosis (C), alopecia (R), morbilliform drug eruption (R), lichenoid reaction (R), psoriasis (R), angioedema (U)

2. Penicillins/cephalosporins. Morbilliform drug eruption (R), fixed drug eruption (R), pemphigus (R), urticaria (R), acute generalized exanthematous pustulosis (U), angioedema (U), erythema multiforme (U), TEN (U), Stevens–Johnson syndrome (U)

3. Tetracyclines. Fixed drug eruption (R), morbilliform drug eruption (R), photosensitivity (R), lichenoid eruption (R), angioedema (U), vasculitis (U), pseudoporphyria (U)

4. ACE inhibitors. Alopecia (R), angioedema (R), morbilliform drug eruption (R), lichenoid reaction (R), psoriasis (R), urticaria (R), vasculitis (U)

5. Calcium channel blockers. Acne (R), morbilliform drug eruption (R), lichenoid reaction (R), psoriasis (R), xerostomia (R), angioedema (U), vasculitis (U)

6. Diuretics. Lichenoid eruption (R), morbilliform drug eruption (R), photosensitivity (R), urticaria (R), acute generalized exanthematous pustulosis (U), bullous eruption (R), vasculitis (U), erythema multiforme (U), TEN (U), Stevens–Johnson syndrome (U), pseudoporphyria (U)

7. Sulfonamides. Morbilliform drug eruption (R), photosensitivity (R), bullous eruption (R), vasculitis (U), erythema multiforme (U), TEN (U), Stevens–Johnson syndrome (U), erythema nodosum (U)

8. Aspirin/NSAIDs. Alopecia (R), angioedema (R), bullous eruptions (R), fixed drug eruption (R), lichenoid eruption (R), morbilliform drug eruption (R), urticaria (R), acute generalized exanthematous pustulosis (U), erythema nodosum (U)

9. Anticonvulsants (phenytoin/carbamaze-pine/phenobarbital). Acne (R), bullous eruption, gingival hyperplasia (R), lichenoid eruption (R), morbilliform drug eruption (R), urticaria (R), erythema multiforme (U), TEN (U), Stevens–Johnson syndrome (U), acute generalized exanthematous pustulosis (U), vasculitis (U)

H. Unique dermatologic reactions associated with specific medications

1. Bleomycin. Flagellate hyperpigmentation, radiation recall, Raynaud phenomenon

2. Penicillamine. Elastosis perforans serpiginosa

3. Aspirin/NSAIDs. Pseudoporphyria

4. Hydralazine. Lupus-like eruption

5. **Procainamide.** Lupus-like eruption
6. **Methotrexate.** "Flag" sign, radiation recall, UV recall, folliculitis
7. **Cytarabine.** Acral erythema, neutrophilic eccrine hidradenitis, radiation recall, eccrine squamous syringometaplasia, leg ulcers
8. **5-FU.** Acral erythema
9. **Doxorubicin.** Acral erythema, radiation recall, "sticky" skin
10. **Dactinomycin.** Radiation recall, folliculitis, serpentine supravenous hyperpigmented eruption
11. **Hydroxyurea.** Dermatomyositis-like eruption, leg ulcers, lichenoid eruption
12. **Vancomycin.** "Red Man" syndrome, Linear IgA bullous dermatosis
13. **Heparin.** Heparin-induced thrombocytopenia
14. **Warfarin.** Skin necrosis
15. **Captopril.** Bullous pemphigoid, vasculitis, lichenoid eruption
16. **Minocycline.** Hyperpigmentation, acute generalized exanthematous pustulosis, lupus-like syndrome, Sweet syndrome, vasculitis
17. **Phenytoin.** Erythema multiforme, TEN, Stevens–Johnson syndrome
18. **Phenobarbital.** Erythema multiforme, TEN, Stevens–Johnson syndrome
19. **Carbamazepine.** Erythema multiforme, TEN, Stevens–Johnson syndrome
20. **Sulfonamides.** Erythema multiforme, TEN, Stevens–Johnson syndrome, vasculitis, fixed drug eruption, acute generalized exanthematous pustulosis
21. **Progesterone.** Autoimmune progesterone dermatosis
22. **Calcium channel blockers, terbinafine, furosemide, hydrochlorothiazide.** Acute generalized exanthematous pustulosis
23. **Pravastatin, simvastatin, atorvastatin.** Lichenoid eruption
24. **Acetylsalicylic acid, NSAIDs, pseudoephedrine, omeprazole, fluconazole, sulfonamides, protease inhibitors, antibiotics.** Fixed drug eruption
25. **Amoxicillin.** Epstein–Barr virus–associated purpuric eruption, flexural exanthem
26. **Hydrochlorothiazide, glipizide, progesterone.** Pigmented purpuric dermatosis

Summary

Drug eruptions can result from almost any systemic medications. Patients often are on numerous medications, making the identification of the causative agent difficult in many cases. Therefore, it is important for clinicians to be aware of specific patterns of drug eruption in order to identify potential offending medications. Eruptions such as Stevens–Johnson syndrome and toxic epidermal necrolysis are severe, life threatening, and often have limited therapeutic options. Therefore, early identification of the causative agent and its discontinuation are essential. Also, there are no good biological tests for identifying the cause of a drug eruption in an individual patient. In this chapter, an outline of important medications and their associated drug eruptions is presented. This information, combined with a careful chronology of medication use, may help narrow down the list of potential offending medications in many cases.

Selected Readings

Ehrlich M. *Drug eruptions. eMedicine Journal* March 4, 2002,Vol. 3, No. 3.

Litt J. *Drug eruption reference manual.* Boca Raton, FL: CRC Press— Parthenon Publishing, 2001.

Susser W. Mucocutaneous reactions to chemotherapy. *J Am Acad Dermatol* 1999;40:367–398.

Bigby M. Rates of cutaneous reactions to drugs. *Arch Dermatol* 2001;137:765–770.

12.2. REACTIONS TO SYSTEMIC MEDICATIONS USED IN DERMATOLOGY

Many dermatologic disorders, including vasculitides, cutaneous T-cell lymphoma, SLE, dermatomyositis, scleroderma, severe cystic acne, severe psoriasis, and parasitic infestations, require systemic medications for optimal control or cure. Oncologists and rheumatologists also use many of the medications used to manage these conditions. These medications also carry significant and severe side effects that require close monitoring during therapy. It is imperative that the treating physician be aware of these important side effects. In this section, a summary of important clinical side effects of systemic medications used by dermatologists is presented. This chapter is meant only as an outline of these effects, and clinicians should consult the complete medication insert for all potential side effects and monitoring requirements for specific medications.

I. **Immunosuppressive agents**
   A. **Azathioprine (Imuran)**
      1. **Contraindications.** Pregnancy, prior hypersensitivity, active infection, reduced activity of thiopurine methyltransferase, drug interactions (allopurinol, alkylating agents, captopril, coumadin, and pancuronium).
      2. **Allergic (immune-related) reactions.** Hypersensitivity (R).
      3. **Pseudoallergic (idiosyncratic) reactions.** Gastrointestinal distress (C), immunosuppression carcinogenesis (R), pancytopenia (R), infection (R).
   B. **Mycophenolate mofetil (Cellcept)**
      1. **Contraindications.** Pregnancy, prior hypersensitivity, severe hepatic or renal disease, drug interactions (including azathioprine and cholestyramine).
      2. **Allergic (immune-related) reactions.** Hypersensitivity (R).
      3. **Pseudoallergic (idiosyncratic) reactions.** Gastrointestinal distress (C), urinary distress (C), headache (C), infection (R), carcinogenesis (U).

II. Injectable agents
A. Interferon-α (Intron, Roferon, Alferon)
  1. **Contraindications.** Prior hypersensitivity, pregnancy (relative), cardiac arrhythmias, depression, leukopenia.
  2. **Allergic (immune-related) reactions.** Hypersensitivity (C), anaphylaxis (R).
  3. **Pseudoallergic (idiosyncratic) reactions.** Flulike symptoms (C), gastrointestinal distress (C), depression (C), cardiac arrhythmia (R), spastic diplegia (R), rhabdomyolysis (U).
B. Botulinum toxin (Botox)
  1. **Contraindications.** Prior hypersensitivity, myasthenia gravis.
  2. **Allergic (immune-related) reactions.** Hypersensitivity (R), anaphylaxis (U).
  3. **Pseudoallergic (idiosyncratic) reactions.** Ptosis (from periorbital injections) (R).
III. Miscellaneous
A. Thalidomide (Thalomid)
  1. **Contraindications.** Pregnancy, prior hypersensitivity, women of childbearing potential, severe hepatic or renal disease, peripheral neuropathy, congestive heart failure, severe hypertension, hypothyroidism, drug interactions (including alcohol, barbiturates, and other CNS depressants).
  2. **Allergic (immune-related) reactions.** Hypersensitivity (R).
  3. **Pseudoallergic (idiosyncratic) reactions.** Sedation (C), mood changes (C), brittle nails (C), increased appetite (C), gastrointestinal distress (C), peripheral neuropathy (C), teratogenicity (C), hypothyroidism (R), hypoglycemia (R), leukopenia (R), erythroderma (U).
B. Spironolactone (Aldactone)
  1. **Contraindications.** Prior hypersensitivity, renal disease, hyperkalemia, pregnancy, breast cancer, gynecologic malignancy, drug interactions (including potassium, digoxin, and ACE inhibitors).
  2. **Allergic (immune-related) reactions.** Hypersensitivity (R).
  3. Pseudoallergic (idiosyncratic) reactions. Gastrointestinal distress (C), hyperkalemia (C), teratogenicity (C), gynecomastia (R), breast or gynecologic malignancy (U).
C. Ortho-TriCyclen or other oral contraceptives
  1. **Contraindications.** Pregnancy, drug interactions (including anticonvulsants, rifampin, and griseofulvin).
  2. **Allergic (immune-related) reactions.** Hypersensitivity (U).
  3. **Pseudoallergic (idiosyncratic) reactions.** Nausea (C), breast tenderness (C), weight gain (C), headaches (C), deep venous thrombosis (R), thromboemboli (R).
D. Pentoxifylline (Trental)
  1. **Contraindications.** Prior hypersensitivity, severe hepatic or renal disease, pregnancy, severe cardiac disease.
  2. **Allergic (immune-related) reactions.** Hypersensitivity (R).

3. **Pseudoallergic (idiosyncratic) reactions.** Nausea (C), headaches (C), dizziness (C), gastrointestinal disease (C).

E. **Methoxsalen (Oxsoralen) or other psoralens**
   1. **Contraindications.** Prior hypersensitivity, pregnancy, pemphigus, bullous pemphigoid, lupus erythematosus, xeroderma pigmentosum, photosensitivity, personal or family history of melanoma, severe cardiac, hepatic or renal disease, concomitant use of photosensitizing medications (including tetracyclines, fluoroquinolones, and thiazide diuretics).
   2. **Allergic (immune-related) reactions.** Hypersensitivity (R).
   3. **Pseudoallergic (idiosyncratic) reactions.** Erythema (C), gastrointestinal distress (C), freckling (C), photoaging (C), nonmelanomatous skin cancers (C), pruritus (R), photosensitive eruptions (R), photoonycholysis (R), hypertrichosis (R), drug fever (R), exanthem (R), herpes simplex recurrences (R), melanoma (R), cataracts (R), immunosuppression (R).

F. **Finasteride (Propecia, Procar)**
   1. **Contraindications.** Pregnancy, prior hypersensitivity, women of childbearing potential.
   2. **Allergic (immune-related) reactions.** Hypersensitivity (R).
   3. **Pseudoallergic (idiosyncratic) reactions.** Teratogenicity (C), loss of libido (C), erectile dysfunction (R), gynecomastia (R), myopathy (R).

IV. **Psoriasis medications**
   A. **Cyclosporine (Neoral)**
      1. **Contraindications.** Severe renal disease, severe hypertension, prior hypersensitivity, history of malignancy, pregnancy (relative), immunodeficiency, active infection, drug interactions (including macrolide antibiotics, azole antifungals, human immunodeficiency virus (HIV) protease inhibitors, calcium channel blockers, H_2 antihistamines, diuretics, grapefruit juice).
      2. **Allergic (immune-related) reactions.** Hypersensitivity (R).
      3. **Pseudoallergic (idiosyncratic) reactions.** Gastrointestinal distress (C), renal dysfunction (C), hypertension (C), hypertrichosis (C), gingival hyperplasia (C), metabolic abnormalities (C), immunosuppression carcinogenesis (R), infection (R).

   B. **Etanercept (Enbral)**
      1. **Contraindications.** Prior hypersensitivity, pregnancy, active infection, immunodeficiency.
      2. **Allergic (immune-related) reactions.** Hypersensitivity (C), anaphylaxis (R).
      3. **Pseudoallergic (idiosyncratic) reactions.** Flulike symptoms (C), headache (C), infection (R), immunosuppressive carcinogenesis (U), multiple sclerosis (U).

V. **Retinoids (oral)**
   A. **Isotretinoin (Accutane)**
      1. **Contraindications.** Pregnancy, hypertriglyceridemia, uncontrolled hypercholesterolemia, severe depression,

concomitant epilation or resurfacing procedures, leukopenia, hypothyroidism, severe hepatic or renal disease.

2. Allergic (immune-related) reactions. Hypersensitivity (R), anaphylaxis (U).

3. Pseudoallergic (idiosyncratic) reactions. Teratogenicity (C), cheilitis (C), xerosis (C), petechiae (C), gastrointestinal distress (C), bone pain (C), conjunctivitis (C), hypertriglyceridemia (C), hypercholesterolemia (C), mood changes (C), photosensitivity (C), depression (R), pseudotumor cerebri (R), alopecia (R), leukopenia (R), myopathy (R), agranulocytosis (U).

  B. Acitretin (Soriatane)

   1. Contraindications. Pregnancy, hypertriglyceridemia, uncontrolled hypercholesterolemia, severe depression, concomitant epilation or resurfacing procedures, leukopenia, hypothyroidism, severe hepatic or renal disease, alcohol use (in women, due to conversion to etretinate).

   2. Allergic (immune-related) reactions. Hypersensitivity (R), anaphylaxis (U).

   3. Pseudoallergic (idiosyncratic) reactions. Teratogenicity (C), cheilitis (C), xerosis (C), petechiae (C), gastrointestinal distress (C), bone pain (C), conjunctivitis (C), hypertriglyceridemia (C), hypercholesterolemia (C), mood changes (C), photosensitivity (C), depression (R), pseudotumor cerebri (R), alopecia (R), leukopenia (R), myopathy (R), agranulocytosis (U).

  C. Bexarotene (Targretin)

   1. Contraindications. Pregnancy, hypertriglyceridemia, uncontrolled hypercholesterolemia, severe depression, concomitant epilation or resurfacing procedures, leukopenia, hypothyroidism, severe hepatic or renal disease.

   2. Allergic (immune-related) reactions. Hypersensitivity (R), anaphylaxis (U).

   3. Pseudoallergic (idiosyncratic) reactions. Teratogenicity (C), cheilitis (C), xerosis (C), petechiae (C), gastrointestinal distress (C), bone pain (C), conjunctivitis (C), hypertriglyceridemia (C), hypercholesterolemia (C), hypothyroidism (C), mood changes (C), photosensitivity (C), depression (R), pseudotumor cerebri (R), alopecia (R), leukopenia (R), myopathy (R), agranulocytosis (U).

VI. Sulfa medications

  A. Dapsone

   1. Contraindications. Prior hypersensitivity, neutropenia, glucose-6-phosphate dehydrogenase (G6PD) deficiency, severe cardiac disease.

   2. Allergic (immune-related) reactions. Hypersensitivity (C), morbilliform eruption (C), anaphylaxis (R), TEN (U), exfoliative erythroderma (U).

   3. Pseudoallergic (idiosyncratic) reactions. Gastrointestinal distress (C), methemoglobinemia (C), peripheral neuropathy (R), psychosis (R), leukopenia (R), hemolytic anemia (U), agranulocytosis (U).

  B. Sulfapyridine

   1. Contraindications. Prior sulfonamide hypersensitivity, neutropenia, severe cardiac disease, renal disease.

2. Allergic (immune-related) reactions. Hypersensitivity (C), morbilliform eruption (C), anaphylaxis (R), TEN (U), exfoliative erythroderma (U).
3. Pseudoallergic (idiosyncratic) reactions. Gastrointestinal distress (C), peripheral neuropathy (R), psychosis (R), hemolytic anemia (R), methemoglobinemia (R), nephrotoxicity (R), leukopenia (R), agranulocytosis (U).

VII. **Systemic chemotherapy agents**
A. **Methotrexate**
   1. **Contraindications.** Pregnancy, prior hypersensitivity, leukopenia, anemia, thrombocytopenia, active infection, hepatic or renal disease, alcohol use, drug interactions (including NSAIDs, sulfonamides, phenytoin, tetracyclines, and dapsone).
   2. **Allergic (immune-related) reactions.** Hypersensitivity (R), anaphylaxis (U).
   3. **Pseudoallergic (idiosyncratic) reactions.** Nausea (C), gastrointestinal distress (C), dizziness (C), hepatotoxicity (C), teratogenicity (C), myelosuppression (C), pancytopenia (R), pulmonary toxicity (R), nephrotoxicity (R), alopecia (R), phototoxicity (R), acral erythema (U), epidermal necrosis (U), vasculitis (U), ultraviolet recall (U), carcinogenicity (U).
B. **Cyclophosphamide (Cytoxan)**
   1. **Contraindications.** Pregnancy, prior hypersensitivity, leukopenia, anemia, thrombocytopenia, active infection, hepatic or renal disease, drug interactions (including allopurinol, cimetidine, doxorubicin, and digoxin).
   2. **Allergic (immune-related) reactions.** Hypersensitivity (R), Stevens–Johnson syndrome (U), anaphylaxis (U).
   3. **Pseudoallergic (idiosyncratic) reactions.** Teratogenicity (C), gastrointestinal distress (C), leukopenia (C), anagen effluvium (C), hemorrhagic cystitis (C), bladder toxicity (C), thrombocytopenia (C), anemia (C), amenorrhea (C), sterility (C), diffuse hyperpigmentation (R), nail ridging (R), acral erythema (R), carcinogenicity (R), infection (R), cardiomyopathy (U), pneumonitis (U), pulmonary fibrosis (U), syndrome of inappropriate secretion of antidiuretic hormone (U).
C. **Chlorambucil**
   1. **Contraindications.** Pregnancy, prior hypersensitivity, active infection, hepatic disease.
   2. **Allergic (immune-related) reactions.** Hypersensitivity (R), morbilliform eruption (R).
   3. **Pseudoallergic (idiosyncratic) reactions.** Teratogenicity (C), leukopenia (C), thrombocytopenia (R), anemia (R), carcinogenicity (R), gastrointestinal (R), hepatotoxicity (R), infection (R), alopecia (R), mucosal ulcerations (R), peripheral neuropathy (R), myoclonus (R), tonic-clonic seizures (R), aplastic anemia (U), pneumonitis (U), pulmonary fibrosis (U), sterile cystitis (U).
D. **Doxorubicin (Adriamycin)**
   1. **Contraindications.** Pregnancy, prior hypersensitivity, active infection.
   2. **Allergic (immune-related) reactions.** Hypersensitivity (R).

3. **Pseudoallergic (idiosyncratic) reactions.** Alopecia (C), stomatitis (C), onychodystrophy (C), nail and acral hyperpigmentation (C), chemical cellulitis or ulceration (R), radiation recall (R), palmoplantar dysesthesia (R), neutrophilic eccrine hidradenitis (R), infection (R).

E. **Dactinomycin**
1. **Contraindications.** Pregnancy, prior hypersensitivity, active infection.
2. **Allergic (immune-related) reactions.** Hypersensitivity (R), erythema multiforme (U).
3. **Pseudoallergic (idiosyncratic) reactions.** Acneiform eruption (C), folliculitis (C), radiation recall (R), infection (R).

VIII. **Antiparasitic agents**
A. **Thiabendazole**
1. **Contraindications.** Prior hypersensitivity, hepatic or renal disease.
2. **Allergic (immune-related) reactions.** Hypersensitivity (R), Stevens–Johnson syndrome (U).
3. **Pseudoallergic (idiosyncratic) reactions.** Nausea (C), diarrhea (C), tinnitus (R), bradycardia (R), leukopenia (R), hematuria (R).

B. **Diethylcarbamazine**
1. **Contraindications.** Prior hypersensitivity.
2. **Allergic (immune-related) reactions.** Hypersensitivity (R).
3. **Pseudoallergic (idiosyncratic) reactions.** Nausea (C).

C. **Sodium stibogluconate**
1. **Contraindications.** Prior hypersensitivity.
2. **Allergic (immune-related) reactions.** Hypersensitivity (R).
3. **Pseudoallergic (idiosyncratic) reactions.** Nausea (C), hemolysis (C), anemia (C).

D. **Pentamidine**
1. **Contraindications.** Prior hypersensitivity, hepatic or renal disease.
2. **Allergic (immune-related) reactions.** Hypersensitivity (R), TEN (U).
3. **Pseudoallergic (idiosyncratic) reactions.** Nausea (C), diarrhea (C), azotemia (R), megaloblastic anemia (U), acute pancreatitis (U), leukopenia (U), thrombocytopenia (U), cardiac arrhythmia (U), hyperkalemia (U).

E. **Ivermectin**
1. **Contraindications.** Prior hypersensitivity.
2. **Allergic (immune-related) reactions.** Hypersensitivity (R).
3. **Pseudoallergic (idiosyncratic) reactions.** Headache (C), dizziness (C), nausea (C), ataxia (R), seizures (R).

Selected Readings
Barranco V. Clinically significant drug interactions in dermatology. *J Am Acad Dermatol* 1998;38:599–612.
Susser W. Mucocutaneous reactions to chemotherapy. *J Am Acad Dermatol* 1999;40:367–98.

Wolverton SE. *Comprehensive dermatologic drug therapy*. Philadelphia: WB Saunders, 2001.

12.3. REACTIONS TO TOPICAL MEDICATIONS

Topical medications are used to manage many dermatological conditions as a first line primarily due to the lower side effect risks in comparison with systemic medications. Almost all topical preparations have the possibility of causing either an irritant or allergic contact dermatitis. Many times the dermatitis is in reaction to the active medication, but in other cases it may due to a component of the vehicle such a preservative ingredient. In this section, a brief summary of the adverse effects of the most commonly used classes of dermatologic medications is presented.

I. **Adverse effects of topical medications**
   A. **Retinoids**
      1. **Tretinoin (Retin-A, Renova), adapalene (Differin), tazarotene (Tazorac), bexarotene (Targretin).** Xerosis, photosensitivity, irritant contact dermatitis, allergic contact dermatitis
   B. **Antibiotics**
      1. **Benzoyl peroxide.** Xerosis, irritant and allergic contact dermatitis
      2. **Neomycin/polymyxin/bacitracin (Neosporin).** Allergic contact dermatitis
      3. **Polymyxin/bacitracin (Polysporin).** Allergic contact dermatitis
      4. **Bacitracin.** Allergic contact dermatitis
      5. **Clindamycin.** Xerosis, irritant contact dermatitis, allergic contact dermatitis
      6. **Mupirocin (Bactroban).** Irritant or allergic contact dermatitis
      7. **Azelaic acid (Azelex).** Irritant or allergic contact dermatitis, hypopigmentation
      8. **Erythromycin.** Irritant or allergic contact dermatitis
      9. **Metronidazole (Metro-Cream, Metro-Lotion, Metro-Gel).** Irritant or allergic contact dermatitis
      10. **Sulfa antibiotics (Plexion, Klaron).** Irritant or allergic contact dermatitis
   C. **Steroids**
      1. See Table 12.1 for a list of topical steroids and their relative potencies. Hypopigmentation, atrophy, telangiectases, striae, allergic contact dermatitis
   D. **Antifungals**
      1. **Amphotericin (Fungizone), butenafine (Mentax), ciclopirox (Loprox, Penlac), clotrimazole (Lotrimin), econazole (Spectazole), itraconazole (Sporonox), ketoconazole (Nizoral), miconazole (Micatin), naftifine (Naftin), nystatin (Mycelex), terbinafine (Lamisil), tolnaftate (Tinactin).** Irritant or allergic dermatitis
   E. **Macrolide anti-inflammatory medications**
      1. **Tacrolimus (Protopic), Pimecrolimus (Elidel).** Irritant or allergic contact dermatitis, folliculitis, acne, herpes zoster, or other skin infections

Table 12.1.   Potency ranking of commonly used topical steroid preparations

Group I (most potent)
Betamethasone [Diprolene] ointment
Diflorasone [Psorcon] ointment
Clobetasol [Temovate] ointment
Halobetasol [Ultravate] ointment

Group II
Halocinonide [Halog] ointment/cream
Fluocinonide [Lidex] ointment/cream
Desoximetasone [Topicort] ointment/cream

Group III
Amcinonide [Cyclocort] cream/lotion
Mometasone [Elocon] ointment

Group IV
Mometasone [Elocon] cream
Triamcinolone [Kenalog] ointment
Fluocinolone [Synalar] ointment
Hydrocortisone valerate [Westcort] ointment

Group V
Hydrocortisone butyrate [Locoid] cream
Fluticasone [Cutivate] cream
Triamcinolone [Kenalog] cream/lotion
Fluocinolone [Synalar] cream
Hydrocortisone valerate [Westcort] cream

Group VI
Alclometasone [Aclovate] ointment/cream
Desonide [DesOwen] ointment/cream/lotion

Group VII (least potent)
Hydrocortisone [Hytone] ointment/cream

F. **Antiparasitic agents**
1. **Permethrin (Elimite, Rid, Nix).** Irritant or allergic contact dermatitis, paresthesias
2. **Lindane (Kwell).** Irritant or allergic contact dermatitis, dizziness, neurotoxicity, seizures
3. **Malathion.** Irritant or allergic contact dermatitis, hyperhidrosis, bradycardia, shortness of breath
G. **Antiviral agents**
1. **Acyclovir (Zovirax), penciclovir (Denavir), docosanol (Abreva).** Irritant or allergic contact dermatitis
H. **Chemical (hydroquinone) bleaching agents**
1. **Lustra, Glyquin, Tri-Luma.** Irritant or allergic contact dermatitis, exogenous ochronisis (with overuse), atrophy (Tri-Luma), telangiectases (Tri-Luma), striae (Tri-Luma)
I. **Agents affecting hair growth**
1. **Minoxidil (Rogaine).** Irritant or allergic contact dermatitis, hirsutism, dizziness, hypotension, tachycardia

   2. Eflornithine (Vaniqa). Irritant or allergic contact dermatitis
J. Anesthetics
   1. EMLA, Ela-Max, Lida-Mantle. Allergic contact dermatitis, methemoglobinemia (EMLA)
K. Chemotherapy agents
   1. 5-FU (Efudex, Carac). Irritant or allergic contact dermatitis, severe peeling and erosions, photosensitivity
   2. Nitrogen mustard, carmustine (BCNU). Irritant or allergic contact dermatitis, increased risk of skin cancer
L. Miscellaneous topical agents
   1. Imiquimod (Aldara). Irritant or allergic contact dermatitis, pruritus, burning, peeling, erosions
   2. Diclofenac (Solaraze). Irritant or allergic contact dermatitis, xerosis, peeling
M. Preservatives used in topical preparations
   1. Parabens, Kathon CG, Euxyl-K400, imidazolidinyl urea, propylene glycol, quaternium-15, formaldehyde. Allergic contact dermatitis
N. UV protections from sun-screening ingredients
   1. Paraaminobutyric acid. Partial UVB and no UVA protection
   2. Benzophenones. Full UVB and partial UVA protection
   3. Cinnamates. Full UVB and partial UVA protection
   4. Salicylates. Full UVB and no UVA protection
   5. Avobenzone. Full UVA and no UVB protection
   6. Parsol 1789. Full UVA and no UVB protection
   7. Titanium dioxide. Full UVA and full UVB protection
O. Cross-reactions of topical and systemic medications
   1. Topical ethylenediamine may cross-react with systemic aminophylline.

Summary

As reviewed in this section, topical medications in dermatology have limited side effects. Most commonly, they cause irritant or allergic contact dermatitis. Thus, topical medications are first-line agents for numerous skin conditions. Systemic medications are generally reserved for cutaneous diseases with extensive body surface area involvement or with internal organ involvement. New topical medications are being developed and approved for an increasing number of clinical indications. Topical medications, therefore, will continue to have an important role in the therapy of cutaneous disease.

SELECTED READINGS

Arndt KA. *Manual of dermatologic therapeutics,* Philadelphia: Lippincott Williams and Wilkins, 1995.
Scheman AJ, Severson DL. *Medications used in dermatology,* Philadelphia: Lippincott Williams and Wilkins, 2001.

Endocrinology

Whitney S. Goldner and Janet Schlechte

I. Diabetes medications

A. Indication. Management of type 1 and type 2 diabetes.

1. **Human insulin (NPH, Regular, Ultralente)**
   a. **Contraindications/precautions.** None.
   b. **Allergic reactions**
      (1) Immediate local (pruritic, erythematous skin wheals) or generalized (nausea, pruritus, tachycardia, wheezing, shortness of breath, flare reaction at other injection sites) (C). Incidence: 10% to 56% of diabetics who have been exposed to human insulin.
         (a) **Treatment.** (1) Substitution of synthetic insulin analogs for human insulin. (2) Coadministration of antihistamines or steroids for severe reactions. (3) Continuous insulin infusion. (4) Tolerance induction with escalating doses of human insulin (see Table 13.1).
      (2) **Leukocytoclastic vasculitis** (U). Incidence: case report.
         (a) **Treatment.** Corticosteroids, azathioprine, methotrexate, or a combination.
      (3) **Cross-reactivity.** Any human insulin.
      (4) **Future precautions.** If insulin therapy is interrupted, reinitiation of human insulin may require repeat tolerance induction.

2. **Synthetic insulin (Humalog, Aspart, Glargine)**
   a. **Contraindications.** None reported.
   b. **Allergic reactions.** None reported.

B. Indication. Management of type 2 diabetes

1. **Insulin.** See discussion of type 1 diabetes.
2. **Sulfonylureas (glipizide, glyburide, glimepiride)**
   a. **Contraindications/precautions.** Prolonged hypoglycemia in elderly patients and patients with impaired renal or liver function. Drugs that may potentiate the action of sulfonylureas: salicylates, phenylbutazone, sulfonamides, warfarin, clofibrate, monoamine oxidase inhibitors, chloramphenicol, fenfluramine, alcohol, probenecid.
   b. **Allergic reactions**
      (1) Skin rash, pruritus, erythema multiforme, pemphigus vulgaris (glyburide), pigmented purpuric dermatosis (glipizide) (R). Incidence: 3%.
         (a) **Treatment.** Discontinuation of the drug.
      (2) Cholestatic jaundice (U). Incidence: case report.
         (a) **Treatment.** Discontinuation of the drug.
      (3) Angioedema, arthralgia, myalgia, vasculitis (U). Incidence: case report.
         (a) **Treatment.** Discontinuation of the drug.
      (4) **Cross-reactivity.** Sulfa-containing drugs.

Table 13.1. **Insulin desensitization protocol**

Time (min)	Insulin Dose (U)^a
0	0.004
30	0.01
60	0.04
90	0.1
120	0.2
150	0.5
180	1.0

^{a}The insulin dose should be slowly titrated up at 30-min intervals until the goal insulin dosage is attained. Dosages will vary.
Reprinted from Wessbecher R, Kiehn M, Stoffel E, et al. Management of insulin allergy. *Allergy* 2001;56:919.

   c. Idiosyncratic reactions
      (1) Leukopenia, agranulocytosis, hemolytic anemia, pancytopenia (U). Incidence: case report.
         (a) Treatment. Discontinuation of the drug.
3. Insulin secretagogues (repaglinide, nateglinide)
   a. Contraindications/precautions. Contraindicated in type 1 diabetes and diabetic ketoacidosis. Hypoglycemia, especially when combined with insulin or other oral hypoglycemics. Should be used cautiously with hepatic or renal impairment.
   b. Allergic reactions. Anaphylaxis (U). Incidence: case report.
      (1) Treatment. Discontinuation of the drug and supportive therapy.
4. Biguanides (metformin)
   a. Contraindications/precautions. Lactic acidosis can occur with renal impairment (serum creatinine >1.5 mg/dL), hepatic impairment, alcoholism, chronic obstructive pulmonary disease, states of increased tissue lactate production (coronary artery disease, congestive heart failure, peripheral vascular disease, sepsis, and diabetic ketoacidosis). Metformin should be discontinued prior to receiving contrast dye and should not be resumed for 48 to 72 hours.
      (1) Incidence. Zero to 0.08 cases per 1,000 patient-years.
   b. Allergic reactions. Leukocytoclastic vasculitis and pneumonitis (U). Incidence: case report.
      (1) Treatment. Corticosteroids and discontinuation of drug.
5. Thiazoladinediones (rosiglitazone, pioglitazone)
   a. Contraindications. Liver dysfunction (alanine aminotransferase > 2.5 upper limit of normal), diabetic ketoacidosis, type 1 diabetes will cause plasma volume expansion, so should be used with caution in patients with congestive heart failure [New York Heart Association (NYHA) class III and IV] or lower extremity edema.

    b.   Allergic reactions. Angioneurotic edema (pioglita-
zone) (U). Incidence: case report.
      (1)   Treatment. Discontinuation of the drug and corti-
costeroids.
  6.   α-Glucosidase inhibitors (acarbose, miglitol)
    a.   Contraindications. Malabsorption syndromes, in-
flammatory bowel disease, intestinal obstruction, cirrhosis
(acarbose), diabetic ketoacidosis, type 1 diabetes.
    b.   Allergic reactions
      (1)   Skin rash (miglitol) (R). Incidence: 4.3%.
        (a)   Treatment. Discontinuation of drug.
      (2)   Erythema multiforme (acarbose) (U). Incidence:
case report.
        (a)   Treatment. Discontinuation of drug and corti-
costeroids.
    c.   Idiosyncratic reaction. Hepatic toxicity (acarbose)
(U) Incidence: 3 case reports.
      (1)   Treatment. Discontinuation of drug.
II.   Osteoporosis medications
  A.   Indication. Prevention and management of osteoporosis.
    1.   Calcium.
      a.   Contraindications. Hypercalcemia.
      b.   No allergic or pseudoallergic reactions reported (U).
    2.   Vitamin D
      a.   Contraindications. Hypercalcemia.
      b.   Allergic reactions
        (1)   Calcipotriol, topical
          (a)   Allergic contact dermatitis (R) Incidence: 1% to
10% (R).
          (b)   Treatment. Discontinuation of drug, corticos-
teroids.
        (2)   Calcitriol , oral and intravenous.
          (a)   Urticaria, pruritus, angioedema, generalized hi-
ves, erythema multiforme (U). Incidence: case reports.
          (b)   Treatment. Discontinuation of drug, oral anti-
histamines.
          (c)   Desensitization protocol. Oral and intra-
venous desensitization in an intensive care unit setting or monitored bed before reinitiation of drug.
        **(3)   Ergocalciferol, cholecalciferol, doxercalcif-
erol, paricalcitriol, and dihydrotachysterol**
          (a)   No reported allergic or pseudoallergic reactions
(U).
    3.   Estrogen. See Chapter 17.
    **4.   Selective estrogen receptor antagonists (ralox-
ifene).** See Chapter 17.
    **5.   Bisphosphonates (alendronate, pamidronate, clo-
dronate, risedronate).**
      a.   Contraindications/precautions. Esophageal dys-
motility, esophageal stricture, achalasia, inability to stand
or sit upright for 30 minutes, hypocalcemia, and a creatinine clearance <35 mL/min.
      b.   Allergic reactions
        (1)   Urticaria, hives, pruritus, erythema multiforme,
vasculitis (R). Incidence: 6 case reports.

(a) **Treatment.** Discontinuation of drug, oral antihistamines. Corticosteroids for severe reaction.

(2) Bronchoconstriction in aspirin-sensitive patients (U). Incidence: 4 case reports.

(a) **Treatment.** Inhaled corticosteroids and β agonists and discontinuation of drug.

(3) Anterior uveitis, conjunctivitis, episcleritis, and scleritis (pamidronate) (R). Incidence: 23 case reports.

(a) **Treatment.** Discontinuation of drug. Depending on severity of reaction, treatment can range from no therapy, to topical corticosteroids and cycloplegics, to oral corticosteroids.

6. **Salmon calcitonin**
   a. **Contraindications/precautions.** None.
   b. **Allergic reactions**
      (1) **Anaphylaxis** (U). Incidence: case report.
      (a) **Treatment.** Discontinuation of drug and supportive therapy.
      (b) **Cross-reactivity.** Eel calcitonin, no cross-reactivity with human calcitonin.
      (2) Skin rash, urticaria (R). Incidence: 10% (injection), 1% to 3% (nasal).
      (a) **Treatment.** Oral antihistamines and discontinuation of drug.

7. **Parathyroid hormone.** No data, recently approved by the U.S. Food and Drug Administration.

III. **Medications for hypogonadism**
   A. **Indication.** Hypogonadism.
      1. **Estrogen.** See Chapter 17.
      2. **Progesterone.** See Chapter 17.
      3. **Testosterone.**
         a. **Contraindications.** Men with breast or prostate cancer, benign prostatic hypertrophy, or suspicion of prostate cancer.
         (1) **Androderm, Andropatch**
            (a) **Allergic reactions.** Contact allergy (R). Incidence: 4%.
            (b) **Treatment.** Removal of patch, application of topical corticosteroids, rotation of patch sites, or switch to intramuscular injection.
         (2) **Nandrolone decanoate**
            (a) Subcutaneous/intramuscular pseudotumor formation (U). Incidence: case report.
            (b) **Treatment.** Discontinuation of drug.
         (3) **Methyltestosterone, oral**
            (a) Peliosis hepatis, hepatic neoplasms, cholestatic hepatitis (R).
            (b) **Treatment.** Discontinuation of the drug.
         (4) **Testosterone enanthate and AndroGel**
            (a) No allergic or pseudoallergic reactions reported (U).

IV. **Glucocorticoids.** Skin testing to corticosteroid preparations and their diluents can be helpful in determining which steroid preparation is suitable for future administration. If the initial reaction was severe, administration of skin test must be performed with caution due to risk of recurrence of anaphylaxis.

  A. Indication. Management of adrenal insufficiency, inflammatory conditions, and various dermatologic and hematologic disorders.

    1. Topical steroids. Hydrocortisone, betamethasone, triamcinolone.

        a. Allergic reactions. Contact dermatitis (R). Incidence: 2% to 6%.

            (1) Treatment. Discontinuation of the drug. Fluorinated steroids (betamethasone and triamcinolone) are less allergenic than nonfluorinated steroids (hydrocortisone).

        b. Cross-reactivity. Other topical steroids.

    2. Systemic steroids. Hydrocortisone, methylprednisolone, prednisolone, cortisone acetate, and dexamethasone.

        a. Allergic reactions. Urticaria, angioedema, bronchospasm, and anaphylaxis (R). Incidence: 0.3%.

            (1) Treatment. Discontinuation of drug and supportive therapy.

V. Thyroid medications

  A. Indication. Management of hypothyroidism.

    1. T$_4$ (levothyroxine, L-thyroxine, Synthroid, Levoxyl, Levothroid, Levotec, Eltroxin, Levo-7) and T$_3$ (liothyronine, Cytomel) .

        a. Contraindications. None.

        b. Allergic reactions. Hypersensitivity: fever, urticaria, rash, liver injury (U). Incidence: case report.

            (1) Treatment. Discontinuation of drug, desensitization before restarting therapy.

  B. Indication. Management of hyperthyroidism and thyrotoxicosis.

    1. Thionamides (methimazole, propylthiouracil).

        a. Idiosyncratic reactions

            (1) Hepatotoxicity (R). Incidence: 1% to 5%.

                (a) Treatment. Discontinuation of drug.

            (2) Agranulocytosis (R) Incidence: 1% to 5%.

                (a) Treatment. Discontinuation of drug.

            (3) Systemic hypersensitivity. Polyarthritis, cutaneous vasculitis, fever, and sensorineural deafness. (U) Incidence: case report.

                (a) Treatment. Discontinuation of drug and supportive therapy.

            (4) Skin rash, urticaria, hives (R). Incidence: unknown.

                (a) Treatment. Discontinuation of drug, topical/oral corticosteroids, and oral antihistamines for severe cases.

            (5) Cross-reactivity. All thionamides.

    2. Iodine (radioactive iodine, Lugol solution)

        a. Contraindications. Pregnant or lactating women.

        b. No allergic or pseudoallergic reactions reported (U).

VI. Lipid-lowering agents

  A. Indication. Management of hypertriglyceridemia.

    1. Niacin

        a. Contraindications. Hepatic dysfunction.

b. Allergic reactions (U).

c. Idiosyncratic reactions. Hepatic necrosis: (R) Incidence: unknown. When converting to Niaspan from crystalline niacin, start at 500 mg qd and titrate slowly. Should not exceed 2 g/day.

(1) **Treatment.** Discontinuation of drug and supportive care.

2. **Fibrates**

a. **Contraindications.** Hepatic impairment (alanine aminotransferase > three times upper limit normal), renal impairment, primary biliary cirrhosis, gallbladder disease.

b. **Allergic reactions.**

(1) Eosinophilic gastroenteritis (gemfibrozil) (U). Incidence: case report.

(a) **Management of reactions.** Discontinuation of drug and oral corticosteroids.

(2) Skin rash, urticaria, Stevens–Johnson syndrome, toxic epidermal necrolysis (fenofibrate) (U). Incidence: <1% to 6%.

(a) **Treatment.** Discontinuation of drug and supportive care.

B. **Management of hypercholesterolemia and elevated low-density lipoproteins.**

1. **3-Hydroxy-3-methylglutaryl coenzyme A reductase inhibitors (statins).**

a. **Contraindications.** Acute liver disease, persistent elevation of alanine aminotransferase > three times upper limit of normal.

b. No allergic or pseudoallergic reactions reported (U).

c. Idiosyncratic reactions: myositis, myalgias (R). Treatment: discontinuation of drug and supportive therapy.

2. **Cholestyramine**

a. No contraindications, allergic or pseudoallergic reactions reported.

3. **Omega-3 fatty acids**

a. No contraindications, allergic reactions, or pseudoallergic reactions reported (U).

VII. **Pituitary hormones**

A. **Indication.** Growth hormone deficiency.

1. **Growth hormone**

a. No contraindications, allergic reactions, or pseudoallergic reactions reported (U).

B. **Indication.** Management of diabetes insipidus.

1. **1-Deamino-8-D -arginine vasopressin (DDAVP)**

a. **Contraindications.** None.

b. **Allergic reactions.** Anaphylaxis with injection (U). Incidence: unknown.

(1) **Treatment.** Discontinuation of drug and supportive therapy.

C. **Indication.** Management of acromegaly, carcinoid tumors, gastrinoma, and other neuroendocrine tumors.

1. **Somatostatin (octreotide)**

a. No contraindications, allergic or pseudoallergic reactions (U).

D. Indication. Management of hyperprolactinemia.

    1. Dopamine agonists (bromocriptine, cabergoline, pergolide)

        a. Contraindications. Uncontrolled hypertension, sensitivity to ergot derivatives.

        b. Idiosyncratic reactions. Pleuritis, pleural fibrosis, pericarditis, retroperitoneal fibrosis (pergolide) (U). Incidence: case reports.

            (1) Treatment. Discontinuation of drug.

            (2) Cross-reactivity. Ergot derivative drugs.

VIII. Drugs used to test for endocrine hypofunction

  A. Indication. Test for primary or secondary adrenal insufficiency.

    1. Cosyntropin

        a. Contraindications. None.

        b. Allergic reactions. Anaphylaxis (U). Incidence: unknown.

            (1) Treatment. Discontinuation of drug and supportive therapy.

  B. Indication. Test for adrenocorticotropic hormone deficiency

    1. Corticotropin-releasing hormone

        a. No contraindications, allergic reactions, or pseudoallergic reactions reported (U).

    2. Metyrapone

        a. No contraindications, allergic reactions, or pseudoallergic reactions reported (U).

  C. Indication. Test for central hypothyroidism.

    1. Thyrotropin-releasing hormone

        a. No contraindications, allergic reactions, or pseudoallergic reactions reported (U).

IX. Miscellaneous endocrine drugs

  A. Indication. Inhibit peripheral conversion of testosterone to estrogen.

    1. Aromatase inhibitors

        a. Anastrozole

            (1) Contraindications/precautions. Use with caution in patients with a history of thromboembolic disease.

            (2) Allergic reactions

                (a) Skin rash (R). Incidence: 6%.

                (b) Treatment. Discontinuation of drug.

        b. Letrozole

            (1) Contraindications. Renal or hepatic impairment.

            (2) No allergic or pseudoallergic reactions reported (U).

  B. Indication. Test for growth hormone deficiency.

    1. Arginine

        a. Contraindications. Persons with allergic tendency or predisposition.

        b. Allergic reactions. Anaphylaxis (U). Incidence: case report.

            (1) Treatment. Discontinuation of drug and supportive therapy.

SELECTED READINGS

Adams BB, Gadenne AS. Glipizide-induced pigmented purpuric dermatosis. *J Am Acad Dermatol* 1999;41:827–829.

Amandeep S, Lomaestro B, Meuwissen H. Hypersensitivity to intravenous and oral calcitriol with successful desensitization. *J Allergy Clin Immunol* 1999;103:176.

Bandyopadhyay U, Biswas K, Banerjee RK. Extrathyroidal actions of antithyroid thionamides. *Toxicol Lett* 2002;128:117–127.

Borja JM, Galindo PA, Feo F, et al. Urticaria to methylprednisolone sodium hemisuccinate. *Allergy* 2001;56:791.

Buckley DA, Wilkinson SM, Higgins EM. Contact allergy to a testosterone patch. *Contact Dermatitis* 1997;39:91–92.

Butany L. Corticosteroid-induced hypersensitivity reactions. *Ann Allergy Immunol* 2002;89:439–445.

Ernst EJ, Egge JA. Celecoxib-induced erythema multiforme with glyburide cross-reactivity. *Pharmacotherapy* 2002;22:637–640.

Fong PC, Pun KK, Tai YT, et al. Propylthiouracil hypersensitivity with circumstantial evidence for drug-induced reversible sensorineural deafness: a case report. *Hormone Res* 1991;35(3-4):132-6.

Frosch PJ, Rustemeyer T. Contact allergy to calcipotriol does exist. *Contact Dermatitis* 1999;40:66–71.

Gallacher SJ, Anderson K, Banham SW, et al. Bisphosphonate-induced bronchoconstriction in aspirin-sensitive asthma. *Lancet* 1994;343:924.

Khankhanian NK, Hammers YA. Exuberant local tissue reaction to intramuscular injection of nandrolone decanoate (Deca-Durabolin)—a steroid compound in a sesame seed oil base-mimicking soft tissue malignant tumors: a case report and review of the literature. *Military Med* 1992;157:670–673.

Klapholz L, Leitersdorf E, Weinrauch L. Leucocytoclastic vasculitis and pneumonitis induced by metformin. *Br Med J* 1986;293:483.

Kono T, Hayami M, Kobayashi H, et al. Acarbose-induced generalized erythema multiforme. *Lancet* 1999;354:396–397.

Krentz AJ, Ferner RE, Bailey CJ. Comparative tolerability profiles of oral antidiabetic agents. *Drug Safety* 1994;11:223–241.

Lee JY, Medellin MV, Tumpkin C. Allergic reaction of gemfibrozil manifesting as eosinophilic gastroenteritis. *S Med J* 2000;93:807–808.

Lutz ME, el-Azhary RA. Allergic contact dermatitis due to topical application of corticosteroids: review and clinical implications. *Mayo Clin Proc* 1997;72:1141–1144.

Mandrup-Poulsen T, Molvig J, Pildal J, et al. Leukocytoclastic vasculitis induced by subcutaneous injection of human insulin in a patient with type 1 diabetes and essential thrombocythemia. *Diabetes Care* 2002;25:242–243.

Macarol V, Fraunfelder FT. Pamidronate disodium and possible ocular adverse drug reactions. *Am J Ophthalmol* 1994;118:220–224.

McCleskey PE, Swerlick RA. Clinical review: thioureas and allergic contact dermatitis. *Cutis* 2001;68:387–396.

Nagai Y, Mori T, Abe T, et al. Immediate-type allergy against human insulin associated with marked eosinophilia in type 2 diabetic patient. *Endocr J* 2001;48:311–316.

Paterson AJ, Lamey PH, Lewis MA, et al. Pemphigus vulgaris precipitated by glibenclamide therapy. *J Oral Pathol Med* 1993;22:92–95.

Phillips E, Knowles S, Weber E, et al. Skin reactions associated with bisphosphonates: a report of 3 cases and an approach to management. *J Allergy Clin Immunol* 1998;102:697–698.

Porcel SL, Cumplido JA, de la Hoz B, et al. Anaphylaxis to calcitonin. *Allergologia Immunopathologia* 2000;28:243–245.

Queille-Roussel C, Duteil L, Parneix-Spake A, et al. The safety of calcitriol 3 microg/g ointment. Evaluation of cutaneous contact sensitization, cumulative irritancy, photoallergic contact sensitization and phototoxicity. *Eur J Dermatol* 2001;11:219–224.

Resnick DJ, Softness BS, Murphy AR, et al. Case report of an anaphylactoid reaction to arginine. *Ann Allergy Asthma Immunol* 2002;88:67–68.

Rodriguez A, Trujillo MJ, Herrero T, et al. Allergy to calcitonin. *Allergy* 2001;56:801.

Shibata H, Hayakawa H, Hirukawa M, et al. Hypersensitivity caused by synthetic thyroid hormones in a hypothyroid patient with Hashimoto's thyroiditis. *Arch Intern Med* 1986;146:1624–1625.

Thomson KF, Wilkinson SM, Powell S, et al. The prevalence of corticosteroid allergy in two U.K. centres: prescribing implications. *Br J Dermatol* 1999;141:863–866.

Van der Klauw MM, Goudsmit R, Halie MR, et al. A population-based case-cohort study of drug-associated agranulocytosis. *Arch Intern Med* 1999;159:369–374.

Wessbecher R, Kiehn M, Stoffel E, et al. Management of insulin allergy. *Allergy* 2001;56:919.

14

Gastroenterology

Bradley B. Rowberry

I. **Antiulcer and antigastroesophageal reflux drugs**

   A. **Antacids** (aluminum hydroxide, magnesium hydroxide, aluminum phosphate, calcium carbonate; Maalox, Mylanta, Gaviscon). Antacids work by neutralizing stomach acid.

   1. **Contraindications.** None.

   2. **Allergic reactions** (U). One case report of immunoglobulin E (IgE)–mediated anaphylaxis to antacid.

   3. **Pseudoallergic reactions.** None.

   B. **H_2 blockers.** Ranitidine (Zantac), cimetidine (Tagamet), famotidine (Pepcid), nizatidine (Axid). H_2 blockers are synthetic analogs of histamine that bind reversibly with the H_2 receptor, which inhibits the accumulation of intracellular cyclic AMP thereby suppressing parietal cell acid secretion.

   1. **Contraindications.** H_2 blockers are contraindicated in individuals known to have a hypersensitivity to any of the products listed above.

   2. **Allergic reactions.** Anaphylactic reactions to H_2 blockers appear to be extremely rare, but case reports are noted in the literature of reactions to ranitidine, nizatidine, and cimetidine. Studies by Lazaro et al. indicate that this a type I hypersensitivity. There also is evidence that the combination of steroids, phenytoin, and H_2 blockers can lead to anaphylaxis (R).

   3. **Pseudoallergic reactions** (U)

   C. **Sucralfate (Carafate).** Sucralfate works by forming a viscous, adhesive gel that bonds to damaged epithelium.

   1. **Contraindications.** None.

   2. **Allergic reactions.** (U)

   3. **Pseudoallergic reactions.** None.

   D. **Misoprostol (Cytotec).** Misoprostol is a prostaglandin analog with gastric cytoprotective activity at low doses and gastric antisecretory activity at higher doses.

   1. **Contraindications.** Misoprostol is absolutely contraindicated in pregnancy.

   2. **Allergic reactions.** (U)

   3. **Pseudoallergic reactions.** None.

   E. **Proton pump inhibitors (PPIs).** Omeprazole (Prilosec), lansoprazole (Prevacid), rantoprazole (Protonix), rabeprazole (Aciphex), esomeprazole (Nexium). Proton pump inhibitors inhibit gastric acid secretion by noncompetitive inhibition of the H^+-K^+-ATPase proton pump of the parietal cell.

   1. **Contraindications.** Hypersensitivity.

   2. **Allergic reactions** (R). Anaphylactic reactions to PPIs have been reported. The Uppsala Monitoring Centre has received a total of 42 reports of anaphylactic reactions or shock in association with PPIs. There are data to suggest

cross-reactivity, by skin tests, between omeprazole and lansoprazole. Skin testing was performed using intravenous omeprazole (4 mg/mL), omeprazole capsules diluted in saline serum (20 mg/mL), and lansoprazole (30 mg/mL) (R). There was one case report of allergic contact dermatitis due to lansoprazole (R).

   3. Pseudoallergic reactions (R).

II. Prokinetic agents

   A. Metoclopramide (Reglan). The exact mechanism of action of metoclopramide is unknown; however, research suggests that it is a potent dopamine receptor antagonist with cholinomimetic properties.

   1. Contraindications. Suspected or known mechanical obstruction, gastrointestinal (GI) perforation, known sensitivity or intolerance, epilepsy, extrapyramidal disorders, or pheochromocytoma.

   2. Allergic reactions. Four case reports of respiratory failure or anaphylaxis after administration of metoclopramide are described. One theory suggests that respiratory failure may be due to anaphylaxis or bronchoconstriction from metoclopramide-induced cholinergic activity of the vagus nerve, possibly through inhibition of acetylcholinesterase (R). Rash and urticaria have been reported frequently (C).

   3. Pseudoallergic reactions. Pseudotetanus (R).

   B. Cisapride (Propulsid). This drug facilitates the release of acetylcholine via an indirect cholinergic mechanism mediated by an unknown receptor on postganglionic nerve endings at the myenteric plexus.

   1. Contraindications. Hypersensitivity.

   2. Allergic reactions. Rash and rhinitis (C).

   3. Pseudoallergic reactions. None.

   C. Domperidone. Acts on the smooth muscle of the gastrointestinal tract by antagonizing the effects of dopamine. The drug has upper GI tract prokinetic and antiemetic properties similar to metoclopramide but without the CNS side effects.

   1. Contraindications. None.

   2. Allergic reactions. One case report of erythema-type drug eruption (U).

   3. Pseudoallergic reactions. None.

III. GI anti-inflammatory agents

   A. Corticosteroids (topical, oral, intravenous). Stabilize lysosomal membranes, reduce capillary permeability, function as inhibitors of chemotaxis and phagocytosis, and impair immunity.

   1. Contraindications. Colonic perforation, peritonitis and abscess formation.

   2. Allergic reactions. None reported to topical use (enemas). See Chapter 13.

   3. Pseudoallergic reactions. None.

   B. Sulfasalazine (5-ASA, Azulfidine). Mechanism of action unknown. 5-ASA metabolite may have effect on connective tissue. Possible antibacterial properties.

   1. Contraindications. Hypersensitivity to sulfonamides, salicylates, or the drug itself.

2. Allergic reactions. Numerous reports of hypersensitivity reactions, including Stevens–Johnson syndrome, photosensitivity, hepatotoxicity, pancreatitis, pulmonary alveolitis and hypersensitivity pneumonitis, agranulocytosis, thrombocytopenia (C).

3. Pseudoallergic reactions. None.

C. 5′-ASA compounds—Mesalamine (Asacol, Pentasa), olsalazine (Dipentum). Mechanism of action unknown. May inhibit cyclooxygenase as well as neutrophil and monocyte chemotaxis. Possible oxidation of short-chain fatty acids. Possible inhibition of synthesis of leukotrienes B_4 and C_4.

1. Contraindications. Patients with hypersensitivity to salicylates or hypersensitivity to the drug.

2. Allergic reactions. Case reports of skin hypersensitivity, pustular drug eruption, hypersensitivity pneumonitis, alveolitis, pancreatitis, hepatotoxicity, pericarditis, and interstitial nephritis (R).

3. Pseudoallergic reactions. None.

D. Anti-tumor necrosis factor: infliximab (Remicade). See Chapter 21.

E. Colchicine (generic). See Chapter 21.

IV. Bile solubility agents

A. Ursodiol (Urso, Actigall). 7β-Hydroxy epimer of chenodeoxycholate. Drug surrounds cholesterol stones with a cholesterol and phospholipid ionophase that enhances cholesterol solubilization from the stone.

1. Contraindications. None.

2. Allergic reactions (U).

3. Pseudoallergic reactions. None.

B. Chenodiol, chenodeoxycholic acid (Chenix). Impairs endogenous cholesterol synthesis by decreasing the activity of 3-hydroxy-3-methylglutaryl coenzyme A reductase and impairs bile synthesis.

1. Contraindications. None.

2. Allergic reactions. One case report of atopic dermatitis-like reaction with elevated IgE levels (U).

3. Pseudoallergic reactions. None.

C. Monoctanoin (Moctanin). Semisynthetic vegetable oil shown in vivo to dissolve common cholesterol bile duct stones.

1. Contraindications. Preexisting jaundice or liver disease, duodenal ulcer, inflammation of the jejunum and ischemic bowel.

2. Allergic reactions. None (U).

3. Pseudoallergic reactions. None.

V. Pancreatic enzymes

A. Lipase, protease, amylase (Pancrease, Viokase, Creon, Kutrase). Pancreatic enzymes derived from porcine sources with standardized enzyme activity.

1. Contraindications. Must be used with caution in patients allergic to pork.

2. Allergic reactions. Several case reports of asthma induced from the enzyme after gel capsules are opened and contents (in powder form) inhaled (C).

3. Pseudoallergic reactions (R).

VI. Laxatives
A. Lactulose (generic). Synthetic disaccharide analog of lactose, which acts as a laxative by stimulating colonic peristalsis.
   1. **Contraindications.** Galactosemia.
   2. **Allergic reactions** (U).
   3. **Pseudoallergic reactions.** None.
B. Psyllium (Metamucil, Perdiem), methylcellulose (Metamucil). These medications are bulk-forming agents that increase colonic motility through distention of the colonic wall.
   1. **Contraindications.** Hypersensitivity.
   2. **Allergic reactions.** Numerous reports of IgE-induced anaphylaxis, asthma, and rhinitis due to psyllium (R).
   3. **Pseudoallergic reactions.** None.
C. Contact laxatives. Stimulate fluid and electrolyte secretion and inhibit sodium absorption. All are contraindicated in cases of acute abdominal pain, undiagnosed abdominal pain, nausea, vomiting, or suspected GI obstruction.
   1. **Docusate (dioctyl sulfosuccinate) (Colase, Surfak, Dialose, Kasof)**
      a. **Allergic reactions.** Single case report of atopic dermatitis from dioctyl sulfosuccinate in a corticosteroid (U).
      b. **Pseudoallergic reactions.** None.
   2. **Anthraquinones.** Cascara (generic), senna (Senokot).
      a. **Allergic reactions.** Several reports of IgE mediated occupational asthma with both medications (R). One report of hypersensitivity reaction to oral and topical aloe.
      b. **Pseudoallergic reactions.** None.
   3. **Diphenylmethane derivatives.** Bisacodyl (Dulcolax, Fleet), phenolphthalein (Correctol, Doxidan, Ex-Lax, Modane).
      a. **Allergic reactions.** Numerous reports of fixed drug eruptions to phenolphthalein with several case reports of toxic epidermal necrolysis.
      b. **Pseudoallergic reactions.** None.
   4. **Ricinoleic acid (castor oil).**
      a. **Allergic reaction.** Isolated reports of contact dermatitis (R). Asthma induced by aerosol released in manufacturing.
      b. **Pseudoallergic reactions.** None.
D. Polyethylene glycol (Golytely, Nulytely, Colyte). Isosmotic solution used for cleansing of the lower GI tract prior to lower GI evaluation (endoscopic or radiologic) or surgery.
   1. **Contraindications.** Bowel obstruction, unexplained or undiagnosed abdominal pain, ileus, bowel perforation, toxic colitis.
   2. **Allergic reactions.** One case report of anaphylactic reaction to polyethylene glycol electrolyte solution (U).
   3. **Pseudoallergic reaction.** None.
VII. Antidiarrheal medications
A. Loperamide (Imodium). Decreases gut motility and gut secretion; has opiate agonist properties.
   1. **Contraindications.** Pseudomembranous colitis, toxic colitis, diarrhea due to organisms that penetrate the intestinal mucosa.

2. **Allergic reactions** (U).

3. **Pseudoallergic reactions.** None.

B. Belladonna and related antimuscarinics (Lomotil, Urised, Donnatal, atropine, Donnagel, Bellergal). Antagonize the muscarinic effects of acetylcholine.

1. **Contraindications.** Pseudomembranous colitis, obstructive jaundice, diarrhea due to organisms that penetrate the intestinal mucosa.

2. **Allergic reactions.** Several case reports of IgE-mediated anaphylaxis resulting from inhaled, oral, and intravenous administered atropine (R).

3. **Pseudoallergic reactions.** None.

C. Glucagon (generic). Inhibits colonic, gastric, and duodenal motility (mechanism unknown).

1. **Contraindications.** None.

2. **Allergic reactions.** (U)

3. **Pseudoallergic reactions.** None.

D. Kalin and pectate (Kaopectate): Nonspecific adsorbent.

1. **Contraindications.** Hypersensitivity to the drug or bowel obstruction.

2. **Allergic reactions.** None (U).

3. **Pseudoallergic reactions.** None.

E. Cholestyramine (Questran). Bile salt–binding resin used in bile salt diarrhea.

1. **Contraindications.** Cholestasis or bile duct stricture.

2. **Allergic reactions.** None (U).

3. **Pseudoallergic reactions.** None.

VIII. Hormones

A. Octreotide acetate (Sandostatin). Somatostatin analog that inhibits the release of serotonin, gastrin, vasoactive intestinal polypeptide, secretin, motilin, and pancreatic polypeptide.

1. **Contraindications.** Sensitivity to the drug.

2. **Allergic reactions.** None (U).

3. **Pseudoallergic reactions.** None.

IX. Sclerosing and hemostatic agents

A. Sodium tetradecyl sulfate (Sotradecal). Synthetic anion detergent that causes blood vessel thrombosis and is utilized in sclerosing esophageal varices.

1. **Contraindications.** Hypersensitivity to the drug.

2. **Allergic reactions.** Anaphylactic reactions have been reported (R).

3. **Pseudoallergic reactions.** None.

B. Sodium morrhuate. Mixture of unsaturated fatty acids derived from cod liver oil that cause endothelial injury and subsequent thrombosis in blood vessels.

1. **Contraindications.** Hypersensitivity to the drug or fatty acids derived from cod liver oil.

2. **Allergic reactions** (U).

3. **Pseudoallergic reactions.** Fever, chest pain, pleural effusion, and respiratory distress may occur.

C. Vasopressin (Pitressin). Splanchnic bed vasoconstrictor.

1. **Contraindications.** Liver disease, coronary artery disease, congestive heart failure (CHF), seizures, severe liver disease, asthma, migraine.

   2. Allergic reactions (U).
   3. Pseudoallergic reactions. None.
X. Immunomodulators
   A. Azathioprine (Imuran). Imidazole derivative of 6-mercaptopurine with antimetabolite and immunosuppressive actions that result in inhibition of purine ring formation and subsequent cellular division.
      1. Contraindications. Hypersensitivity to the drug, pregnancy.
      2. Allergic reactions. Anaphylactic shock has been reported in one case followed by a positive challenge (R).
      3. Pseudoallergic reactions. None.
   B. 6-Mercaptopurine (Purenthol). Same mechanism of action as azathioprine.
      1. Contraindications. Renal failure, pregnancy.
      2. Allergic reactions. Anaphylaxis (R).
      3. Pseudoallergic reactions. None.

SELECTED READINGS

Wyngaarden JB, MD, ed. Cecil Textbook of Medicine. Philadelphia: W.B. Saunders Company, 2000.

Anderson PO, Troutman WG, Knoben JE, eds. Handbook of Clinical Drug Data. New York: McGraw-Hill/Appleton & Lange, 2001.

Meyers FH, Jawetz E, Goldfien A. Review of Medical Pharmacology. Los Altos, CA: Lange Medical Publications, 1980.

Feldman M, Scharschmidt BF, Sleisenger MH, Fordtran JS, Zorab R, eds. Gastrointestinal and Liver Disease: Pathophysiology/Diagnosis/Management, 6th Edition. Philadelphia: W.B. Saunders and Company, 1998.

15

Hematology and Oncology

Mary Rachel Faris and John Redmond III

I. **Antiemetic drugs.**
 A. **Serotonin antagonists: granisetron (Kytril), ondansetron (Zofran), dolasetron mesylate (Anzemet).**
  1. **Contraindication.** Prolonged cardiac conduction intervals (dolastron mesylate) (R).
  2. **Allergic reaction.** (R).
  3. **Adverse drug effects.** Headache (C), diarrhea (R), abdominal pain (R).
 B. **Metoclopramide (Reglan)**
  1. **Contraindication.** Bowel obstruction, Parkinson disease, seizures, impaired renal function.
  2. **Allergic reaction.** (R).
  3. **Adverse drug effects.** Akathisia (R), acute dystonia (R), diarrhea (R), tremor (C), sedation (C). Urinary retention (C).
 C. **Prochlorperazine (Compazine)**
  1. **Contraindication.** Caution in the elderly.
  2. **Allergic reaction.** (R).
  3. **Adverse drug effects.** Mild sedation (C), akathisia (R), agranulocytosis (R), blurred vision (C), dry mouth (C), orthostatic hypotension (C).
 D. **Dexamethasone (Decadron)**
  1. **Contraindication.** Use with caution in diabetes, hypertension, infection, impaired liver function.
  2. **Allergic reaction.** (R).
  3. **Adverse drug effects.** Hiccoughs (C), dyspepsia (C), increased appetite (C), fluid retention (R) with short course. Long term associated with immunosuppression (C), osteoporosis (C).
II. **Supportive drugs**
 A. **Filgrastim (Neupogen)**
  1. **Contraindication.** Known hypersensitivity to *Escherichia coli*-derived proteins.
  2. **Allergic reaction.** Skin rash, hypotension (R).
  3. **Adverse drug effects.** Medullary bone pain (C).
 B. **Epoetin alfa (Epogen, Procrit)**
  1. **Contraindication.** Uncontrolled hypertension, known sensitivity to mammalian cell–derived products and albumin.
  2. **Allergic reaction.** Skin rash and urticaria (R).
  3. **Adverse drug effects.** Thrombotic events (R), hypertension (R).
 C. **Cyanocobalamin (vitamin B_{12})**
  1. **Contraindication.** None.
  2. **Allergic reaction.** (R).
  3. **Adverse drug effects.** Pruritus (R), diarrhea (R), urticaria (R).

D. Ferrous sulfate
1. **Contraindication.** Hemachromatosis/hemosiderosis.
2. **Allergic reaction.** (R).
3. **Adverse drug effects.** Constipation (C), nausea and vomiting (R), dyspepsia (C), dark stools (C).

E. Folic acid
1. **Contraindication.** None.
2. **Allergic reaction.** (R).
3. **Adverse drug effects.** (R).

F. Fluoxymesterone (Halotestin)
1. **Contraindication.** Prostate cancer, hepatic dysfunction, cardiac insufficiency.
2. **Allergic reaction.** Anaphylaxis (R).
3. **Adverse drug effects.** Erythrocytosis (C), priapism (R), hirsutism (C), irregular menses (C), acne (C), deepened voice (C), cholestatic hepatitis (R), clitoral enlargement (C), fluid retention (C).

G. Warfarin (Coumadin)
1. **Contraindication.** Pregnancy, bleeding, thrombocytopenia, underlying coagulopathy, surgery, invasive procedure, vitamin K deficiency. Warfarin not distributed into milk.
2. **Allergic reaction** (R).
3. **Adverse drug effects.** Blue toe syndrome/skin necrosis (R), bleeding (C), and ecchymosis (C). Many drug interactions, which increase or decrease effect of warfarin (C).

H. Heparin sodium
1. **Contraindication.** Bleeding, surgery/invasive procedure, central nervous system (CNS) metastases. May be given during pregnancy or to lactating mothers.
2. **Allergic reaction.** Generalized chills, fever, urticaria, asthma (R).
3. **Adverse drug effects.** Transient increase in aspartate aminotransferase, alanine aminotransferase (C), osteoporosis with long-term use (C), bleeding (C), Heparin-induced thrombocytopenia may be associated with thrombosis (R).

III. Alkylating drugs
A. Carboplatin (Paraplatin)
1. **Contraindications.** Allergy to cisplatin. Dosing based on renal function.
2. **Allergic reaction.** Immediate rash, urticaria, chest tightness, bronchospasm, hypotension (C). Occurs after multiple courses of treatment.
3. **Adverse drug effects.** Thrombocytopenia (C), neutropenia (C), alopecia (C), renal (R), electrolyte abnormalities (R), nausea, vomiting (C), paresthesias (R).

B. Chlorambucil (Leukeran)
1. **Contraindications.** Barbiturates may increase toxicity. Dose adjustment with concomitant allopurinol or colchicine.
2. **Allergic reaction.** (R).
3. **Adverse drug effects.** Myelosuppression (C), secondary malignancies: acute myelogenous leukemia (AML) and myelodysplasia with prolonged administration (R).

C. Cisplatin (Platinol)

1. **Contraindications.** Hypersensitivity to cisplatin. Other drugs causing nephrotoxicity.
2. **Allergic reactions.** Immediate anxiety, cough, bronchospasm hypotension (R). Usually occurs after multiple cisplatin doses.
3. **Adverse drug effects.** Ototoxicity (C), renal failure is dose dependent with renal tubular damage and with potassium, calcium, and magnesium wasting (C). Myelosuppression (C), severe nausea and vomiting—acute and delayed (C).

D. **Cyclophosphamide (Cytoxan, Neosar)**
1. **Contraindications.** Multiple drug interactions with drugs that increase or decrease P450 enzyme hepatic metabolism (i.e., corticosteroids, barbiturates).
2. **Allergic reactions** (R).
3. **Adverse drug effects.** Myelosuppression (C), mild nausea and vomiting (C), hemorrhagic cystitis (R), pulmonary toxicity (R), alopecia (C). Secondary malignancies with high cumulative doses (R). Sterility (C).

E. **Ifosfamide (Ifex)**
1. **Contraindications.** Multiple drug interactions: allopurinol, cimetidine, phenobarbital, phenytoin, phenothiazides, succinylcholine.
2. **Allergic reactions.** (R).
3. **Adverse drug effects.** Myelosuppression (C), CNS (C), bladder toxicity (C). Use with uroprotectant (Mesna). Nausea (C), alopecia (C), infertility (C).

F. **Melphalan (Alkeran)**
1. **Contraindications.** H_2 antagonists decrease absorption of melphalan. High-dose melphalan increases cyclosporine nephrotoxicity.
2. **Allergic reactions.** Acute anaphylaxis (R): more common with intravenous than with oral melphalan.
3. **Adverse drug effects.** Myelosuppression (C), mild nausea (C), alopecia (C). AML and myelodysplasia with long-term use (R).

IV. **Antimetabolites**
A. **Cytosine arabinoside (Cytarabine, Ara-C)**
1. **Contraindications.** Monitor digoxin levels.
2. **Allergic reactions.** Fever, rash (C), hypotension (R).
3. **Adverse drug effects.** Myelosuppression (C). CNS (particularly in elderly) (R).

B. **Capecitabine (Xeloda)**
1. **Contraindications.** Antacids administered concurrently.
2. **Allergic reactions.** 5-Fluorouracil (5-FU) hypersensitivity (R).
3. **Adverse drug effects.** Myelosuppression (C), hepatic. Palmar-plantar erythrodysia (hand–foot syndrome), may be dose-limiting toxicity (C). Diarrhea (C), eye irritation (C).

C. **5-FU**
1. **Contraindications.** Photosensitivity. Radiation sensitizer. Dihydropyrimidine dehydrogenase deficiency with severe and prolonged GI toxicity (R).
2. **Allergic reactions.** (R).

   3. Adverse drug effects. Diarrhea and mucositis (C).
 D. Gemcitabine (Gemzar)
   1. Contraindications. Concurrent radiation.
   2. Allergic reactions. Bronchospasm (R). Rash (C).
   3. Adverse drug effects. Myelosuppression (C), GI (C), rash (C), dyspnea (R), flulike syndrome (R).
 E. Methotrexate (MTX, Mexate)
   1. Precaution. Accumulates in effusions, which prolongs toxicity.
   2. Allergic reactions. Acute urticaria, bronchospasm, hypotension (R).
   3. Adverse drug effects. Myelosuppression (C), nausea (C), renal (R), pulmonary (R), CNS (R), alopecia (C), rash (R), photosensitivity (R).
V. Antibiotics
 A. Bleomycin (Blenoxane)
   1. Precaution. Requires test dose prior to first administration.
   2. Allergic reactions. Fever, hypotension, confusion, chills (C). Anaphylaxis (R).
   3. Adverse drug effects. Pulmonary fibrosis (C) fever (C), pain (C), mucocutaneous (C).
 B. Doxorubicin (Adriamycin)
   1. Contraindications. Congestive cardiomyopathy.
   2. Allergic reactions. Vesicant. Immediate urticaria, angioedema, bronchospasm (R). Urticaria at drug injection site (C).
   3. Adverse drug effects. Myelosuppression (C), nausea (C), cardiac (R), alopecia (C).
VI. Microtubular agents
 A. Docetaxel (Taxotere)
   1. Contraindication. Hypersensitivity to docetaxel or polysorbate 80.
   2. Allergic reactions. Angioedema, rash, hypotension (R). Most common with the first or second dose.
   3. Adverse drug effects. Myelosuppression (C), fluid retention (may be prevented with steroids) (C), mucositis (C), diarrhea (C), nail changes (C).
 B. Paclitaxel (Taxol)
   1. Contraindication. Hypersensitivity to paclitaxel or cremophor.
   2. Allergic reactions. Acute hypersensitivity reactions. Requires steroid, antihistamine, H_2 blocker pretreatment. Severe reactions (immediate hypotension, bronchospasm, dyspnea) 2%; mild (rash or flushing) 40% of patients. 50% of severe reactions occur with first treatment.
   3. Adverse drug effects. Myelosuppression (C), peripheral neuropathy (C), myalgias (C).
 C. Vincristine (Oncovin)
   1. Contraindications. Vesicant. Intrathecal administration is fatal.
   2. Allergic reactions (R).
   3. Adverse drug effects. Peripheral and autonomic neurotoxicity (C), constipation (C).
 D. Vinorelbine (Navelbine)

    1. Contraindications. Mild vesicant. Hypersensitivity to vinka alkaloids.

    2. Allergic reactions. Acute anaphylactic-like reactions (R).

    3. Adverse drug effects. Myelosuppression (C), peripheral and autonomic neuropathy (R).

  E. Vinblastine sulfate (Velban)

    1. Contraindications. Vesicant. Intrathecal administration is fatal.

    2. Allergic reactions. (R).

    3. Adverse drug effects. Jaw pain (C), peripheral and autonomic neurotoxicity (C), constipation (C), neutropenia (C).

VII. Topoisomerase inhibitors

  A. Etoposide (VP-16, Vepesid)

    1. Precaution. Hypotension with rapid administration.

    2. Allergic reactions. Fever, chills, and bronchospasm (R).

    3. Adverse drug effects. Myelosuppression (C), nausea (C), alopecia (C), mucositis (C).

  B. Irinotecan (Camptosar, CPT-11)

    1. Precaution. Toxicity increased with pelvic radiation or hepatic dysfunction.

    2. Allergic reactions (R).

    3. Adverse drug effects. Diarrhea (may be severe) (C), myelosuppression (C), alopecia (C).

VIII. Purine antagonists

  A. Fludarabine (Fludara)

    1. Precaution. Tumor lysis syndrome.

    2. Allergic reaction (R).

    3. Adverse drug effects. Myelosuppression (C) including leukopenia, lymphocytopenia and thrombocytopenia, neurotoxicity (R), dyspnea (R), chest pain (R).

  B. Pentostatin, 2′-deoxycoformycin (Nipent)

    1. Precaution. Cutaneous irritant with erythema and burning (C). Maintain hydration and precautions for tumor lysis syndrome (R).

    2. Allergic reactions. Severe allergic reactions may occur (R).

    3. Adverse drug effects. Leukopenia (C), thrombocytopenia (C), renal insufficiency (R), neurotoxicity (R), conjunctivitis (R).

  C. Chlorodeoxyadenosine, 2-Cladribine, 2-CdA (Leustatin)

    1. Precaution. Caution in patients with renal or hepatic insufficiency. Cutaneous irritant with erythema and pain at injection site. Precaution for acute tumor lysis syndrome.

    2. Allergic reactions. Maculopapular rash (R).

    3. Adverse drug effects. Myelosuppression (C) neutropenia and lymphocytopenia, Renal failure (R), hepatic failure (R).

IX. Antibodies

  A. Rituximab (Rituxan)

    1. Precaution. Avoid in patients with history of hypersensitivity.

    2. Allergic reactions. Acute fever, rigors, dyspnea (C), hypotension (R).

  3. Adverse drug effects. Monitor for acute tumor lysis syndrome, particularly in patients with high circulating malignant cell count such as in chronic lymphocytic leukemia (CLL) (R.).
 B. Ibritumomab tiuxetan (Zevelin)
  1. Precaution. Rituximab hypersensitivity.
  2. Allergic reactions. Fever, rigors, bronchospasm (R).
  3. Adverse drug effects. Neutropenia (C), thrombocytopenia (C).
 C. Trastuzumab (Herceptin)
  1. Precaution. Baseline cardiac evaluation. Risk of cardiac dysfunction increased for trastuzumab with an anthracycline.
  2. Allergic reactions. Bronchospasm, rash, hypotension (R).
  3. Adverse drug effects. Increased risk of cardiac dysfunction and clinical congestive heart failure (R), increased with anthracycline (C).
X. Hormonal therapy
 A. Tamoxifen citrate (Nolovadex)
  1. Precautions. May enhance coumadin anticoagulant effect. Regular gynecologic surveillance for endometrial cancer.
  2. Allergic reactions. Stevens–Johnson syndrome (R).
  3. Adverse drug effects. Increased risk of endometrial cancer (R), thromboembolic events (R), flare of bone pain in patients with bone metastases (C).
 B. Anastrozole (Armidex)
  1. Precaution. Monitor hepatic enzymes.
  2. Allergic reactions. (R).
  3. Adverse drug effects. Hot flashes (C), mild dizziness (C).
 C. Letrozole (Femara)
  1. Allergic reactions. (R).
  2. Adverse drug effects. Arthralgia, headache, fatigue (C), hot flashes (C).

SELECTED READINGS

Anti-neoplastic agents. In: McKevoy GK, ed. *American hospital formulary service drug information 2002,* 44th ed. Bethesda: American Society of Health-System Pharmacists: 886–1179.

Chabner BA, Longo DL, eds. *Cancer chemotherapy and biotherapy: principles and practice,* 3rd ed. Baltimore: Lippincott Williams & Wilkins, 2001.

Perry MC, ed. *The chemotherapy sourcebook,* 3rd ed. Baltimore: Lippincott Williams & Wilkins, 2001.

Weiss RB. Hypersensitivity reactions. *Semin Oncol* 1992;19:458–477.

Neurology

Olga Bessmertny and Lauren M. Robitaille

I. Antiepileptics (aromatic). Antiepileptics are responsible for either isolated cutaneous reactions or cutaneous reactions as a component of antiepileptic hypersensitivity syndrome (AHS). AHS is a severe, dose-independent, immune-mediated, idiosyncratic cutaneous reaction to aromatic anticonvulsants that can potentially result in end-organ damage and death. Numerous case reports in the literature describe AHS related to administration of phenytoin, phenobarbital, carbamazepine, primidone, and lamotrigine. A common feature of the above-mentioned drugs is their aromatic ring structure. Despite the inconsistency in the literature classifying lamotrigine as an aromatic anticonvulsant, lamotrigine should be grouped with the classic aromatic anticonvulsants as a potential cause of AHS due to the large number of case reports describing AHS in association with this agent. The incidence of AHS ranges between 1 in 1,000 to 1 in 10,000 new exposures to aromatic anticonvulsants. The classic constellation of symptoms associated with AHS includes a triad of fever, rash, and lymphadenopathy or internal organ involvement (Table 16.1). The usual onset of AHS is 7 days up to 3 months after therapy initiation, with the majority of cases reported within 2 to 8 weeks. Management of patients with presumptive diagnosis of AHS is described in Table 16.2. The risk of cross-reactivity between aromatic anticonvulsants ranges from 40% to 80%.

  A. Carbamazepine (Tegretol, Tegretol-XR, Carbatrol)

    1. Contraindications: hypersensitivity to carbamazepine, hypersensitivity to tricyclic antidepressants, concomitant therapy with monoamine oxidase inhibitors (MAOIs), bone marrow suppression

    2. Allergic reactions: rash (C), urticaria, photosensitivity, erythema multiforme (R), Stevens–Johnson syndrome (R), toxic epidermal necrolysis (R), antiepileptic hypersensitivity syndrome (R), eosinophilia (R)

    3. Adverse drug effects: aplastic anemia (R), agranulocytosis (R), leukopenia (R), pancytopenia (R), thrombocytopenia (R), acute intermittent porphyria (R), leukocytosis (R), tinnitus (R), lymphadenopathy (R), hepatitis (R), pancreatitis (U), hyponatremia (R), syndrome of inappropriate secretion of antidiuretic hormone (SIADH) (R)

    4. Comments: Must be discontinued immediately in patients with presumptive diagnosis of AHS. Should not be used in patients with history of AHS caused by carbamazepine or other anticonvulsants.

  B. Fosphenytoin (Cerebyx)

    1. Contraindications: hypersensitivity to fosphenytoin or phenytoin

    2. Allergic reactions: see Phenytoin

Table 16.1.   Clinical features of antiepileptic hypersensitivity syndrome

Manifestation	Frequency (%)[a]
Fever	100
Skin rash	100
Lymphocytosis	71
Lymphadenopathy	70
Hepatic involvement	64
Atypical lymphocytes	50
Eosinophilia	42
Coagulopathy	42
Renal involvement	11
Pneumonitis	9

[a] Frequency based on highest reported value in the literature.
Adapted from Bessmertny O, et al. *Curr Allergy Asthma Rep* 2002;2:34–39, with permission.

   3.   **Adverse drug effects:** see Phenytoin
   4.   **Comments:** see Phenytoin
 C.   **Lamotrigine (Lamictal)**
   1.   **Contraindications:** hypersensitivity to lamotrigine
   2.   **Allergic reaction:** rash (11%) (C), Stevens–Johnson syndrome/toxic epidermal necrolysis (up to 1.1% in children) (R), AHS (R), angioedema (R)
   3.   **Adverse drug effects:** disseminated intravascular coagulation with rhabdomyolysis (mostly reported in children)

Table 16.2.   Suggested management of antiepileptic hypersensitivity syndrome

1.   Discontinue anticonvulsant immediately.
2.   Patients receiving anticonvulsants for seizure control can be switched to lorazepam, topiramate, gabapentin, tiagabine, or levetiracetam.
3.   Obtain a complete blood count with differential, hepatic enzymes panel, and basic metabolic panel.
4.   Examine the patient for the presence of lymphadenopathy, hepato- or splenomegaly; perform a thorough skin exam.
5.   Give supportive care with hydration, antihistamines, H_2 receptor antagonists (especially in patients with mucositis), and topical corticosteroids.
6.   In patients with life-threatening disease or severe end-organ involvement (e.g., transaminases more than five times upper limits of normal and rising), consider systemic corticosteroids with or without intravenous immune globulin.
7.   If desquamation or mucous membrane involvement is present, consider obtaining dermatology consult.
8.   Consider skin biopsy in patient with pustules or blistering.
9.   Avoid cross-reacting anticonvulsants (phenytoin, carbamazepine, oxcarbazepine, phenobarbital, primidone, lamotrigine), and educate patients and family about the risk of cross-reactivity.
10.   Counsel family members about increased risk of this syndrome in first-degree relatives.
11.   Label the patient's chart with allergy to phenytoin, carbamazepine, oxcarbazepine, phenobarbital, primidone, and lamotrigine.

Adapted from Bessmertny O, et al. *Curr Allergy Asthma Rep* 2002;2:34–39, with permission.

(R), thrombocytopenia (U), neutropenia (U), anemia (U), hepatic failure (R)

4. **Comments:** The rashes are usually maculopapular or morbilliform in appearance and occur generally within 2 to 8 weeks of initiating therapy. Risk factors for rash are young age (children), concurrent valproic acid therapy, high starting dose, and rapid dose escalation. Lamotrigine-induced rash can also be accompanied by systemic signs and symptoms consistent with AHS. Must be discontinued immediately in patients with presumptive diagnosis of AHS. Should not be used in patients with history of AHS caused by lamotrigine or other anticonvulsants.

D. **Oxcarbazepine (Trileptal)**
  1. **Contraindications:** hypersensitivity to oxcarbazepine
  2. **Allergic reactions:** rash (R), purpura (R), Stevens–Johnson syndrome (R), erythema multiforme (R), toxic epidermal necrolysis, AHS (R)
  3. **Adverse drug effects:** hyponatremia (R), SIADH (R)
  4. **Comments:** Oxcarbazepine is better tolerated and is associated with less cutaneous rashes than carbamazepine. Hyponatremia may be more common with oxcarbazepine than carbamazepine. The risk of hyponatremia development is mainly within the first 90 days of treatment. Oxcarbazepine should be used with extreme caution in patients with history of AHS.

E. **Phenobarbital (Luminal)**
  1. **Contraindications:** hypersensitivity to phenobarbital or primidone, severe central nervous system (CNS) depression or respiratory distress with dyspnea or obstruction, porphyria
  2. **Allergic reaction:** rash (R), exfoliative dermatitis (R), Stevens–Johnson syndrome (R), AHS (R)
  3. **Adverse drug effects:** paradoxical CNS excitation (R), hematologic toxicity (thrombocytopenia, agranulocytosis, megaloblastic anemia) (R), hepatitis (R)
  4. **Comments:** Must be discontinued immediately in patients with presumptive diagnosis of AHS. Should not be used in patients with history of AHS caused by phenobarbital or other anticonvulsants.

F. **Phenytoin (Dilantin)**
  1. **Contraindications:** hypersensitivity to phenytoin or fosphenytoin, heart block, sinus bradycardia
  2. **Allergic reactions:** rash (C), exfoliative dermatitis (R), Stevens–Johnson syndrome (R), toxic epidermal necrolysis (R), erythema multiforme (R), eosinophilia (R)
  3. **Adverse drug effects:** fever (R), systemic lupus erythematosus (SLE)–like syndrome (R), gingival hyperplasia (C), hirsutism (R), coarsening of facial features (R), hematologic toxicity (agranulocytosis, leukopenia, thrombocytopenia) (R), myositis/arthritis (R), renal failure (R), choreathetoid movements (R), hepatitis (R), pseudolymphoma (R), lymphoma (U)
  4. **Comments:** Must be discontinued immediately in patients with presumptive diagnosis of AHS. Should not be used in patients with history of AHS caused by phenytoin or other anticonvulsants.

G. Primidone (Mysoline)
1. **Contraindications:** hypersensitivity to primidone or phenobarbital, porphyria
2. **Allergic reactions:** see Phenobarbital
3. **Adverse drug effects:** see Phenobarbital
4. **Comments:** see phenobarbital

H. Zonisamide (Zonegran)
1. **Contraindications:** hypersensitivity to sulfonamides or zonisamide
2. **Allergic reactions:** rash (R), Stevens–Johnson syndrome/toxic epidermal necrolysis (R)
3. **Adverse drug effects:** paresthesia (R), nephrolithiasis (R), aplastic anemia (R), agranulocytosis (R), hyperthermia and decreased ability to sweat in children (R), psychosis (2%, R), thrombocytopenia (R), SLE (U), IgA and IgG_2 deficiency (R)
4. **Comments:** Should be used with caution in patients with history of AHS

II. Antiepileptics (nonaromatic). Can be used safely in patients with a history of AHS.

A. Clonazepam (Klonopin)
1. **Contraindications:** hypersensitivity to clonazepam or other benzodiazepines, severe liver disease, acute narrow-angle glaucoma
2. **Allergic reactions:** dermatitis (R), rash (R)
3. **Adverse drug effects:** blood dyscrasias (U), menstrual irregularities (U)

B. Diazepam (Diastat Rectal Delivery System, Valium)
1. **Contraindications:** hypersensitivity to diazepam or other benzodiazepines, severe liver disease, acute narrow-angle glaucoma, respiratory or CNS depression
2. **Allergic reactions:** rash (C), dermatitis (R), tinnitus (R)
3. **Adverse drug effects:** blood dyscrasias (U), menstrual irregularities (U), hiccups (R)

C. Ethosuximide (Zarontin)
1. **Contraindications:** hypersensitivity to ethosuximide
2. **Allergic reactions:** rash (R), urticaria (R), Stevens–Johnson syndrome (R)
3. **Adverse drug effects:** hepatotoxicity (R), hematologic toxicity (leukopenia, aplastic anemia, thrombocytopenia) (R), hiccups (R), SLE (R)

D. Felbamate (Felbatol)
1. **Contraindications:** hypersensitivity to felbamate or other carbamates
2. **Allergic reactions:** rash (R), pruritis (R)
3. **Adverse drug effects:** hematologic toxicity (thrombocytopenia, granulocytopenia, agranulocytosis, aplastic anemia) (R), hepatitis/fulminant hepatic failure (R)
4. **Comments:** The use of felbamate is associated with 100-fold increased risk of aplastic anemia occurring 5 to 30 weeks after therapy initiation. Fulminant hepatic failure can result in death. All patients receiving felbamate must be monitored closely for hepatotoxicity and hematologic toxicity. (Liver enzymes and complete blood count should be obtained before initiation therapy and every 1 to 2 weeks during the first year of therapy).

E. Gabapentin (Neurontin)
   1. **Contraindications:** hypersensitivity to gabapentin
   2. **Allergic reactions:** rash (R), Stevens–Johnson syndrome (U), pruritis (R)
   3. **Adverse drug effects:** (U)
F. Levetiracetam (Keppra)
   1. **Contraindications:** hypersensitivity to levetiracetam
   2. **Allergic reactions:** (U)
   3. **Adverse drug effects:** psychotic symptoms (R), decreased erythrocyte and leukocyte counts (R)
G. Lorazepam (Ativan)
   1. **Contraindications:** hypersensitivity to lorazepam or other benzodiazepines, severe hypotension, acute narrow-angle glaucoma, severe CNS depression
   2. **Allergic reactions:** rash (R)
   3. **Adverse drug effects:** blood dyscrasias (U), menstrual irregularities (U)
   4. **Comments:** Drug of choice for the initial management of epileptic patients with AHS.
H. Tiagabine (Gabitril)
   1. **Contraindications:** hypersensitivity to tiagabine
   2. **Allergic reactions:** (U)
   3. **Adverse drug effects:** thrombocytopenia (U), nonconvulsive status epilepticus (C)
I. Topiramate (Topamax)
   1. **Contraindications:** hypersensitivity to topiramate
   2. **Allergic reaction:** (U)
   3. **Adverse drug effects:** hepatic failure (U), nephrolithiasis (1.5%) (R), flulike symptoms (U), paresthesia (R), word finding difficulties (C), decreased hearing (R), weight loss (C)
J. Valproic acid (Depakote, Depakene, Depacon, Depakote-ER)
   1. **Contraindications:** hypersensitivity to valproic acid, hepatic dysfunction
   2. **Allergic reactions:** rash/pruritis (R), cutaneous vasculitis (R), erythema multiforme (R)
   3. **Adverse drug effects:** pancreatitis (R), encephalopathy (reported in 41% of patients with pancreatitis) (R), fatal hepatotoxicity/Reye-like syndrome (R), Fanconi-like syndrome (R), bone marrow failure (U), myelodysplasia (U), acute promyelocytic leukemia (U)
   4. **Comments:** Most cases of hepatotoxicity occurred in children younger than 2 years receiving valproic acid polytherapy and preexisting metabolic defects (pyruvate dehydrogenase deficiency, primary carnitine deficiency, propionic acidemia, etc.). Valproic acid should be avoided in patients with known or suspected metabolic defects and family history of Reye-like syndrome. Carnitine supplementation may decrease the potential for valproic acid–induced hepatotoxicity in young children. Valproic acid can be used safely in patients with history of AHS as long as liver enzyme abnormalities are not present.
III. Antimigraine agents (ergot alkaloids and derivatives). The use of ergot alkaloids and derivatives has the potential to induce fibrotic syndromes (pleural, cardiac, or

retroperitoneal fibrosis with respiratory distress). Drug holidays do not prevent serious fibrotic reactions.

Persons with cardiovascular impairment (e.g., myocardial infarction, arteriosclerosis) should avoid the use of ergot derivatives due to potential for ergotamine-induced vascular ischemia. Symptoms may include chest pain, abdominal pain, cold extremities, convulsions, peripheral gangrene, headaches, myocardial infarction, numbness, paresthesia, and weak pulses. Complications may be seen in patients within 24 hours of the first dose or may be delayed for many years.

   A. Dihydroergotamine (D.H.E. 45 Injection, Migranal Nasal Spray)

      1. Contraindications: hypersensitivity to dihydroergotamine or derivatives, high-dose aspirin therapy, concomitant use within 2 weeks of MAOIs, concomitant use within 24 hours of serotonin agonists, and pregnancy. Use with caution in patients with cardiovascular disease.

      2. Allergic reactions: rash (R), pruritis (R)

      3. Adverse drug effects: fibrotic syndromes and vascular ischemic complications, subarachnoid/cerebral hemorrhage (<1%) (R), transient tachycardia (R), bowel ischemia (U), discolored urine (C), edema (C), renal failure (U)

   B. Ergotamine (Cafergot, Cafergot-PB, Cafetrate, Ercaf, Ergomar, Phenerbel-S, Wigraine)

      1. Contraindications: hypersensitivity to ergot alkaloids and derivatives or caffeine, peripheral vascular disease, hepatic or renal dysfunction, hypertension, peptic ulcer disease, sepsis, pregnancy

      2. Allergic reactions: (U)

      3. Adverse drug effects: fibrotic syndromes and vascular ischemic complications. Other adverse effects include myocardial infarction (U), ventricular arrhythmias (R), ischemic colitis (U), hallucinations (U), porphyria (R), superinfections (U), acute renal failure (U)

   C. Methysergide (Sansert)

      1. Contraindications: peripheral vascular disease, severe arteriosclerosis, pulmonary disease, severe hypertension, phlebitis, serious infections, pregnancy

      2. Allergic reactions: rash, facial flushing

      3. Adverse drug effects: fibrotic syndromes and vascular ischemic complications. Other adverse effects include myocardial infarction, perceptual disorders and psychosis (U), akathisia (U), weight gain, chronic pleural effusion, arthralgia, myalgia, telangiectasia, alopecia, hemolytic anemia (U), neutropenia (R), thrombocytopenia (R)

IV. Antimigraine agents (serotonin agonists). Serotonin (5-hydroxytryptamine, 5-HT$_1$) agonists are commonly associated with "triptan sensations" that include tightening of throat and chest, paresthesia, and warmth. These symptoms occur most commonly with sumatriptan subcutaneous injection.

Serotonin syndrome (altered mental status, dysautonomia, neuromuscular changes) may occur when combining 5-HT$_1$ agonists and selective serotonin reuptake inhibitors.

   A. Naratriptan (Amerge)

      1. Contraindications: use in patients with ischemic heart disease or signs/symptoms of ischemic heart disease, cerebrovascular or peripheral vascular syndromes, uncontrolled hypertension; use within 24 hours of ergotamine derivatives or another 5HT$_1$ agonist, concurrent administration or within 2 weeks of discontinuation of MAOI, hypersensitivity to naratriptan, severe hepatic or renal impairment, prophylactic treatment for migraine, management of hemiplegic or basilar migraine

2. Allergic reactions: hypersensitivity reactions (U)

3. Adverse drug effects: arrhythmias (R), elevated liver enzyme tests (R), convulsions (U), eye hemorrhage (R), hypothyroidism (R), hyperglycemia (R), cerebrovascular accidents (U), myocardial infarction (R)

B. Rizatriptan (Maxalt, Maxalt-MLT)

1. Contraindications: use in patients with ischemic heart disease or signs/symptoms of ischemic heart disease, cerebrovascular or peripheral vascular syndromes, uncontrolled hypertension; use within 24 hours of ergotamine derivatives or another 5-HT$_1$ agonist, concurrent administration or within 2 weeks of discontinuation of MAOI, hypersensitivity to rizatriptan, prophylactic treatment for migraine, management of hemiplegic or basilar migraine

2. Allergic reactions: toxic epidermal necrolysis (R), pruritus (R)

3. Adverse drug effects: neurologic/psychiatric abnormalities (R) convulsions (U), tinnitus (R), dysgeusia (R), cerebrovascular accidents (U), myocardial infarction (R)

C. Sumatriptan (Imitrex)

1. Contraindications: intravenous administration, use in patients with ischemic heart disease or signs/symptoms of ischemic heart disease, cerebrovascular or peripheral vascular syndromes, uncontrolled hypertension; use within 24 hours of ergotamine derivatives or another 5-HT$_1$ agonist, concurrent administration or within 2 weeks of discontinuation of MAOI, hypersensitivity to sumatriptan, severe hepatic impairment, prophylactic treatment for migraine, management of hemiplegic or basilar migraine

2. Allergic reactions: rash (U), hypersensitivity reactions (U), pruritus (U), angioedema (U)

3. Adverse drug effects: convulsions (U), acute renal failure (U), hemolytic anemia (U), pancytopenia (U), thrombocytopenia (U), elevated liver function test (LFT) results (U), abdominal aortic aneurysm (U), abnormal menstrual cycle (U), hiccups (U), cerebrovascular accidents (R), myocardial infarction (R)

D. Zolmitriptan (Zomig)

1. Contraindications: use in patients with ischemic heart disease or signs/symptoms of ischemic heart disease, cerebrovascular or peripheral vascular syndromes, uncontrolled hypertension; use within 24 hours of ergotamine derivatives or another 5-HT$_1$ agonist, patients with Wolff–Parkinson–White syndrome or arrhythmias associated with other cardiac conduction pathways disorders, concurrent administration or within 2 weeks of discontinuing of MAOI, hypersensitivity to zolmitriptan, prophylactic treatment for migraine, management of hemiplegic or basilar migraine

2. **Allergic reactions:** rash (R)
3. **Adverse drug effects:** renal calculi (R), dysmenorrhea (R), hiccups (R), dyspnea (R), thirst (R), cerebrovascular accidents (U), myocardial infarction (R)

V. **Antimigraine agents (other).** Anticholinergics frequently cause side effects such as xerostomia, constipation, urinary retention, and blurred vision. They have also been known to increase ocular pressure, induce hyperpyrexia, and affect the cardiovascular system (hypotension, palpitations, tachycardia, arrhythmias) and the CNS (dizziness, drowsiness, confusion, hallucinations). Medications with anticholinergic properties should be avoided in patients with advanced age, cardiovascular disease, narrow-angle glaucoma, reactive airway disease, obstructive gastrointestinal (GI) or genitourinary (GU) disease, and seizure disorders.

A. **Cyproheptadine (Periactin)**
  1. **Contraindications:** hypersensitivity to cyproheptadine, narrow-angle glaucoma, bladder neck obstruction, acute asthmatic attack, stenosing peptic ulcer, GI tract obstruction, concomitant use of MAOIs, use in neonates
  2. **Allergic reactions:** skin rash (R), urticaria (R), photosensitivity (R)
  3. **Adverse drug effects:** convulsions (R), cholestasis (R), hyperbilirubinemia (R), hallucinations (more common in children), central anticholinergic syndrome (consists of altered mental status, agitation, confusion, visual hallucinations) (U), angioedema (R), appetite stimulation and weight gain (C), hemolytic anemia, thrombocytopenia, leukopenia (R).
  4. **Comments:** Use in premature and term infants may be associated with sudden infant death syndrome (SIDS)

B. **Isometheptene (Midrin, Migratane, Isocom, Isopap, Midchlor—often in combination with dichloralphenazone and acetaminophen)**
  1. **Contraindications:** narrow-angle glaucoma, severe renal, hepatic or heart disease, or concomitant use of MAOI
  2. **Allergic reactions:** skin rash (R)
  3. **Adverse drug effects:** none
  4. **Comments:** transient dizziness and skin rash may appear in sensitive patients, which can usually be eliminated by reducing the dosage.

VI. **Antiparkinson agents (dopaminergic agents; nonergot derivatives)**

A. **Amantadine (Symmetrel)**
  1. **Contraindications:** hypersensitivity to amantadine
  2. **Allergic reactions:** rash (R), eczematoid dermatitis (C)
  3. **Adverse drug effects:** nightmares (R), livedo reticularis (C), SIADH (R), myasthenia gravis (R), psychosis (R), hallucinations (C), amnesia (R), peripheral neuropathy (R), dyskinesias (R), myoclonus (R), neutropenia (R), leukopenia (R)

B. **Carbidopa/levodopa (Sinemet)**
  1. **Contraindications:** hypersensitivity to levodopa or carbidopa, narrow-angle glaucoma, MAOIs
  2. **Allergic reactions:** phlebitis (R)
  3. **Adverse drug effects:** depression, delirium, dementia, psychosis, dyskinesia, choreoathetosis, oculogyric crisis,

agranulocytosis, hemolytic anemia, thrombocytopenia, leukopenia, arrhythmias, chest pain, hypertension, palpitations, pseudotumor cerebri, hyperuricemia, SIADH, GI bleed, dysguesia, priapism, alopecia, dyspepsia, blepharospasm, on–off phenomenon

C. Pramipexole (Mirapex)
1. **Contraindications:** hypersensitivity to pramipexole
2. **Allergic reactions:** (U)
3. **Adverse drug effects:** sleep attacks (C), orthostatic hypotension (C), abnormal dreams (C), hallucinations (C), extrapyramidal symptoms (C), edema (C), chest pain (C), hyperesthesia (C), hypertonia (C), tachycardia (C), akathisia (C), dystonias (C), gait abnormalities (C), myoclonus (C), paranoia (C), anorexia (C), weight loss (C), xerostomia (C), impotence (C), arthritis (C), bursitis (C), leg cramps (C), vision changes (C), dyspnea (C), elevated liver function test results (R)
4. **Comments:** Sleep attacks occur more often with pramipexole than with ropinirole.

D. Ropinirole (Requip)
1. **Contraindications:** hypersensitivity to ropinirole.
2. **Allergic reactions:** urticaria (R), photosensitivity (R)
3. **Adverse drug effects:** syncope (C), sleep attacks (C), viral infection (C), dependent edema (C), flushing (C), orthostasis (C), hypertension (C), chest pain (C), palpitations (C), tachycardia (C), hallucinations (C), hypoesthesia (C), amnesia (C), vertigo (C), dyspepsia (C), abdominal pain (C), anorexia (C), urinary tract infection (C), impotence (C), abnormal vision (C), pharyngitis (C), rhinitis (C), diaphoresis (C), dyskinesias (C), neuralgias (C), asthma (R), cardiac arrest (R), cholecystitis (R), extrapyramidal symptoms (EPS) (R), pancreatitis (R), pulmonary edema (R), acute renal failure (R), seizures (R), SIADH (R)
4. **Comments:** Sleep attacks occur more often with pramipexole than with ropinirole.

VII. Antiparkinson agents (dopaminergic agents; ergot derivatives) The use of ergot alkaloids and derivatives has been known to cause fibrotic syndromes (pleural, cardiac, or retroperitoneal fibrosis with respiratory distress) and peripheral vascular complications. Drug holidays do not prevent serious fibrotic reactions. Persons with cardiovascular impairment (e.g., myocardial infarction, arteriosclerosis) should avoid ergot derivatives due to potential for vasoconstriction and thrombus formation.

High doses or prolonged use of ergot alkaloids and derivatives may cause ergotism. Symptoms arise due to vasoconstriction and thrombus formation and include cold skin, severe muscle pain, vascular stasis, dry peripheral gangrene, miosis, peripheral artery insufficiency, paresthesias, and weak pulses.

A. Bromocriptine (Parlodel)
1. **Contraindications:** hypersensitivity to bromocriptine, severe ischemic heart disease, peripheral vascular disorders, pregnancy
2. **Allergic reactions:** edema (R), cutaneous pseudolymphoma (U)
3. **Adverse drug effects:** hypotension (C), Raynaud phenomenon (R), hallucinations (C), anorexia (C), leg cramps

(C), hypertension (R), myocardial infarction (R), seizures (R), syncope (R)

B. Pergolide (Permax)

1. Contraindications: hypersensitivity to pergolide or other ergot derivatives

2. Allergic reactions: rash (C)

3. Adverse drug effects: dystonia (C), hallucinations (C), dyskinesia (C), arrhythmias (R), chest pain (C), myocardial infarction (R), hypertension (C), peripheral edema (C), syncope (C), vasodilation (C), EPS (C), psychosis (C), myalgia (C), diplopia (C), dyspnea (C), epistaxis (R), leukopenia or leukocytosis, thrombocytopenia, megaloblastic anemia (R)

4. Comments: Neuroleptic malignant syndrome may occur with rapid dose decreases.

VIII. Antiparkinson agents (catecholamine *O*-methyl-transferase inhibitors)

A. Entacapone (Comtan)

1. Contraindications: hypersensitivity to entacapone

2. Allergic reactions: purpura (2%) (R)

3. Adverse drug effects: dyskinesia (C), orthostatic hypotension (C), syncope (C), hallucinations (C), hyperpyrexia and confusion (similar to neuroleptic malignant syndrome) (R), pulmonary or retroperitoneal fibrosis (U), rhabdomyolysis (R)

4. Comments: Hepatotoxicity has not yet been demonstrated with entacapone as it has with tolcapone. It may be prudent to check liver function periodically.

B. Tolcapone (Tasmar)

1. Contraindications: hypersensitivity to tolcapone; liver dysfunction; elevated LFTs while taking tolcapone; history of rhabdomyolysis, hyperpyrexia, or confusion possibly related to a medication

2. Allergic reactions: (U)

3. Adverse drug effects: acute, fulminant hepatic failure (R), increased LFTs (C), delayed-onset diarrhea (C), hallucination (C), orthostasis (C), sleep disorders (C), chest pain (C), syncope (C), arthritis (R), hyperkinesia (R), dyspnea (C), hallucinations (C)

4. Comments: Due to the potential for severe liver toxicity, it is recommended to check aspartate aminotransferase (AST) and alanine aminotransferase (ALT) at baseline and then weekly for one year. For the following 6 months AST and ALT should be checked every 4 weeks, then every 6–8 weeks thereafter until discontinuation of therapy. Tolcapone-associated diarrhea will likely occur 6 to 12 weeks after initiation of therapy. Hallucination will commonly occur within the first 2 weeks of treatment and will diminish with a decrease in the dose of levodopa.

IX. Antiparkinson agents (monoamine oxidase type-B inhibitors)

A. Selegiline (Eldepryl)

1. Contraindications: hypersensitivity to selegiline. At doses greater than 10 mg/day there is an increased risk of nonselective MAO inhibition. Typical treatment doses should not have an interaction with tyramine-containing foods/products

   2. Allergic reactions: rash, photosensitivity (R)
   3. Adverse drug effects: angina (R), arrhythmias (R), hypertension (R), orthostatic hypotension (C), palpitations (R), peripheral edema (R), syncope (R), tachycardia (R), mood changes, delusions, hallucinations (C), anorexia, xerostomia, prostatic hypertrophy (R), urinary retention (R), bradykinesia (R), chorea (R), blepharospasm, diaphoresis (R)

X. **Antiparkinson agents (anticholinergics).** Anticholinergics frequently cause side effects such as xerostomia, constipation, urinary retention, and blurred vision. They have also been known to increase ocular pressure, induce hyperpyrexia, and affect the cardiovascular system (hypotension, palpitations, tachycardia, arrhythmias) and the CNS (dizziness, drowsiness, confusion, hallucinations). Medications with anticholinergic properties should be avoided in patients with advanced age, cardiovascular disease, narrow-angle glaucoma, reactive airway disease, obstructive GI/GU disease, and seizure disorders.

  A. Benztropine (Cogentin)
    1. Contraindications: hypersensitivity to any component, narrow-angle glaucoma, pyloric/duodenal obstruction, stenosing peptic ulcers, bladder neck obstructions, achalasia, myasthenia gravis, age less than 3 years
    2. Allergic reactions: rash (R)
    3. Adverse drug effects: diaphoresis (C), increased sensitivity to light (C), ataxia (R), coma (U), hallucination (R), amnesia (R), increased intraocular pain (R)

  B. Trihexyphenidyl (Artane)
    1. Contraindications: hypersensitivity to trihexyphenidyl, narrow-angle glaucoma, pyloric/duodenal obstruction, stenosing peptic ulcers, bladder neck obstructions, achalasia, myasthenia gravis, age less than 3 years
    2. Allergic reactions: rash (R)
    3. Adverse drug effects: diaphoresis (C), increased sensitivity to light (C), ataxia (R), amnesia (R), increased intraocular pain (R)

SELECTED READINGS

Bessmertny O, Hatton RC, Gonzalez-Peralta RP: Antiepileptic hypersensitivity syndrome in children. *Ann Pharmacother* 2001;35:533–8.

Bessmertny O, Pham T. Antiepileptic hypersensitivity syndrome: clinicians beware and be aware. *Current Allergy and Asthma Reports* 2002;2(1):34–39.

Hebert AA, Ralston JP: Cutaneous reactions to anticonvulsant medications. *J Clin Psychiatry* 2001;62(suppl 14):22–6.

Knowles SR, Shapiro LE, Shear NH: Anticonvulsant hypersensitivity syndrome: incidence, prevention, management. *Drug Saf* 1999;17:503–6.

Rzany B, Correia O, Kelly JP, et al: Risk of Steven-Johnson syndrome and toxic epidermal necrolysis during first weeks of antiepileptic therapy: a case-control study. *Lancet* 1999;353:2190–4.

Tennis P, Stern R: Risk of serious cutaneous disorders after initiation of the use of phenytoin, cabamazepine, or sodium valproate: a record linkage study. *Neurology* 1997;49:542–6.

Moore KL, Noble SL. Drug treatment of migraine: Part I. Acute therapy and drug-rebound headache. *Am Fam Phys* 1997 Nov;56(8):2039–48, 2051–4.

Noble SL, Moore KL. Drug treatment of migraine: Part II. Preventative therapy. *Am Fam Phys* 1997 Dec;56(9):2279–86.

Tepper SJ. Safety and rational use of the triptans. *Medical Clinics of North America.* 2001;85(4):959–70.

Management of parkinson's disease: an evidence-based review. *Mov disord.* 2002 Jul:17(S4)

Obstetrics and Gynecology

Howard Wadstrom and Tony Ogburn

There are a limited number of drugs specifically used in obstetrics and gynecology. These have been separated into three categories: obstetrics, gynecology, and reproductive endocrinology and infertility. Antibiotics used for generalized or surgical infectious illnesses are covered in Chapter 1 and 2. Oncology drugs used for obstetric and gynecologic oncology disorders are found in Chapter 15.

I. **Obstetrics**
   A. **Tocolytics**
      1. **Magnesium sulfate**
         a. **Precautions.** Should not be used in conjunction with calcium channel blockers.
         b. **Allergic reactions.** Urticaria (R).
         c. **Adverse drug effects.** Flushing and sweating are common at usual doses (C). Significant reactions are usually due to magnesium toxicity resulting from overdosage and include hypotension, depressed reflexes, flaccid paralysis, hypothermia, circulatory collapse, cardiac depression, and central nervous system depression progressing to respiratory paralysis (U). Hypocalcemia has been reported without signs of tetany (R).

         Treatment for respiratory depression is 1 g calcium gluconate given intravenously over 3 minutes. Response may be short lived and may require respiratory support and/or dialysis.
      2. **β-Mimetics: terbutaline sulfate (Brethine), ritadrine (Yutopar)**
         a. **Precautions.** Avoid in patients with significant cardiovascular disease. May cause significant rise in blood glucose in diabetics with rare hyperglycemic ketoacidosis.
         b. **Allergic reactions.** Rash with prolonged use. Anaphylaxis reported (R).
         c. **Adverse drug effects.** Tremor, nervousness, palpitations, and tachycardia are common (C). Minor reactions such as dizziness, headache, drowsiness, dyspnea, chest discomfort, nausea, vomiting, weakness, sweating, and flushing have been reported (U). Pulmonary edema is most common major adverse reaction and is associated with concomitant fluid overload and/or steroid use (R). Cardiac arrhythmias, myocardial ischemia, liver dysfunction, and neutropenia reported (R).
      3. **Prostaglandin inhibitors: indomethacin (Indocin)**
         a. **Precautions.** Avoid in patients with gastrointestinal conditions such as peptic ulcer disease or gastroesophageal reflux disease. Contraindicated in patients allergic to aspirin or other nonsteroidal anti-inflammatory agents.
         b. **Allergic reactions.** Similar to aspirin.

c. **Adverse drug effects.** Associated with premature closure of the ductus arteriosis and oligohydramnios (U).
4. **Calcium channel blockers: nifedipine (Procardia)**
   a. **Precautions.** Avoid using in combination with $MgSO_4$.
   b. **Allergic reactions** (U).
   c. **Adverse drug effects.** Mild edema, headache (U). Significant hypotension may occur if used in conjunction with $MgSO_4$ (U).
B. **Oxytocic agents**
1. **Oxytocin** (Pitocin, Syntocinon)
   a. **Precautions.** Avoid antepartum use in patients with nonreassuring fetal surveillance or previous classical caesarean section.
   b. **Allergic reactions.** Anaphylaxis—extremely rare—few cases presented in literature (R).
   c. **Adverse drug effects.** Uterine hyperstimulation resulting in fetal compromise (U). Water intoxication with prolonged use (R). Cardiac arrhythmias, fatal afibrinogenemia reported (R).
2. **Methylergonovine (Methergine)**
   a. **Precautions.** Avoid in patients with hypertension (preeclampsia or essential).
   b. **Allergic reactions.** No major reactions reported.
   c. **Adverse drug effects.** Minor reactions include transient hypertension, headache, dizziness, nausea, vomiting, and uterine cramping (C). Rare reactions include myocardial infarction, seizure, transient chest pain, dyspnea, hematuria, thrombophlebitis, leg cramps, tinnitus, nasal congestion, diarrhea, palpitation, foul taste, and diaphoresis (R).
3. **Prostaglandins.** Carboprost (Hemabate), misoprostol (Cytotec)
   a. **Precautions.** Avoid in patients with significant reactive airway disease.
   b. **Allergic reactions** (U).
   c. **Adverse drug effects.** Minor reactions include transient fever, nausea/vomiting, diarrhea, uterine cramping, flushing, and sweating (C). Major reactions included severe bronchospasm, uterine rupture, and pulmonary edema (R).
C. **Ripening agents**
1. **Dinoprostone** (Cervidil, Prepidil, prostaglandin E_2), misoprostol (Cytotec)
   a. **Precautions.** Use with caution in patients with nonreassuring fetal surveillance. Avoid in patients with previous uterine surgery or significant reactive airway disease. May potentiate the action of oxytocin.
   b. **Allergic reactions** (U).
   c. **Adverse drug effects.** Minor reactions include nausea, fever, diarrhea and abdominal cramping (C). Significant reactions include uterine hyperstimulation resulting in fetal distress, and uterine rupture, especially in the previously scarred uterus (U). Tocolytic agents can be used to counteract hyperstimulation.

II. Gynecology
  A. **Contraceptives**
    1. **Oral contraceptive pills**
      a. **Progesterone-only pills**
        (1) **Precautions.** Should not be used in patients with undiagnosed genital bleeding. Not as effective as combination pills.
        (2) **Allergic reactions.** No significant reactions have been reported (U).
        (3) **Adverse drug effects.** Breakthrough bleeding is common (C). Weight gain, acne, and nervousness may occur (U). Significant reactions have not been reported.
      b. **Combination pills** (estrogen and progesterone containing)
        (1) **Precautions.** Avoid in patients with history of thromboembolic disease, significant vascular disease, uncontrolled hypertension, active liver disease, and smokers over age 35. Use caution in patients with functional heart disease as fluid retention may result in heart failure. May mask symptoms of a prolactin-secreting tumor. Contraceptive efficacy may be reduced in patients on certain medications, including rifampin and anticonvulsants. Concerns have been raised about decreased efficacy with common antibiotics though clinical studies have not demonstrated this effect.
        (2) **Allergic reactions.** Rash reported relatively frequently (U). Case reports of photosensitivity reactions, erythema nodosa, herpes gestationis, and urticaria (R). No severe allergic reactions have been reported.
        (3) **Adverse drug effects.** Common minor reactions include breakthrough bleeding, nausea/vomiting, breast tenderness and minimal weight gain secondary to fluid retention, particularly during the first few months of use (C). Melasma may occur and may take a long time to resolve after discontinuation of pills (U). May worsen symptoms in patients with migraines (U). Causes transient decrease in milk production in lactating women but impact on breast-feeding continuation is unclear. The most common major reaction is an approximate fourfold increase in the incidence of venous thromboembolic events (relative to a sixfold increase with pregnancy) (R). The risk of myocardial infarction is increased in smokers, especially over age 35 (U).
    2. **Injectables**
      a. **Depo-Provera (medroxyprogesterone acetate injection)**
        (1) **Precautions.** Should be avoided in patients with undiagnosed abnormal genital bleeding. May exacerbate depressive illness.
        (2) **Allergic reactions.** Minor reactions including rash and urticaria have been reported (U). Case reports of anaphylaxis, possibly due to polyethylene glycol, a solubilizing agent in the drug (R).
        (3) **Adverse drug effects.** Irregular bleeding is common, especially in the first 6 to 12 months (C).

Amenorrhea occurs in many long-term users (C). Weight gain of 1 to 4 kg per year of usage has been reported as well as alopecia, mood changes, and headache (U). Return to fertility may take a year or longer after the last injection. Decrease in bone density has been reported with return to baseline after discontinuation. May decrease milk production in lactating mothers although effect on breast-feeding continuation is unclear.

b. Lunelle (medroxyprogesterone acetate and estradiol cypionate)

(1) Precautions. (Same as combination pills) Avoid in patients with history of thromboembolic disease, significant vascular disease, uncontrolled hypertension, active liver disease, and smokers over age 35. Use with caution in patients with functional heart disease as fluid retention may result in heart failure. May mask symptoms of a prolactin-secreting tumor. Contraceptive efficacy may be reduced in patients on certain medications, including rifampin and anticonvulsants.

(2) Allergic reactions. Local skin reactions have been reported (U). Serious allergic reactions such as anaphylaxis have been reported with the individual components of Lunelle but not with Lunelle itself (R).

(3) Adverse drug effects. Initial studies indicate there may an increase in gallbladder disease (U). Alteration of menses is common, especially in the first few months of use (C). Local injection site irritation (U). May have similar reactions to combination pills but more data are needed.

3. Seminal fluid

a. Allergic reactions. Human seminal hypersensitivity described with local burning and redness as well as systemic reactions, including hives, angioedema, and wheezing (U). Anaphylaxis reported (R). May cause severe allergic reactions if whole semen is used for intrauterine insemination (U).

b. Adverse drug effects. Burning semen syndrome described in some Gulf War veterans with partners complaining of local burning and irritation.

4. Spermicides. Nonoxynol-9, octoxynol-9, benzalkonium chloride, menfegol

a. Allergic reactions. Minor local allergic reactions occur either to the vehicle or to the agent itself (R). No severe or systemic reactions reported.

b. Adverse drug effects. Alters vaginal flora and may result in higher incidence of urinary tract infections (R). Protects against sexually transmitted diseases to some degree. May cause local inflammation and irritation of vaginal mucosa (R).

5. Intrauterine devices (IUDs). Paragard (copper containing), Mirena (progestin containing).

a. Precautions. Should be avoided in patients with acute pelvic infection, undiagnosed genital bleeding, or documented allergy to copper (Paragard).

b.   Allergic reactions. Multiple reports of rash and other allergic-type reactions, including interstitial nephritis with copper-containing IUDs (R). However, in studies where patients had follow-up testing allergy to copper usually was not confirmed. Reactions may be due to allergy to other metals present in trace amounts in the Paragard, such as nickel. If reaction felt to be possibly related to IUD, then IUD should be removed.

c.   Adverse drug effects. Alteration in menstrual flow (C). Typically, increased flow with copper-containing devices and irregular flow with progestin-containing devices. May cause dysmenorrhea. Symptoms typically improve with duration of IUD use. Pregnancy occurring with IUD in place may result in higher incidence of ectopic pregnancy, spontaneous or septic abortion (R).

6.   Implantable devices. Progesterone containing (Norplant). No longer marketed in the United States.

a.   Precautions. Should not be used in patients with undiagnosed genital bleeding. May exacerbate mood disorders. Patients must have access to health care for removal.

b.   Allergic reactions. Several reports of postinsertion "collapse" (R). Likely due to reaction to xylocaine as opposed to Norplant device.

c.   Adverse drug effects. Irregular bleeding, amenorrhea, alopecia, mood alteration, breast tenderness, acne, insertion site infection, and weight gain (C/U).

B.   Estrogens

1.   Oral preparations

a.   Conjugated equine estrogens (Premarin)

(1)   **Precautions.** Should not be used in patients with undiagnosed genital bleeding, breast cancer, coronary artery disease, stroke, or thromboembolic disease.

(2)   **Allergic reactions.** Multiple reports of minor reactions such as rash and pruritus (R). Major reactions, such as anaphylaxis, have been rarely reported with oral and parenteral preparations (R). With pills likely due to dye in pills, not estrogen.

(3)   **Adverse drug effects.** Minor reactions include abnormal bleeding, bloating, and breast tenderness (C). Increases incidence of endometrial hyperplasia without concomitant progestin use (R). Recent studies indicate increased risk of breast cancer and myocardial infarction (R).

b.   Others including estradiol, estropipate, esterified estrogens

(1)   **Precautions.** Assumed to be same as Premarin; much less information to confirm.

(2)   **Allergic reactions.** Several reports of minor reactions with previous sensitization to transdermal estradiol (R). Reports of systemic dermatitis (R).

(3)   **Adverse drug effects.** Assumed to be same as Premarin; much less information to confirm.

c.   Estratest. Esterified estrogen and methyltestosterone. Same as estrogens "plus."

(1) **Precautions.** Use with caution in patients with significant liver disease.

(2) **Allergic reactions.** Minor reactions such as rash are reported (U). No major reactions reported.

(3) **Adverse drug effects.** Cholestatic jaundice, fluid retention (R). May cause virilization in high doses (R).

2. **Transdermal preparations**

a. **Allergic reactions.** In estradiol-containing preparations local skin rash has been reported, which may be an irritant as opposed to a type 4 immune-mediated reaction (C). Systemic contact dermatitis reported (R).

3. **Topical preparations** (vaginal creams)

a. **Precautions.** All are absorbed to some degree; thus, same precautions as with oral preparations.

b. **Allergic reactions.** Local skin rashes reported (R). No severe reactions reported.

c. **Adverse drug effects.** Same as systemic preparations. In addition, may cause local discomfort with application. May weaken condoms and result in decreased contraceptive efficacy.

4. **Estring**

a. **Precautions.** Minimal systemic absorption so can be used in patients with contraindications to other types of estrogen.

b. **Allergic reactions.** None reported (U).

c. **Adverse reactions.** Vaginal discomfort with insertion (R).

C. **Progestins**

1. **Oral preparations.** Medroxyprogesterone acetate (Provera), norethindrone, micronized progesterone (Prometrium)

a. **Precautions.** Should be avoided in patients with undiagnosed abnormal genital bleeding.

b. **Allergic reactions.** Case reports of reactions including anaphylaxis with oral agents as well as endogenous progesterone (R). Can be controlled with gonadotropin-releasing hormone agonists or cured with oophorectomy.

c. **Adverse drug effects.** Alteration in menstrual pattern, bloating, breast tenderness, water retention and acne (R).

2. **Progesterone gel** (Crinone)

a. **Precautions.** Should be avoided in patients with undiagnosed abnormal genital bleeding.

b. **Allergic reactions.** Minor reactions, such as rash and pruritus, have been reported (R). No major allergic reactions reported.

c. **Adverse drug effects.** Nausea, bloating, breast tenderness, acne, and water retention (R). No major adverse reactions reported.

D. **Aci-jel vaginal cream** (acetic acid/hydroxyquinoline/ ricinoleic acid)

1. **Precautions.** None reported.

2. **Allergic reactions.** Local reactions have been reported to propylhydroxybenzoate, a preservative in Aci-jel (R).

3. Adverse drug effects. May increase incidence of some types of vaginitis in some patients (R). Local irritation may occur (R).

E. Other vaginal creams (AminoCerv, Trimo-San)
  1. Precautions. None.
  2. Allergic reactions. None reported (U).
  3. Adverse drug effects. May cause local irritation (R).

F. Antifungal vaginal creams/ointments (including miconazole, terconazole, clotrimazole, butoconazole)
  1. Precautions. None.
  2. Allergic reactions: Contact dermatitis infrequently (R). No major reactions reported.
  3. Adverse drug effects: Local discomfort with insertion (R).

G. Imiquimod (Aldara)
  1. Precautions. Should be avoided in tissue that is acutely inflamed or recently operated on until completely healed.
  2. Allergic reactions. Contact dermatitis reported (U). No major reactions reported.
  3. Adverse drug effects. Local erythema, flaking and edema, excoriation, and erosion are common (C). Serious skin irritation can occur and treatment should cease until the area has healed (R). Systemic reactions are rare and include headache, flu-like symptoms, and myalgias (R). Distant skin irritation has been reported (R).

H. Metronidazole vaginal cream (Metrogel)
  1. Precautions. Theoretically same as oral preparations though absorption is minimal.
  2. Allergic reactions. Major allergic reactions have been reported with oral metronidazole but not vaginal preparations. Eczema-type reactions and wheal formation have been reported (R). Hypersensitivity reactions to paraben contained in the gel have been reported rarely (R). Sensitization may occur with vaginal preparations with severe reactions when oral preparations are taken (R).
  3. Adverse drug effects. Local skin irritation is uncommon (R).

I. Clindamycin vaginal cream (Cleocin)
  1. Precautions. May weaken condoms, diaphragms, and cervical caps, thus reducing contraceptive efficacy.
  2. Allergic reactions. Major allergic reactions have not been reported with vaginal preparations but should not be used in patients with a history of allergic reaction to oral or parenteral preparation (U).
  3. Adverse drug effects. Local skin irritation is uncommon (R).

J. Urinary tract medications
  1. Oxybutinin (Ditropan), **tolterodine** (Detrol)
    a. Precautions. Should not be used in patients with glaucoma, urinary retention, myasthenia gravis, or significant gastrointestinal disorders (e.g., bowel obstruction, ulcerative colitis, and severe constipation).
    b. Allergic reactions. Minor reactions such as rash have been reported (R). Anaphylaxis has been reported rarely (R).

    c. **Adverse drug effects.** Dry mouth is very common (C). Constipation, dry eyes, blurred vision, and drowsiness are common (C). Rare reports of heat prostration especially in older patients in hot climates (R).

  2. **Pentosan** (Elmiron)

    a. **Precautions.** Acts as an anticoagulant so caution should be exercised in patients at risk for bleeding or undergoing procedures.

    b. **Allergic reactions.** Minor rashes and pruritus (R). Case reports of delayed immunoallergenic thrombocytopenia with similar compounds (R).

    c. **Adverse drug effects.** Minor reactions such as nausea, dizziness, diarrhea, and headache (R). Alopecia has been reported (R).

K. Mifepristone (RU-486)

  1. **Precautions.** Should not be used to terminate advanced pregnancy. Intrauterine pregnancy should be confirmed as not effective treatment for ectopic pregnancy. Patients must have access to appropriate follow-up.

  2. **Allergic reactions.** No major reactions reported (U).

  3. **Adverse drug effects.** Bleeding and cramping are expected though bleeding requiring transfusion is rare (R). Common reactions include abdominal pain, nausea, vomiting, and diarrhea (C). Fainting, headache, and dizziness are rare (R).

L. Topical agents for human papillovirus (HPV): podophyllin resin, podophilox lotion

  1. **Allergic reactions.** Contact dermatitis reported.(R) No major allergic reactions reported.

  2. **Adverse drug effects.** Local inflammatory dermatitis with burning, pain, erosion, and pruritus is common (C). Systemic effects have been reported rarely with application to large areas for prolonged time periods and include paresthesia, polyneuritis, leukopenia, thrombocytopenia, and death (R).

M. Selective estrogen receptor modulators (SERMS)

  1. **Raloxiphene** (Evista)

    a. **Precautions.** Avoid in patients with history or current thromboembolic disease or who are immobilized. Should not be used in premenopausal women, as safety has not been assessed.

    b. **Allergic reactions.** Major reactions have not been reported (U).

    c. **Adverse drug effects.** Leg cramps and hot flashes occur in approximately 5% more patients relative to placebo and improve usually within 6 months (C). Fourfold increase in venous thromboembolic events (R).

  2. **Tamoxifen.** See Chapter 15.

III. Reproductive endocrinology and infertility

A. Gonadotropins. Human menopausal gonadotropins (Pergonal, Humegon), follicle-stimulating hormone (Metrodin, Puregon, Gonal-F, Follistim), human chorionic gonadotropin (Pregnyl, Profasi)

  1. **Precautions.** Must monitor serum estradiol levels and follicle development prior to administration to minimize

hyperstimulation syndrome. Patients with polycystic ovaries may be more sensitive to these agents.

2. Allergic reactions. Case reports of significant systemic reactions most likely due to contaminants in urine derived products (R). Less common with recombinant products.

3. Adverse drug effects. Local skin reactions, fever, generalized edema, flulike symptoms, photophobia reported (U). Multiple gestations are common (C). The risk of ectopic pregnancy is increased (R). Ovarian hyperstimulation syndrome reported (R) and can be life threatening (R).

B. Clomiphene citrate (Clomid)

1. Precautions. Patients should be warned of possible visual changes, which may affect their ability to perform usual activities, including driving.

2. Allergic reactions. A case report of a neutrophilic drug reaction with petechiae and palpable purpura (R).

3. Adverse drug effects. Minor reactions including nausea, breast engorgement, headache, abdominal bloating, visual changes, and hot flashes (C). Functional ovarian cyst formation may occur and usually resolves spontaneously (R). Multiple gestations, usually twins, are common (C). Hyperstimulation syndrome can occur but is rare (R).

C. Danazol (Danocrine)

1. Precautions. Should not be used during pregnancy or in patients with undiagnosed genital bleeding.

2. Allergic reactions. Diffuse maculopapular rash, urticaria, pruritus, and, rarely, nasal congestion have been reported (U).

3. Adverse drug effects. Androgen-like effects, including fluid retention, weight gain, acne, and seborrhea, are common (C). Hirsutism, edema, hair loss, and voice changes may occur (R). Thrombotic events such as sagittal sinus thrombosis and fatal stroke have been associated with use (R). Several reports of intracranial hypertension (pseudotumor cerebri), peliosis hepatis, and benign hepatic adenoma with long-term use (R).

D. Bromocriptine- See Chapter 13, section on dopamine agonists.

E. Gonadotropin-releasing hormone agonists: leuprolide (Lupron Injection) and **nafarelin sulfate** (Synarel Nasal Spray).

1. Precautions. Avoid in pregnancy and breast-feeding patients. Do not use in patients with undiagnosed vaginal bleeding.

2. Allergic reactions. Case reports of anaphylaxis. Reports of hypersensitivity to benzyl alcohol, an ingredient of the drug's vehicle (R).

3. Adverse drug effects. May cause formation of ovarian cysts in first 1 to 2 months of treatment (R). Side effects related to estrogen deprivation are to be expected, including hot flashes and vaginal dryness (C). Osteopenia or osteoporosis in long-term use (>6 months) (C).

SELECTED READINGS

Cunningham FG, Gant NF, Leveno KJ, et al., eds. *Williams' Obstetrics,* 21st ed. New York: McGraw-Hill, 2001.

Speroff L, Glass RH, Kase NG, eds. *Clinical gynecologic endocrinology and infertility,* 6th ed. Philadelphia: Lippincott Williams & Wilkins, 1999.

Stenchever MA, Droegemueller W, Herbst AL, et al., eds. *Comprehensive gynecology,* 4th ed. St. Louis: Mosby, 2001.

Ophthalmology

Daniel E. Hutter and Bill K. Nika

I. **Topical Anti-infectives**
   A. **Chloramphenicol**
      1. **Allergic reactions (U)**
      2. **Adverse drug effects.** Bone marrow hypoplasia with long-term use (R).
   B. **Aminoglycosides (gentamicin and tobramycin)**
      1. **Allergic reactions (U)**
      2. **Adverse drug effects.** Ocular toxicity, especially punctate keratopathy after prolonged use (R).
   C. **Neomycin**
      1. **Allergic reactions.** Contact sensitivity with punctate keratitis, conjunctivitis, burning, erythema, rash, and urticaria (C).
   D. **Trifluridine**
      1. **Allergic reactions (U)**
      2. **Adverse drug effects.** Ocular toxicity, especially punctate keratopathy after prolonged use (>21 days) (C).
   E. **Sulfacetamide**
      1. **Allergic reactions.** Hypersensitivity reactions including Stevens–Johnson syndrome, bone marrow suppression, toxic epidermal necrolysis, and fulminant hepatic necrosis (R).
      2. **Adverse drug effects (U).**
   F. **Fluoroquinolones** (ciprofloxacin, ofloxacin, levofloxacin)
      1. **Allergic reactions.** Stevens–Johnson syndrome reported in one patient who was using ofloxacin (R).
      2. **Adverse drug effects.** Crystalline precipitates in the cornea with ciprofloxacin (C).
II. **Topical anesthetics**
   A. **Proparacaine and tetracaine**
      1. **Allergic reactions (U)**
      2. **Adverse drug effects.** Corneal epithelial erosions and delayed healing with prolonged use (C).
III. **Topical anti-inflammatories**
   A. **Corticosteroids** (prednisolone, dexamethasone, fluorometholone, rimexolone, loteprednol etabonate)
      1. **Contraindications.** Keratitis in eyes with herpes simplex or fungal infections can worsen.
      2. **Allergic reactions (U)**
      3. **Adverse drug effects**
         a. Increased intraocular pressure (less risk with loteprednol etabonate) (C).
         b. Posterior subcapsular cataracts (C)
         c. Increased risk for infections (C)
         d. Decreased corneal wound healing (C)
   B. **Nonsteroidal anti-inflammatory drugs** (flurbiprofen, ketorolac, diclofenac)

    1. Contraindications
      a. Potential cross sensitivity with aspirin
      b. Potential for increased bleeding time
    2. Allergic reactions (U)
    3. Adverse drug effects
      a. May slow corneal wound healing (C)
      b. May be associated with corneal thinning and perforation with prolonged use of diclofenac (R).

IV. Topical glaucoma drugs

  A. Carbonic anhydrase inhibitors (dorzolamide, brinzolamide)
    1. Contraindications
      a. Sulfa allergy
      b. Severe renal and hepatic impairment
    2. Allergic reactions
      a. All allergic reactions due to sulfonamides are possible (R). See Chapter 2

  B. α_2-Adrenergic agonists (brimonidine, apraclonidine)
    1. Contraindications
      a. Concurrent monoamine oxidase inhibitor use.
      b. Children due to reports of apnea and bradycardia.
    2. Allergic reactions: (U)
    3. Adverse drug effects
      a. Hyperemia, burning and stinging, pruritus (C)
      b. Dry mouth (C)

  C. β-Adrenergic blockers (timolol, betaxolol, carteolol, levobunolol, metipranolol)
    1. Contraindications
      a. Asthma and chronic obstructive pulmonary disease (less risk of exacerbations with betaxolol due to its β_1 cardioselective activity)
      b. Sinus bradycardia, second- and third-degree heart block
      c. Cardiac failure and cardiogenic shock
    2. Allergic reactions (U)

  D. Prostaglandins (latanoprost, travoprost, bimatoprost, unoprostone)
    1. Allergic reactions (U)
    2. Adverse drug effects
      a. Increased pigmentation of the iris and eyelid (C)
      b. Increased pigmentation and growth of eyelashes (C)
      c. Intraocular inflammation (R)

  E. Pilocarpine
    1. Contraindications
      a. Iritis
      b. Angle-closure glaucoma due to pupillary block
    2. Allergic reactions (U)

V. Topical mydriatics and cycloplegics

  A. Mydriatics (phenylephrine)
    1. Contraindications
      a. Narrow occludable angles at risk for angle-closure glaucoma.
      b. Significant cardiovascular disease.
    2. Allergic reactions: (U)

   3. **Adverse drug effects**
      a. Elevation of blood pressure (R)
B. Cycloplegics (atropine, homatropine, scopolamine, cyclopentolate, tropicamide).
   1. **Contraindications.** Narrow occludable angles at risk for angle-closure glaucoma
   2. **Allergic reactions (U)**
   3. **Adverse drug effects.** All side effects from anticholinergic drugs are possible (C)
VI. **Topical antiallergy drugs**
   A. **Topical vasconstrictors** (naphazoline, oxymetazoline, tetrahydrozoline)
      1. **Contraindications.** Narrow occludable angles at risk for angle-closure glaucoma
      2. **Allergic reactions (U)**
      3. **Adverse drug effects.** Rebound congestion with prolonged use (C)
   B. **Topical antihistamines (levocabastine, olapatadine)**
      1. **Allergic reactions (U)**
VII. **Topical drug inactive ingredients**
   A. **Preservatives** (benzalkonium chloride)
      1. **Allergic reactions (R)**
      2. **Adverse reactions.** Can cause diffuse punctate keratopathy with prolonged use (U).

SELECTED READINGS

Albert D, Jakobiec F, eds. *Principles and practice of ophthalmology,* 2nd ed. Philadelphia: WB Saunders, 2000.

American Hospital Formulary Service. *Drug information 2001.* Bethesda: American Society of Health-System Pharmacists, 2000.

Lacy CL, Armstrong LL, Goldman MP, et al. *Drug information handbook 2001–2002.* Hudson, OH: Lexi-Comp, 2000.

Ophthalmic drug facts. St. Louis: Facts and Comparisons, 2000.

Physicians' desk reference for ophthalmic medicines, 30th ed. Montvale, NJ: Medical Economics, 2002.

19

Psychiatry

Howard C. Margolese and Emmanuelle Lévy

I. Antidepressants
A. Tricyclic antidepressants
   1. Imipramine (Tofranil), desipramine (Norpramin, Pertofrane), nortriptyline (Pamelor, Aventyl), amitriptyline (Elavil, Endep), and others.
   a. Contraindications. Monoamine oxidase inhibitor (MAOI) use within 14 days, glaucoma, acute myocardial infarction (MI).
   b. Allergic reactions (U).
   c. Adverse drug effects. Anticholinergic side effects (C), seizures (R), MI (R), stroke (U), agranulocytosis (R), thrombocytopenia (R).
B. Monoamine oxidase inhibitors (MAOI)
   1. Tranylcypromine (Parnate), phenelzine (Nardil), moclobemide (Aurorix, Manerix).
   a. Contraindications. Congestive heart failure (CHF), hypertension, pheochromocytoma, liver failure, general anesthesia or cocaine use within 10 days, selective serotonin reuptake inhibitors (SSRI) or tricyclic antidepressant within 14 days, bupropion use.
   b. Allergic reactions (U).
   c. Adverse drug effects. Hypertensive crisis (avoid tyramine-rich foods) (C), hypermetabolic syndrome (R), leukopenia (C), seizures (R), anticholinergic side effects (C).
C. Selective serotonin reuptake inhibitors (SSRI)
   1. Fluoxetine (Prozac), fluvoxamine (Luvox), paroxetine (Paxil), citalopram (Celexa), escitalopram (Lexapro), sertraline (Zoloft).
   a. Contraindications. MAOI within 14 days, thioridazine use (Paxil), cisapride astemizole or terfenadine use (Luvox). *Caution:* Impaired liver function, medications with narrow therapeutic index metabolized by the CYP450 system.
   b. Allergic reactions. Rash (R), pruritus (R), urticaria (R), vasculitis (U), toxic epidermal necrolysis (U).
   c. Adverse drug effects. Serotonin syndrome (Table 19.1) (R), SSRI withdrawal syndrome (C), syndrome of inappropriate secretion of antidiuretic hormone (SIADH) (R), hyponatremia (Paxil, Celexa) (R), bleeding (R), extrapyramidal symptoms (Paxil) (R), bradycardia (R), hepatoxicity (Luvox) (U), nausea and other gastrointestinal (GI) symptoms (C), tremor (C), sexual dysfunction (C).
D. Serotonin norepinephrine reuptake inhibitors (SNRIs)

Table 19.1.   Serotonin syndrome versus neuroleptic malignant syndrome

Feature	SS	NMS
Serotonin syndrome		
Serotonimimetic drug	+++	0
Rapid onset	+++	0
Mental state changes—agitation[a]	+	Akathisia
Mental state changes—hyperactivity	+++	0
Clonus/myoclonus	+++	0
Ocular oscillations	+++	0
Shivering	+++	0
Tremor	+++	+
Hyperreflexia	+++	0
Neuroleptic malignant syndrome		
Antipsychotic (neuroleptic)	0	++
Slow onset	0	++
Bradykinesia/stupor	0	+++
Leaden rigidity	0	+++
Autonomic instability	+[b]	++
Nonspecific		
Confusion	++	+++[c]
Hyperpyrexia	++	++
Diaphoresis	++	+++
Tachypnea	++	+++
Tachycardia	++	+++
Hypertension	++	++
Raised creatinine phosphokinase	+	+++

[a]Distinguishing between akathisia and agitation may be difficult.
[b]Autonomic instability may only occur in severe cases.
[c]Confusion probably more severe in NMS.
SS, serotonin syndrome; NMS, neuroleptic malignant syndrome.
Adapted from Gillman PK. The serotonin syndrome and its treatment. *J Psychopharmacol* 1999;13:100–109, with permission.

    1. Venlafaxine (Effexor), duloxetine
      a. Contraindications. MAOI within 14 days, impaired liver or renal function (caution).
      b. Allergic reactions. Rash (R).
      c. Adverse drug effects. Serotonin syndrome (Table 19.1) (R), seizures (R), hypertension (C), sweating (C), anticholinergic side effects (R), sexual dysfunction (C).
  E. Norepinephrine dopamine reuptake inhibitors (NDRIs)
    1. Bupropion (Wellbutrin, Zyban)
      a. Contraindications. Seizure disorder, bulimia or anorexia nervosa (current or past), MAOI within 14 days.
      b. Allergic reactions. Stevens–Johnson syndrome (U), rash (R).
      c. Adverse drug effects. Seizures (R at dose <450 mg/day; C at doses >600 mg/day), arrhythmia (R), third-degree atrioventricular block (R), rhabdomyolysis (R), headache (C), tremor (C), insomnia (C), sweating (C), weight loss (C).

F. Norepinephrine and selective serotonin (NaSSa)
1. Mirtazapine (Remeron)
   a. Contraindications. MAOI within 14 days. *Caution:* cardiovascular/cerebrovascular disease, impaired liver/renal function, seizures, dehydration, hypotension.
   b. Allergic reactions. Agranulocytosis (R).
   c. Adverse drug effects. Torsade de pointes (R), orthostatic hypotension (R), somnolence (C), increased appetite (C), weight gain (C), hypercholesterolemia, hypertriglyceridemia (U), elevated liver transaminases (U), myalgia (R), tremor (C).

G. Serotonin antagonist and reuptake inhibitor (SARI)
1. Nefazodone (Serzone)
   a. Contraindications. Hepatic disease, elevated liver transaminases, cisapride use, MAOI within 14 days, caution with drugs metabolized by CYP450 3A4.
   b. Allergic reactions (U).
   c. Adverse drug effects. Liver failure (R), hepatoxicity (R), seizures (R), priapism (R), headache (C), dry mouth (C), GI side effects (C), blurred vision (C), infection (R), somnolence (C), paresthesias (U).
2. Trazodone (Desyrel)
   a. Contraindications. MAOI within 14 days, acute MI, pregnancy. *Caution:* CNS depressants, antihypertensives, receiving electroconvulsive therapy, arrhythmias.
   b. Allergic reactions (U).
   c. Adverse drug effects. Hypotension (R), syncope (R), priapism (R), dizziness (C), sedation (C), dry mouth (C), headache (C), GI and sexual side effects (C).

H. Norepinephrine reuptake inhibitor (NRI).
1. Reboxetine (Edronax, Vestra, Norebox, Prolift, Vestra)
   a. Contraindications. MAOI within 14 days, pregnancy. *Caution:* tachycardia; with medications inhibiting CYP450 3A4.
   b. Allergic reactions (U).
   c. Adverse drug effects. Tachycardia (C), urinary hesitancy/retention (C), impotence (U), constipation (C), dry mouth (C), insomnia (C), increased sweating (C), vertigo (U).

II. Antipsychotics (neuroleptics)
A. Typical antipsychotics: low potency
1. **Phenothiazines: aliphatic.** Chlorpromazine (Thorazine, Largactil), triflupromazine (Vesprin), promazine (Sparine) and **Piperidine:** thioridazine (Mellaril), mesoridazine (Serentil).
   a. Contraindications. Severe hypotension, hepatic dysfunction, bone marrow depression, hypersensitivity to drug/class, seizure disorder.
   b. Allergic reactions. Photosensitivity and allergic dermatitis (C), agranulocytosis (U).
   c. Adverse drug effects
      (1) **Anticholinergic.** Blurred vision, constipation, urinary retention, drowsiness, mydriasis (C).
      (2) **Cardiovascular.** Prolonged QT and PR intervals, blunted T waves, depressed ST segment (R), orthostatic

hypotension (C), reflex tachycardia (C), malignant arrhythmias (D), torsade de pointes–sudden death (R).

(3) Endocrine and sexual. Breast enlargement, galactorrhea, decreased libido, erectile and ejaculatory disturbances, impotence, priapism, anorgasmia, amenorrhea, increased appetite, weight gain (C).

(4) Gastrointestinal. Cholestatic jaundice (reversible if RX d/c) (U).

(5) Hematologic. Transient leukopenia (U).

(6) Ophthalmologic. Lenticular pigmentation, retinitis pigmentation (C).

(7) Dermatologic. Photosensitivity reaction and blue–gray skin discoloration (sunlight) (U).

(8) Neurologic. Sedation (C), seizures (U), tardive dyskinesia (TD) (C), acute (R) or tardive dystonia (C), parkinsonism (C), acute or tardive akathisia (C), neuroleptic malignant syndrome (NMS) (Table 19.1) (R).

B. **Typical antipsychotics: high potency**

   1. Thioxanthenes: zuclopenthixol, flupenthixol, thiothixene (Navane).

   2. Butyrophenone: haloperidol (Haldol), droperidol (Inapsine).

   3. Diphenylbutylpiperidine: pimozide (Orap), fluspirilene (Imap).

   4. Phenothiazine-piperazine: trifluoperazine (Stelazine), fluphenazine (Prolixin, Permitil, Moditen).

   a. **Contraindications.** Same as for low potency.

   b. **Allergic reactions.** Same as for low potency but photosensitivity and anticholinergic effects less common.

   c. **Adverse drug effects.** Same as for low potency but parkinsonism, akathisia, and acute dystonia more common; SIADH (especially with depot haloperidol) (C).

C. **Atypical antipsychotics**

   1. Benzisoxazole: risperidone (Risperidal)

   a. **Precautions (same for all atypicals)**

   (1) Decreased vigilance and sedation: avoid driving or using heavy machinery.

   (2) Orthostatic hypotension and tachycardia, particularly in elderly.

   (3) *Caution:* hypotension, diabetes mellitus, MI; if on antihypertensives, increased risk of hypotension and syncope.

   b. **Allergic reactions** (U).

   c. **Adverse drug effects.** Sedation (C), dizziness (C), somnolence (C), weight gain, (C); insomnia (U), agitation (U), anxiety (U), nausea (U), anticholinergic effects (U), headache (C), NMS (Table 19.1) (R), seizures (R), prolactin elevation (U), sexual side effects (U), tachycardia and postural hypotension (C), extrapyramidal symptoms (C, if >6 mg/day dosage), akathisia (C), TD (U), rhinitis (C).

   2. Thienobenzodiazepine: olanzapine (Zyprexa)

   a. **Precautions.** See "Risperidone." Also caution if hepatic disorders.

   b. **Allergic reactions.** Transient eosinophilia (U).

   c. **Adverse drug effects.** Sedation (C), weight gain (C),

anticholinergic: dry mouth, constipation (C), extrapyramidal symptoms (U), TD (R), akathisia (U), prolactin elevation (U), transient prolactin elevation (C), sexual dysfunction (U), transient transaminase elevation (U), orthostatic hypotension (U), dizziness (U); headache (C), rhinitis (C), NMS (Table 19.1) (R), seizures (R).

3. Dibenzodiazepine. Clozapine (Clozaril)

   a. **Contraindications.** If WBC < 3,500, history of bone marrow disorder, history of clozapine-induced agranulocytosis.

   b. **Precautions.** Cardiac disease, seizure disorder, or history or risk of diabetes.

   c. **Allergic reactions.** Agranulocytosis (U), fever (R).

   d. **Adverse drug effects.** Transient temperature elevation (first 3 weeks) (C); eosinophilia (U), neutropenia (U), leukopenia (U); transient leukocytosis (R); weight gain (C), sedation (C), somnolence (C); hypersalivation (C); dizziness (C), syncope (U), seizures (U), NMS (Table 19.1) (risk increased if given with lithium) (R), toxic delirium (R), cholestatic jaundice (R), reflex tachycardia (C), orthostatic hypotension (C); paradoxical hypertension (U); nausea (C), vomiting (C); anticholinergic: mainly constipation (C); SIADH (U), hyperglycemia (U); obsessive-compulsive symptoms (R); urinary frequency or urgency (U), urinary retention (U), enuresis (C); transient transaminase elevation (first 3 months) (U); akathisia (U); TD (R), extrapyramidal symptoms (R).

4. Arylpiperidylindole. Sertindole (Serlect).

   a. **Precautions.** See "Risperidone." Prolongation of QT interval (U).

   b. **Allergic reactions** (U).

   c. **Adverse drug effects.** Nasal congestion (U); decreased ejaculatory volume (U); akathisia (U), extrapyramidal symptoms (U), TD (R), tremor (U); weight gain (U); tachycardia (U), seizures (R), NMS (Table 19.1) (U).

5. Dibenzothiazepine. Quetiapine (Seroquel)

   a. **Precautions.** *See "Risperidone." Caution:* If known/suspected hepatic disease; monitor transaminases.

   b. **Allergic reactions** (U).

   c. **Adverse drug effects.** Somnolence (C), sedation (C), orthostatic hypotension (U), tachycardia (U), dizziness (U); weight gain (C); constipation (U), transient rise in liver transaminases (first 3 months) (U); decreased concentration of thyroxine (R); increase in cholesterol (C); akathisia (U), extrapyramidal symptoms (U), TD (R), cataracts and lens opacities (U), seizures (R), NMS (Table 19.1) (U).

6. Benzisothizolyl. Ziprasidone (Geodon)

   a. **Precautions.** See "Risperidone." Cardiac conduction abnormalities (ziprasidone can prolong QT).

   b. **Allergic reactions** (U).

   c. **Adverse drug effects.** Somnolence (C), headache (C), dizziness (U), light-headedness (U); nausea (C), dyspepsia (U); transient elevation of liver enzymes, triglycerides, and cholesterol (R); akathisia (U), extrapyramidal symptoms (U), TD (R), seizures (R), NMS (Table 19.1) (U).

III. Anxiolytics

A. Benzodiazepines. Diazepam (Valium), chlordiazepoxide (Librium), alprazolam (Xanax), oxazepam (Serax), midazolam (Versed), lorazepam (Ativan), clorazepate (Tranxene), flurazepam (Dalmane), and others.

　　1. Contraindications. Glaucoma (Xanax, Versed, Ativan, Tranxene, Valium), CNS depression, pregnancy. *Caution:* elderly, liver disease, impaired pulmonary function.

　　2. Allergic reactions. Rash (R), injection site (If intramuscular) (R).

　　3. Adverse drug effects. Respiratory depression (R), coma (U), pancytopenia or thrombocytopenia or neutropenia (U), hypotension (C), dependency (C), ataxia (R), drowsiness (C), depression (R), blurred vision (R), dizziness (C), elevated liver function test results (R), jaundice (R).

B. Azaspirone: buspirone (BuSpar)

　　1. Contraindications. MAOI within 14 days.

　　2. Precautions. Impaired liver or renal function

　　3. Allergic reactions (U).

　　4. Adverse drug effects. Dizziness (C), drowsiness (C), headache (C), GI side effects (C), numbness (R), weakness (R), dry mouth (R).

C. Nonbenzodiazepine anxiolytics. Zolpiden (Ambien), zaleplon (Sonata), zoplicone (Imovane)

　　1. *Caution:* elderly, pulmonary disease, pregnancy, impaired liver, alcohol/drug abuse, depression.

　　2. Allergic reactions (U).

　　3. Adverse drug effects. Dependency (R), ataxia (R), hallucinations (R), headaches (C), amnesia (R), drowsiness (C), dizziness (C), myalgias (R).

SELECTED READINGS

Gillman PK. The serotonin syndrome and its treatment. *J Psychopharmacol* 1999;13:100–109.

Kapur S. Remington G. Atypical antipsychotics: new directions and new challenges in the treatment of schizophrenia. *Annu Rev Med* 2001;52:503–517.

Kent JM. SNaRIs, NaSSAs, and NaRIs: new agents for the treatment of depression. *Lancet* 2000;355:911–918.

Stahl SM. Selecting an antidepressant by using mechanism of action to enhance efficacy and avoid side effects. *J Clin Psychiatry* 1998;59(Suppl 18):23–29.

Teboul E, Chouinard G. A guide to benzodiazepine selection. II: Clinical aspects. *Can J Psychiatry* 1991;36:62–73.

Radiology

John B. Hagan and James T. Li

I. **Radiocontrast media (RCM)** (high-osmolar ionic contrast media, low-osmolar ionic contrast media, low-osmolar nonionic contrast media, and iso-osmolar nonionic contrast media) have various x-ray and computed tomography scanning applications.

    A. **Allergic reactions.** Although reactions to radiocontrast media are common, they do not meet the criteria for immunologically mediated events (U). There is no cross-reactivity with seafood allergy or iodine sensitivity.

    B. **Adverse drug effects.** RCM contrast reactions may cause vasomotor, vagal-type, or anaphylactoid reactions (C).

        1. Vasomotor effects include self-limited warmth, nausea, and emesis.

        2. Vagal-type reactions include hypotension associated with bradycardia.

        3. Anaphylactoid reactions (clinically indistinguishable from anaphylactic reaction but without documented IgE-mediated mechanism) have been classified as minor, moderate, and severe.

            a. Minor reactions involve nausea and/or vomiting (limited) associated with urticaria (limited), pruritus, and diaphoresis.

            b. Moderate anaphylactoid reactions involve faintness, vomiting (severe), urticaria (profound), facial edema, laryngeal edema, bronchospasm (mild).

            c. Severe anaphylactoid reactions may include hypotensive shock, pulmonary edema, respiratory arrest, cardiac arrest, and convulsions.

        4. Anaphylactoid reactions usually occur within 30 minutes. Severe or fatal reactions usually develop rapidly, with 94% within 20 minutes and 60% in the first 5 minutes following administration of contrast. Respiratory decompensation caused 40% of anaphylactoid deaths from RCM.

II. **Incidence of RCM reactions**

    A. The average historical risk of RCM reaction is 4.73%.

    B. A Japanese study of 337,647 case administrations showed an overall prevalence of adverse reactions of 12.66% (0.22% severe) in the ionic contrast group as opposed to 3.13% (0.04% severe) in the nonionic contrast group.

    C. In other studies, risk of RCM reaction requiring hospitalization was approximately 0.69% (38 in 5,546).

    D. Life-threatening reactions occurred in approximately 0.03% (1 in 3,000) in one study and 0.02% (1 in 4,530) in another.

III. **Risk factors for RCM reactions**

    A. Significant risk factors for RCM reaction include a history of asthma/bronchospasm (by a factor of 10); previous RCM reaction (by a factor of 5); history of allergy or atopy (by a factor of 3).

B. Other significant risk factors for RCM reactions include cardiac disease; dehydration; hematologic conditions such as sickle cell anemia, thrombotic tendencies, e.g., polycythemia, multiple myeloma, pheochromocytoma; renal disease; anxiety and apprehension; and use of ionic as opposed to nonionic contrast media.

C. Possible risk factors for RCM reactions include medications such as β-blockers, interleukin-2, aspirin, and nonsteroidal anti-inflammatory drugs, although there is no consensus regarding the deleterious effects of these medications.

D. Although age 20 to 50 years is associated with more frequent reactions, severe reactions are associated with debilitated, unstable, and/or elderly age groups.

IV. Pretreatment of RCM reactions for patients with elevated risk

  A. Pretreatment for elective RCM–requiring procedures

  1. Nonionic contrast agent.

  2. Prednisone 50 mg PO 13, 7, and 1 hour prior to procedure.

  3. Diphenhydramine 50 mg PO or IM 1 hour prior to procedure.

  4. Ephedrine sulfate 25 mg PO 1 hour prior to procedure may provide additional protective benefit. However, potential risks in patients with underlying heart disease, hypertension, or hyperthyroidism must be considered. For this reason, ephedrine is not commonly used.

  5. H_2 blockers are adjunctive agents with marginal benefit.

  B. Pretreatment for emergent RCM–requiring procedures

  1. Nonionic contrast agent.

  2. Hydrocortisone 200 mg IV immediately and q4h until procedure completed.

  3. Diphenhydramine 50 mg IV 1 hour before procedure.

  4. Ephedrine sulfate 25 mg PO 1 hour prior to procedure may provide additional protective benefit. However, potential risks in patients with underlying heart disease, hypertension, or hyperthyroidism must be considered. For this reason, ephedrine is not commonly used.

  5. H_2 blockers are adjunctive agents with marginal benefit.

V. Management of RCM reactions (Table 20.1)

  A. Reassurance is appropriate management for vasomotor effects although the clinician and radiology technologist must be alert to progression of these symptoms.

  B. Emergent treatment for vagal reactions may include intravenous fluids and/or atropine.

  C. Emergent treatment for anaphylactoid reactions would parallel that of anaphylactic reaction with maintenance of an adequate airway, breathing, and circulation with the appropriate pharmacologic use of intravenous fluids and epinephrine.

VI. General preparation should include the following:

  A. Assess necessity of test.

  B. Assess risk(s) of reaction.

  C. All staff cardiopulmonary resuscitation trained.

Table 20.1. Prophylactic treatment for patients at risk for radiocontrast media reactions

Elective Treatment	Emergent Treatment
Nonionic contrast agent	Nonionic contrast agent
Prednisone 50 mg PO 13, 7, and 1 hr prior to procedure	Hydrocortisone 200 mg IV immediately and every 4 hr until procedure completed
Diphenhydramine 50 mg PO or IM 1 hr prior to procedure	Diphenhydramine 50 mg IV 1 hr prior to procedure
Ephedrine sulfate 25 mg orally 1 hr before procedure (not commonly used because of potential risks)	Ephedrine sulfate 25 mg orally 1 hr before procedure (not commonly used because of potential risks)

D. Available supplies.

E. Consider maintaining the intravenous access required for administration of the RCM agent. This access may be used for management of an immediate RCM reaction.

VII. Intravenous Gd-DTPA reactions. Gadolinium-containing contrast media, such as gadopentetate dimeglumine (Gd-DTPA), gadoteridol, gadodiamide, and gadoversetamide) are used frequently as contrast agents in magnetic resonance imaging.

A. Severe anaphylactoid and fatal reactions to gadolinium chelates have been reported (R).

B. Frequency and severity of reactions.

1. Clinical trials of up to 2,540 adult and pediatric patients have suggested up to a 15.1% to 19.8% overall incidence of adverse events associated with Gd-DTPA. The overwhelming majority were mild, transient, and resolved spontaneously.

2. Approximately 1.0% to 2.6% involved headache, local reaction, nausea, dysgeusia, and/or vasodilation (flushing). Only 5 of 2,540 (0.2%) were reported as severe.

3. Postmarketing surveillance of approximately 100,000 doses revealed an overall adverse reaction incidence of less than 0.03% and with serious adverse reactions reported for less than 0.005% of patients.

C. There are no data to suggest that the risk associated with use of a specified type of gadolinium chelate is greater than that associated with another specified type of gadolinium chelate.

VIII. Risk of lactic acidosis with radiocontrast media and metformin

A. Metformin (dimethylbiguanide) is contraindicated in patients with renal disease or dysfunction by an abnormal creatinine clearance or serum creatinine level ≥ 1.5 mg/dL (male) or ≥ 1.4 mg/dL (female). RCM may reduce renal function, causing retention of metformin, lactic acidosis, and death.

B. Serum creatinine level should be measured in all patients receiving metformin, and low-osmolality contrast should always be used.

C. Consensus guidelines suggest that metformin should be stopped and not resumed until 48 hours after the administration of RCM and until renal function and serum creatinine has been confirmed as within the normal range.

D. For emergent procedures with an elevated prestudy creatinine, the physician must weigh the risks and benefits of the procedure. If RCM is administered, metformin should be discontinued. Hydration should be given at approximately 100 cm^3/hr PO/IV with clinical and laboratory assessments of serum creatinine and lactic acid.

E. Prompt hemodialysis has been recommended to correct the acidosis and remove the accumulated metformin.

IX. Radiocontrast nephropathy

A. Frequency and risk of RCM nephrotoxicity

1. RCM nephrotoxicity is the third leading cause of new acute renal failure in hospitalized patients.

2. High-risk patients for contrast nephropathy include stable preexisting renal insufficiency (stable creatinine clearance <25 cm^3/min or stable creatinine clearance 25 to 50 cm^3/min plus risk factors of diabetes mellitus, recent administration of RCM, large volume of RCM, or congestive heart failure.

3. Moderate-risk patients include patients with stable creatinine clearance 25 to 50 cm^3/min or patients with stable creatinine clearance 50 to 75 cm^3/min plus risk factors of diabetes mellitus, recent administration of RCM, large volume of RCM, or congestive heart failure.

4. Uncontrolled glucose elevation, decreased effective arterial volume, and current use of nephrotoxic drugs are additional risk factors.

B. Prevention of RCM nephrotoxicity should include:

1. Measurement of serum creatinine in all subjects receiving RCM with estimation of creatinine clearance.

2. Define necessity of RCM study.

3. Consider discontinuation of nonsteroidal anti-inflammatory drugs, angiotensin-converting enzyme inhibitors, diuretics, and metformin prior to study.

4. Furosemide, mannitol, dopamine, and prophylactic hemodialysis have not shown a benefit in reducing the risk of RCM nephrotoxicity.

5. More recent studies have suggested a beneficial effect with hydration, nonionic low-osmolality contrast agent, minimal quantity of contrast agent, and use of either fenoldopam and N-acetylcysteine in patients at risk for RCM nephrotoxicity.

C. Postprocedure monitoring of hydration is performed to maintain a positive fluid balance with high urine flow rate, serum creatinine, and blood urea nitrogen at 24 hours to ensure stability. Atheroembolism should remain in the differential of renal insufficiency following the intraarterial administration of contrast. The presence of urine eosinophilia may provide a clue to the presence of atheroembolism.

D. Management of oliguria, anuria, or progressive increase in serum creatinine should involve consultation with a nephrologist.

X.   Other RCM reaction case reports have included RCM-induced noncardiogenic pulmonary edema, delayed hypersensitivity, iodide mumps, and cardiac arrest.

SELECTED READINGS

Borish L, Matloff SM, Findlay SR. Radiographic contrast media–induced noncardiogenic pulmonary edema: case report and review of the literature. *J Allergy Clin Immunol* 1984;74:104.

Bush WH, Swanson DP. Acute reactions to intravascular contrast media: types, risk factors, recognition, and specific treatment. *AJR Am J Roentgenol* 1991;157:1153.

Greenberger PA, Patterson R, Tapio CM. Prophylaxis against repeated radiocontrast media reactions in 857 cases. Adverse experience with cimetidine and safety of beta-adrenergic antagonists. *Arch Intern Med* 1985;145:2197.

Kalaria VG, Porsche R, Ong LS. Iodide mumps: acute sialadenitis after contrast administration for angioplasty. *Circulation* 2001;104:2384.

Kini AS, Mitre CA, Kim M, et al. A protocol for prevention of radiographic contrast nephropathy during percutaneous coronary intervention: effect of selective dopamine receptor agonist fenoldopam. *Cath Cardiovasc Intervent* 2002;55:169.

Runge VM. Allergic reactions to gadolinium chelates. *AJR Am J Roentgenol* 2001;177:944.

Shehadi WH, Toniolo G. (1980) Adverse reactions to contrast media: a report from the Committee on Safety of Contrast Media of the International Society of Radiology. *Radiology* 1980;137:299.

Tepel M, van der Giet M, Schwarzfeld C, et al. Prevention of radiographic-contrast-agent-induced reductions in renal function by acetylcysteine. *N Engl J Med* 2000;343:180.

Rheumatology

Fredrica E. Smith and Ralph C. Williams Jr.

I. **Disease-modifying antirheumatic drugs**
   A. **Hydroxychloroquine (Plaquenil) sulfate**
      1. **Allergic reactions.** Skin: pruritus (U). Skin eruptions of urticarial, morbilliform, lichenoid, maculopapular, erythema annulare centrifugum types, Stevens–Johnson syndrome, acute generalized exanthematous pustulosis or exfoliative dermatitis may occur from immune-mediated mechanisms (R).
      2. **Adverse drug effects.**
         a. **Idiosyncratic reactions.** (Dose-related—very rare at low doses): Ocular reactions that may produce disturbances of accommodation with blurred vision; a relation to dose occurs and this reverses with cessation of treatment. Other ocular reactions, including transient corneal edema, punctate to lineal corneal opacities, and decreased corneal sensitivity, may occur with or without symptoms of blurred vision, halos around lights, or photophobia, and are fairly common but reversible. Incidence of corneal changes and visual side effects appears to be considerably lower with hydroxychloroquine than with chloroquine. Changes such as edema; atrophy; abnormal pigmentation; loss of foveal reflex; increased macular recovery time after exposure to bright light; elevated retinal threshold to red light in macular, paramacular, and peripheral retinal areas may occur. Visual field defects, including pericentral or paracentral scotoma, central scotoma with decreased visual acuity, or, rarely, field restriction, may occur. The most common eye symptoms related to retinopathy are reading and seeing difficulties, photophobia, blurred distance vision, missing or blacked out areas in the central or peripheral visual field, light flashes, or streaks.

         Retinopathy appears to be dose related and has rarely occurred within several months to several years of daily therapy. A few cases have been reported several years after antimalarial drug therapy was stopped. Retinopathy may progress even after the drug has been discontinued.
         b. **Other adverse reactions.** Myopathy: proximal lower extremity muscle weakness, normal creatine kinase, but abnormal nerve and muscle biopsy results (R). Bleaching of hair; alopecia; skin and mucosal pigmentation (grayish hypopigmentation or blue–black hyperpigmentation) (R). Various blood dyscrasias such as aplastic anemia, agranulocytosis, leukopenia, and hemolysis in individuals with glucose-6-phosphate dehydrogenase deficiency have been observed (R).

Anorexia, nausea and vomiting, abdominal cramps, bloating, and diarrhea may be alleviated by reduction in dose (rare to common depending on dose).
B. Azathioprine (Imuran)
  1. Allergic reactions. Skin rash (R).
  2. Adverse drug effects
  a. Idiosyncratic reactions. Common to uncommon depending on dose. Leukopenia, a decrease in hemoglobin or hematocrit, or thrombocytopenia. Elevation of liver enzymes or bilirubin is sometimes observed, in which case the drug must be stopped.
  b. Other adverse reactions. Because of its immunosuppressive effects, some patients taking azathioprine experience serious and occasionally life-threatening infections. In this instance, the drug must be discontinued or the dose lowered on reinstitution of therapy.
C. Sulfasalazine (Azulfidine EN tablets)
  1. Precautions. There appear to be more adverse reactions in systemic-onset juvenile rheumatoid arthritis with an increased tendency for serum sickness reactions, nausea, vomiting, headache, rash, and abnormal liver function test results. Therefore, management of systemic juvenile rheumatoid arthritis with sulfasalazine is not indicated.
  2. Allergic reactions. Hypersensitivity to sulfasalazine, its metabolites, sulfonamides, or salicylates. Anaphylaxis (R). Skin rash (C). Photosensitization (U). Erythema multiforme (Stevens–Johnson syndrome) (R), exfoliative dermatitis, alopecia. Serum sickness syndrome (R). Pneumonitis with or without eosinophilia; fibrosing alveolitis (R). Vasculitis (R). Pleuritis; pericarditis with or without tamponade (R). Polyarteritis nodosa (R). Systemic lupus erythematosus (SLE)–like syndrome (R). Hepatitis, hepatic necrosis, and fulminant hepatitis, sometimes leading to liver transplantation (R). Rhadomyolysis (R). Arthralgias (R). Periorbital edema; conjunctival and scleral injection (R).
  3. Adverse drug effects. (C or R depending on dose). Anorexia, headache, nausea, vomiting, gastric distress. Apparently reversible oligospermia (C).
  Less common reactions include pruritus, urticaria, rash, fever, Heinz body anemia, hemolytic anemia, and cyanosis, which may occur at a frequency of 1 in 30 patients or less. When the daily dose of sulfapyridine is 4 gm or more (serum concentration) >50 mcg/mL, the incidence of adverse reactions is increased (R).
  Rare adverse reactions include aplastic anemia, agranulocytosis, megaloblastic anemia, purpura, hypoprothrombinemia, methemoglobinemia, congenital neutropenia, and myelodysplastic syndrome. Occasionally transverse myelitis, cauda equina syndrome, Guillain–Barré syndrome, peripheral neuropathy, ataxia, tinnitus, or drowsiness has been recorded (R).
  Other rare adverse events include toxic nephrosis with oliguria and anuria, nephritis, nephrotic syndrome, hematuria, proteinuria, and hemolytic uremic syndrome (R).

D. Methotrexate
1. **Precautions**
   a. Patients *must* agree to forego ingestion of any alcoholic beverages when they are receiving methotrexate therapy.
   b. It is recommended that patients taking weekly methotrexate also take 1 mg of folic acid per day; this generally protects them from induced folate deficiency (C).
2. **Allergic reactions.** Sun-induced skin rashes are sometimes observed after initiation of methotrexate therapy. In some patients, mucous membrane ulcerations or mouth ulcers require reduction in dosage (C).
3. **Adverse drug effects**
   a. **Immunosuppression.** These are usually dose dependent. Leukopenia, decrease in percentage of polymorphonuclear leukocytes on differential, fall in hemoglobin or hematocrit, or decrease in platelet count may indicate drug toxicity; if this occurs, the drug should be discontinued temporarily and the dosage reduced subsequently. Unexpectedly severe (sometimes fatal) bone marrow suppression and gastrointestinal (GI) toxicity have been reported when high doses of methotrexate are given in conjunction with some nonsteroidal anti-inflammatory drugs (NSAIDs).
   b. **Liver.** Methotrexate may cause hepatotoxicity, fibrosis, and cirrhosis, but only after prolonged use. When patients are carefully followed with complete blood counts and liver enzyme determinations performed every 6 to 8 weeks, liver enzyme elevations may often be seen (C), but these are usually transient and do not appear to predict subsequent hepatic damage. In most instances, temporary cessation of therapy and reinitiation of treatment at a lower dose level will suffice and liver enzyme level elevations will subside. If liver function abnormalities persist, liver biopsy is indicated and should be carried out prior to continuation of methotrexate therapy.
   c. **Lung.** In some patients receiving methotrexate, lung inflammation may occur acutely at any time during treatment. This adverse reaction may occur at doses as low as 7.5 mg/week. Pulmonary symptoms, particularly dry nonproductive cough or sudden onset of shortness of breath, may require immediate cessation of therapy and careful evaluation with pulmonary function, diffusion capacities, and radiographic assessment. Methotrexate-induced lung toxicity is uncommon but not always fully reversible.
   d. **Risk of malignancy.** As with all potent cytotoxic or immunosuppressive agents, long-term therapy may increase the risk of eventual malignancy. The increased risk of malignancy is small, but patients who receive this agent for prolonged periods must be made aware of the risk.
   e. **Nodulosis.** Many observers have reported that methotrexate in some patients with rheumatoid arthritis may accentuate the occurrence of rheumatoid nodules often present on extensor surfaces of elbows, hand, and feet (C).
   f. **Macrocytic anemia.** Since methotrexate acts on the folic–folinic acid metabolic pathway, it sometimes induces macrocytosis and macrocytic anemia.

E. Leflunomide (Arava)
   1. Allergic reactions. There are rare cases of Stevens–Johnson syndrome and toxic epidermal necrolysis (R).
   2. Adverse drug effects
   a. Idiosyncratic reactions. Rare reports of pancytopenia. In most of these individuals, patients were receiving concomitant treatment with methotrexate or other immunosuppressant. If evidence of bone marrow suppression occurs in a patient taking leflunomide, the drug should be stopped and cholestyramine or charcoal administered to reduce plasma concentrations of the active metabolite.
   b. Risk of malignancy. As with many immunosuppressive agents, the risk of malignancy, particularly lymphoproliferative disorders, might be increased although no increased incidence of malignancies was reported in the initial trials of leflunomide.
F. Cyclosporine
   1. Allergic reactions. Skin: Abnormal pigmentation, angioedema, dermatitis, dry skin, eczema, nail disorders, pruritus, urticaria (C).
   2. Adverse drug effects.
   a. Idiosyncratic reactions. Nephrotoxicity (common to uncommon depending on dose). Risk increases with increasing doses of cyclosporine. Renal dysfunction including structural kidney damage is a potential consequence of cyclosporine.
   Hepatotoxicity (R).
   Hyperkalemia, hyperchloremic metabolic acidosis, hyperuricemia (R).
   Common to uncommon, depending on dose: encephalopathy: impaired consciousness, convulsions (especially when combined with high-dose methylprednisolone), visual disturbances, loss of motor function, movement disorders, psychiatric disturbances (common, depending on dose).
   b. Risk of malignancy. Development of lymphomas and other malignancies should be considered.
G. Etanercept (Enbrel). See Chapter 27
   1. Precautions.
   a. Tumor necrosis factor (TNF) antagonists administered to patients with multiple sclerosis have been associated with increases in disease activity (R).
   b. Etanercept should not be given to patients with class 3 or 4 heart failure.
   2. Allergic reactions. In controlled trials, 37% of patients treated with etanercept developed injection site reactions. All injection site reactions were felt to be mild or moderate (erythema and/or itching, pain, and swelling) and did not necessitate discontinuation of the drug. Injection site reactions usually were noted in the first month and then decreased considerably in frequency (C).
   Patients with rheumatoid arthritis treated with etanercept had serum samples tested for various autoantibodies at multiple time points. In preliminary studies, the percentage of patients who developed antinuclear antibodies of 1:40 was higher (11%) than in placebo-treated controls,

and the percentage of patients who developed anti-double-stranded DNA antibodies by radioimmunoassay was also higher (15%) than in the placebo controls (4%). No patients treated with etanercept developed clinical signs of lupus-like syndrome.

3. Adverse drug effects.

a. Treatment with etanercept or other agents that inhibit TNF has been associated with rare cases of new onset or exacerbation of central nervous system (CNS) demyelinating disorders, some presenting with mental status changes and some associated with permanent disability (R). Rare cases of transverse myelitis, optic neuritis, and new onset of exacerbation of seizure disorders have been observed (R). The causal relationship to etanercept therapy remains unclear.

b. Rare but serious in some instances, including heart failure, myocardial infarction, cerebral ischemia, hypertension, hypotension, cholecystitis, pancreatitis, dyspnea, deep venous thrombosis, pulmonary embolism, membraous glomerulonephritis, polymyositis.

H. Infliximab (Remicade). See Chapter 27

1. Allergic reactions

a. Anaphylaxis: acute facial and chest wall flushing, chest pain, hypotension (R).

b. Vasculitis: diffuse maculopapular rash with leukocytoclastic vasculitis on biopsy (R). Human chimeric antibody development, usually low titer; incidence lower in patients receiving other immunosuppressive therapy; clinical significance unknown. Development of autoimmune antibodies, such as anti-DNA (U), and development of a lupus-like syndrome (R). Discontinuation of infliximab infusion resulted in resolution of symptoms and antibodies.

c. Not truly a drug reaction but important adverse event: development or reactivation of tuberculosis; reactivation of histoplasmosis also reported.

d. Idiosyncratic reaction R. Demyelinating disease: development of new or exacerbation of preexisting CNS demyelinating disease has been reported with anti-TNF therapy. Relationship is unknown (U).

2. Adverse drug effects

a. Infusion reactions. Common, depending on rate of infusion: urticaria; hypotension; facial, lip, or hand edema; facial flushing; pruritus; dysphagia; headache; chest pain; dyspnea.

b. Delayed reactions. Myalgias, polyarthalgias; rash; fever.

I. Gold

1. Allergic reactions. Anaphylactic shock: facial and mouth swelling, dyspnea, chest tightness, hypotension, and ultimately collapse (R). Angioedema (hives, especially on face, eyelids, mouth, lips, and/or tongue) but without other symptoms of anaphylaxis (R). Hives, itching, papular rash, vesicular dermatitis; may be aggravated by exposure to sunlight (C). Exfoliative dermatitis (R).

2. Adverse drug effects

a. Nitritoid reaction. Difficulty breathing or swallowing, fainting, bradycardia, hivelike swelling of face, eyelids, mouth, lips, and/or tongue. Common with aurothiomalate (Myochrysine); rare with aurothioglucose (Solganol). CNS (R): confusion, convulsions, encephalitis, Guillain–Barré syndrome, hallucinations, peripheral neuropathy.

b. Skin: If chrysiasis (grayish-blue pigmentation) occurs, it is usually after large doses.

c. GI. Enterocolitis, with abdominal pain, cramping, bloody or black tarry stools, hematemesis (R). Cholestatic hepatitis and toxic hepatitis (R). Pancreatitis (R).

d. Hematologic. Anemia (U), aplastic anemia (U), eosinophilia (U). Agranulocytosis (U); leukopenia (U). Thrombocytopenia (U), with or without purpura.

e. Mucus membrane reactions. Gingivitis (C); glossitis (C); stomatitis (C); metallic taste (C); pharyngitis (U); tracheitis (U); vaginitis (U).

f. Ocular. Conjunctivitis; corneal ulcers, iritis (R). Corneal and lens chrysiasis—usually after prolonged use (U).

g. Pulmonary. Bronchitis; fibrosis; interstitial pneumonitis (R).

h. Renal. Hematuria; glomerulonephritis (U). Proteinuria (C). Nephrotic syndrome (U).

i. Joint pain. May occur for 1 or 2 days after injection; common with aurothiomalate; uncommon with aurothioglucose.

J. Penicillamine

1. Allergic reactions. Allergic reaction: fever, joint pain, skin rash, hives, itching, lymphadenopathy (U). Fever, drug induced (U). Pemphigus foliaceus or vulgaris (lesions on face, neck, scalp, or trunk) (U). Stomatitis (C). Toxic epidermal necrolysis (R).

2. Adverse drug effects

a. Hematologic. Agranulocytosis (U); aplastic anemia; hemolytic anemia (U). Leukopenia (C). Thrombocytopenia (C).

b. Renal. Proteinuria, hematuria (C). Membranous nephropathy with immune complex deposition (U). Rapidly progressive glomerulonephritis (R).

c. Lung. Obstructive bronchiolitis (R); Goodpasture-like syndrome.

d. CNS. Optic neuritis, myasthenia gravis syndrome (R).

e. GI. Pancreatitis (R). Loss of taste; diarrhea; anorexia; nausea or vomiting (C).

f. Autoimmune syndromes. SLE; polymyositis (R).

K. Nonsteroidal anti-inflammatory drugs (NSAIDs)

1. Cyclooxygenase-1 (COX-1)

a. Aspirin (acetylsalicylic acid)

b. Proprionic acids. Ibuprofen, naproxen, fenoprofen, flurbiprofen, oxaprozin.

c. Indopyrroles: indomethacin, sulindac, tolmetin, diclofenac.

      d. **Piroxicam**
      e. **Nabumetone**
      f. **Etodolac**
  2. **COX-1/COX-2 behavior depending on dose**
      a. **Meloxicam** (Mobic)
  3. **COX-2**
      a. **Celecoxib** (Celebrex)
      b. **Rofecoxib** (Vioxx)
      c. **Valdecoxib** (Bextra)
      d. **Etoricoxib** (in clinical trials)
  4. **Allergic reactions.** (R).
  5. **Adverse drug effects**
      a. **Asthma (U).** This reaction occurs with aspirin and all other NSAIDs, although it may be rare with the COX-2 drugs. Reactions are usually slow in onset, 30 minutes to 2 hours after ingestion, and may resolve slowly. Wheezing from bronchospasm and laryngospasm is prominent, but patients may also have nasal symptoms, facial flushing, angioedema, and GI symptoms. This reaction occurs more commonly in patients with nasal polyps, sinusitis, and eosinophilia.

      The mechanism is unclear but may result from either or both inhibition of prostaglandin synthesis via the COX pathway or shunting of arachidonic acid into leukotriene production. There is a correlation between bronchoconstriction and in vitro potency of COX inhibition. In the pathway of shunting to leukotriene production, leukotrienes cause bronchoconstriction of airway smooth muscle, attract eosinophils, increase mucous secretions, slow mucociliary clearance, and increase vascular permeability.

      b. **Aspirin sensitivity without asthma (U).** Hives do not usually occur with aspirin-sensitive asthma but in a distinct syndrome called aspirin-induced urticaria and angioedema.

      c. **Pulmonary infiltrates with eosinophilia (R).** This can occur in patients receiving NSAIDs, but it is not known whether it is associated with specific NSAIDs or is an effect of the general class. In one review, the typical presentation consisted of fever, cough, dyspnea, infiltrates on chest x-ray, and absolute peripheral eosinophilia. Corticosteroids and discontinuation of the drug were required to reverse the process.

      d. **Other hypersensitivity reactions**
         (1) **Hepatic injury (R).** The acute hepatic injury from sulindac occurred more often in women than in men, was more prevalent in patients over the age of 50 but occurred in teenagers also, and was usually an idiosyncratic hypersensitivity reaction.
         (2) **Renal (R).** An idiosyncratic reaction accompanied by massive proteinuria and acute interstitial nephritis. Other hypersensitivity phenomena such as fever, rash, and eosinophilia may occur. This syndrome has occurred with most NSAIDs (R). Other renal effects occur with all

NSAIDs but are not allergic or hypersensitivity reactions (C).

(3) CNS: Aseptic meningitis (R). This may be a type of hypersensitivity reaction. It occurs more commonly in patients with SLE and has been reported with ibuprofen, naproxen, sulindac, and tolmetin.

(4) Skin (rare but have all been reported with almost all NSAIDs). Photosensitivity reactions; pseudoporphyria refers to bullous cutaneous eruptions that occur in some patients taking NSAIDs (as well as other medications); erythema multiforme; Stevens–Johnson syndrome; toxic epidermal necrolysis (R).

e. Nonallergic reactions

(1) Hematologic (R). Neutropenia is uncommon, probably occurring in less than 1% of users of NSAIDs. Phenylbutazone, which is no longer available in the United States but is available elsewhere, was the most common cause. Indomethacin has also been the cause of neutropenia. Risks were not associated with any other particular NSAIDs, but the number of patients may be too small to allow detection of differences among them. Antiplatelet effects are due to inhibition of COX-1, leading to decreased production of thromboxane A_2. The only NSAID other than aspirin that has significant cardioprotective effect is naproxen.

(2) Vasculitis (R). This has been reported with celecoxib in a patient with maculopapular and urticarial eruption that progressed to angioedema, then multiorgan failure and death. At necropsy there was intense necrotizing gastritis and ileoenterocolitis. The authors observed that this could have been triggered by a mechanism such as inhibition of endothelial prostacyclin synthesis resulting in a prothrombic state. Celecoxib belongs to the sulfa drug group, and that group has previously been shown to cause potentially fatal adverse skin reactions (See Chapter 2).

(3) GI. Not allergic but common as a consequence of mechanism of action: GI toxicity ranges from serious adverse events such as peptic ulcers, perforations, and bleeds (both upper and lower GI and also rarely small bowel) to less serious events such as nonulcer dyspepsia, heartburn, epigastric pain, nausea, diarrhea, and constipation.

L. Acetaminophen

1. Allergic reactions. Unlikely.

2. Adverse drug effects

a. Bronchospasm. Mild bronchospasm has been reported with acetaminophen in patients with aspirin-sensitive asthma.

b. Hepatotoxicity. This is dose related and potentially fatal, but not an allergic reaction. Effect may be accentuated by interactions with alcohol, aspirin or other NSAIDs, or other hepatotoxic drugs.

c. Renal. Analgesic nephropathy is seen with prolonged

concurrent use of acetaminophen and a salicylate or other NSAID. One study suggested that analgesic nephropathy can occur with prolonged use of high-dose acetaminophen alone.

M. Allopurinol

1. Precautions. Increased incidence of allergic reactions in patients receiving ampicillin.

2. Allergic reactions

a. Skin. Rash, hives, or itching 2% (C). These reactions are increased 10-fold in patients also given ampicillin. Maculopapular rash (most common). Eczema, exfoliative rash, urticaria, vesicular bullous lesions, purpura, lichen planus, and loosening of fingernails, toxic epidermal necrolysis, Stevens–Johnson syndrome have all been reported (R). Hair loss (U).

b. Vasculitis. Very rarely, skin rash may be followed by more severe allergic reactions, usually in patients with renal impairment or patients on thiazide diuretics.

3. Adverse drug effects

a. Hypersensitivity reaction. Hepatitis, acute renal failure, rash, chills, fever, myalgia. Very rare; can occur with or without the vasculitis above.

b. Hematologic. Aplastic anemia, thrombocytopenia (R). Bone marrow failure has occurred 6 weeks to 6 years after starting allopurinol. It is not clear whether this is from allopurinol alone or from allopurinol in combination with other medications.

c. GI. Nausea, with or without vomiting, diarrhea, stomach pain but without other symptoms of hypersensitivity reaction (U).

N. Probenecid

1. Allergic reactions. Very rare: hypersensitivity reaction: fever, hepatic necrosis. Anaphylaxis (R).

2. Adverse drug effects

a. Hematologic: Anemia, hemolytic anemia, aplastic anemia; leukopenia (R).

b. Idiosyncratic. Miscellaneous: headache, anorexia, mild nausea or vomiting, dizziness, facial flushing, urinary frequency, sore gums (R). Urate stone formation, rare but when seen is most common in the first few weeks of therapy (R).

O. Sulfinpyrazone (Anturane)

1. Contraindications. Allergy to aspirin, NSAIDs, dipyrone.

2. Allergic reactions

a. Cross-reaction with hypersensitivity to aspirin and possibly other NSAIDs. Also cross-reaction in patients with hypersensitivity to dipyrone.

b. Skin. Dermatitis (rash) (R).

3. Adverse drug effects

a. Hematologic. Anemia, agranulocytosis, thrombocytopenia; aplastic anemia—all rare. Also rare: renal failure, possibly associated with urate nephropathy, but also associated with hypersensitivity reactions such as acute interstitial nephritis and acute renal tubular necrosis (causal relationship not always clearly established).

P. Colchicine

1. Allergic reactions. Skin rash, hives, angioedema.

2. Adverse drug effects

a. Skin rash. Also rash not associated with hypersensitivity. Alopecia.

b. GI. Diarrhea, nausea, vomiting, stomach pain, anorexia (all usually dose related.)

c. With intravenous administration. Cardiac arrhythmias with administration that is too rapid.

d. Local reactions such as inflammation, thrombophlebitis, median nerve neuritis in the injected arm; necrosis of skin and soft tissues with extravasation.

e. Hematologic. Bone marrow suppression including agranulocytosis, aplastic anemia, thrombocytopenia.

f. Neurologic. Myopathy and neuropathy, especially in patients with impaired renal or hepatic function.

g. Endocrine. Amenorrhea, dysmenorrhea, oligospermia, azoospermia.

SELECTED READINGS

Clements PJ, Paulus HE. Nonsteroidal antirheumatic drugs. In: Kelley WN, Harris ED, Ruddy S, et al., eds. *Textbook of rheumatology,* 5th ed. Philadelphia: WB Saunders, 1997.

Drug information for the health care professional. Micromedex; US Pharmacopeial Convention, Inc., 2000.

Fisher CJ Jr, Agosti JM, Opal SM, et al. Treatment of septic shock with the tumor necrosis factor receptor: Fc fusion protein. The Soluble TNF Receptor Sepsis Study Group. *N Engl J Med* 1996:334: 1697.

Fitzcharles MA, Clayton D, Maynard HA. The use of infliximab in academic rheumatology practice: an audit of early clinical experience. *J Rheumatol* 2002;29:2525–2530.

Gordon, Duncan A. Gold compounds and penicillamine in the rheumatic diseases. In: Kelley WN, Harris ED, Ruddy S, et al., eds. *Textbook of rheumatology,* 5th ed. Philadelphia: WB Saunders, 1997.

Imundo LF, Jacobs JC. Sulfasalazine therapy for juvenile rheumatoid arthritis. *J Rheumatol.* 1996:23:360–366.

Van Ousten BW, Barkhof F, Truyen L, et al. Increased MRI activity and immune activation in two multiple sclerosis patients treated with the monoclonal anti-tumor necrosis factor antibody cA2. *Neurology* 1996;47:1531.

22

Urology

Kimberly S. Jones, Ganesh V. Raj,
and Craig F. Donatucci

1. *Adverse event percentages listed reflect data from both the manufacturer and clinical studies.*
2. *All possible adverse effects are not listed for each drug. This chapter reflects the focus of the book, primarily allergic and allergic-type reactions.*

I. Bladder agents (anticholinergics/antispasmodics). Anticholinergics commonly produce the following side effects: dry mouth, constipation, urinary retention, palpitations/tachycardia, blurred vision, dizziness, drowsiness, other central nervous system (CNS) changes, hyperthermia, increased ocular pressure. Because of these effects, all medications with anticholinergic potential should be used with caution or are contraindicated in obstructive gastrointestinal (GI) or genitourinary (GU) disease, restrictive airway disease, unstable cardiovascular status, seizure disorder, etc.

   A. Belladonna and opium (B&O Supprettes)
      1. Contraindications: hypersensitivity to anticholinergic agents, glaucoma, seizure disorder, severe renal or hepatic disease, premature labor, severe respiratory depression or obstructive airway disease, myasthenia gravis, GI or GU obstruction, unstable cardiovascular status
      2. Allergic reactions: Stevens Johnson syndrome (belladonna) (R)
      3. Adverse drug effects: sedation (C), respiratory depression (R, in low doses), hypotension (R), bradycardia (R), tachycardia (R), excitement (R), agitation (R), hyperthermia (R), biliary spasm (R), myasthenia gravis (R)

   B. Bethanechol (Urecholine, Urecholine SC, Duvoid)
      1. Contraindications: acute GI inflammatory disease, asthma, bradycardia/hypotension, coronary artery disease, bladder neck obstruction, epilepsy, hyperthyroidism, Parkinson's disease, peptic ulcer disease, peritonitis, spastic GI disturbances, vagatonia, vasomotor instability
      2. Allergic reactions: bronchial constriction (R), asthmatic attacks (R)
      3. Adverse drug effects: hypotension (R), heart block (R), headache (R), hypothermia (R), myosis (R), lacrimation (R), iatrogenic miliaria crystalline (U)

   C. Flavoxate (Urispas)
      1. Contraindications: GI or GU obstruction, GI hemorrhage
      2. Allergic reactions: pruritic erythema (R), rash (R), eosinophilia (R), fever (U)
      3. Adverse drug effects: drowsiness (R), confusion (R), blurred vision (R), leukopenia (U)

4. Comments: A case report of an 83-year-old man revealed an allergic reaction to flavoxate verified by a patch test. Symptoms included diffuse pruritic erythema, fever, and loss of appetite, which began 5 months after initiation of therapy.

D. Hyoscyamine (multiple brands including Anaspaz, Cystospaz, Levsin, Levbid, Levsinex, Hyosol, Hyospaz; combinations including Urised, Prosed)

1. Contraindications: hypersensitivity to anticholinergic agents, GI or GU obstruction, severe hepatic, renal, or pulmonary disease, glaucoma, myasthenia gravis, unstable cardiovascular status

2. Allergic reactions: urticaria (R), rash (R)

E. Oxybutinin (Ditropan, Ditropan XL, Urotrol

1. Contraindications: GI or GU obstruction, myasthenia gravis, uncontrolled narrow-angle glaucoma, reflux esophagitis, ulcerative colitis, unstable cardiovascular status

2. Allergic reactions: urticaria (R)

F. Tolterodine (Detrol, Detrol LA)

1. Contraindications: hypersensitivity to tolterodine, GI or GU obstruction or retention, uncontrolled narrow-angle glaucoma

2. Allergic reactions: anaphylactoid reaction (R)

II. Bladder agents (other)

A. Desmopressin (DDAVP, Stimate)

1. Contraindications: Intravenous form contraindicated in children younger than 3 months, type IIB von Willebrand disease

2. Allergic reactions: anaphylaxis (R), erythematous rash (U)

3. Adverse drug effects: anaphylactoid reactions (R), nasal congestion (R), hypotension (R), psychosis (R), thrombocytopenia (U)

4. Desensitization protocol. One case of intranasal desensitization has been reported in a 49-year-old woman with raised erythematous rash to DDAVP. In addition to an antihistamine, DDAVP 1 μg twice daily was given for 1 week, followed by 2 μg twice daily for 1 week, 4 μg twice daily for 3 weeks. Gradually increasing doses at 1- to 3-week intervals were tried until 10 μg twice daily was reached. 4 μg twice daily for 3 weeks. Gradually increasing doses at 1- to 3-week intervals were tried until 10 μg twice daily was reached.

B. Imipramine (Tofranil, Tofranil-PM)

1. Contraindications: hypersensitivity to other tricyclic antidepressants, concurrent monoamine oxidase inhibitor (MAOI) use, pregnancy, cardiovascular disease, arrhythmias, congestive heart failure (CHF)

2. Allergic reactions: rash (R), pruritus (R), photosensitivity (U), eosinophilia (U), pulmonary hypersensitivity (U), hypersensitivity myocarditis (U), hypersensitivity hepatitis (U)

3. Adverse drug effects: nephrotoxicity (R), hepatotoxicity (R), porphyria (R), hepatic necrosis (R), tinnitus/ototoxicity (R), hypertension/hypotension (R), arrhythmias (R), cerebral ischemia (R), psychosis (R), ataxia (R), hyperthyroidism (R), gynecomastia (R), impotence (R); agranulocytosis, thrombocytopenia, purpura (U)

    4. Comments: A few cases of allergic reaction to tartrazine yellow dye in generic imipramine preparations have been reported as urticaria and/or rash.

  C. Methylene blue (Urolene Blue, Methylenblau)

    1. Contraindications: renal failure, glucose-6-phosphate dehydrogenase deficiency

    2. Adverse drug effects: hemolytic anemia (R), methemoglobinemia (R), headache (R), dizziness (R), confusion (R), diaphoresis (R), hypertension/hypotension (R), arrhythmias (R), pulmonary edema (U)

    3. Comments: In select case studies, methylene blue has actually been used to *manage* anaphylactic shock caused by radiocontrast or penicillin, refractory to standard treatment.

    In one case report, methylene blue was administered intravenously, which resulted in severe burning pain of the skin and blue macules on the forearm. The macules and pain resolved over several days.

  D. Pentosan polysulfate (Elmiron)

    1. Contraindications: caution with heparin or dextran products.

    2. Allergic reactions: rash (R)

    3. Adverse drug effects: thrombocytopenia (R), leukopenia (R), anemia (R), hepatotoxicity (elevated liver enzymes) (R), alopecia (4%) (R), peripheral edema (R), dizziness (R)

  E. Phenazopyridine (multiple brands including Pyridium, Urogesic, Azo-Standard, Viridium, Urodol, Baridium, Prodium)

    1. Contraindications: hepatic failure, renal dysfunction

    2. Allergic reactions: reversible hepatitis, jaundice, hepatomegaly (R), rash (R), pruritis (R)

    3. Adverse drug effects: anaphylactoid reaction (R), hemolytic anemia (R), methemoglobinemia (R), renal failure (R), thrombocytopenia (U), neutropenia (U), agranulocytosis (U), sulfmethemoglobinemia (U)

    4. Comments: The cases of allergic hepatitis reported were seen with one or a combination of the following symptoms: elevated aspartate aminotransferase, alanine aminotransferase, or bilirubin; hepatomegaly, jaundice, rash, fever, chills, weakness, vomiting, back pain, and headache. The patients developed hepatotoxicity anywhere from 5 hours to several days after initiation of therapy, and all recovered upon discontinuation of the drug.

III. Prostate agents. The α antagonists (doxazosin, prazosin, and terazosin) are known to cause hypotension, leading to adverse effects such as dizziness, vertigo, headache, fatigue, and visual changes. Because of their cardiac effects, other events reported include angina, palpitations, bradycardia or tachycardia, and edema. These medications are also associated with increases in high-density lipoprotein cholesterol and slight reductions in low-density lipoprotein cholesterol, which improves cardiovascular risk status.

  A. Doxazosin (Cardura)

    1. Contraindications: hypersensitivity to quinazolines

   2. Allergic reactions: pruritus (U), eczema (U)
   3. Adverse drug effects: leukopenia (R), neutropenia (R), thrombocytopenia (R), inhibition of platelet aggregation (R), hepatitis (R), cholestatic hepatitis (R), exacerbation of bronchospasm (R), impotence (R)

B. Finasteride (Proscar, Propecia)
   1. Contraindications: use in women, children, or pregnancy
   2. Allergic reactions: hypersensitivity reaction (urticaria, pruritis, and facial/lip swelling) (R), rash (<1%) (R)
   3. Adverse drug effects: impotence (2% to 9%) (C), dizziness (8%) (C), asthenia (7%) (R), headache (6%) (R), decreased libido (1% to 5%) (R), rhinitis (3%) (R), ejaculatory abnormality (2%) (R), postural hypotension (2%) (R), syncope (1%) (R), sinusitis (1%) (R), gynecomastia (R), myopathy (U)
   4. Comments: One case report of leukocytoclastic vasculitis was found 2 weeks after initiation of finasteride 5 mg qd, managed with discontinuation of finasteride and dapsone 50 mg PO bid. Myopathy and dyspnea were reported after several years of finasteride 5 mg PO qd, which gradually improved over 1 month after cessation of the drug.

C. Prazosin (Minipress)
   1. Contraindications: hypersensitivity to quinazolines
   2. Allergic reactions: rash (1% to 4%) (R); pruritis, alopecia, lichen planus (<1%) (R), systemic lupus erythematous (SLE) (R)
   3. Adverse drug effects: hepatotoxicity (<1%) (R), nephrotoxicity (R), nasal congestion (<4%) (R), impotence (R), urinary incontinence (R), leukopenia (U), priapism (U)
   4. Comments: Two case reports of an SLE-type disorder have been reported. One was questionably related to prazosin; the other was noted after 10 weeks of prazosin 2 mg tid and presented as acute polyarthritis with fever, leukocytosis, and increased plasma viscosity, which resolved soon after cessation of the drug. Rechallenge with prazosin produced the same disorder.
   About 25% of patients on prazosin in one study developed a positive antinuclear factor, which remained elevated in 10 of 12 patients, but with no symptoms of autoimmune disease.
   One case of a 70-year-old woman was reported as recurrent urticaria, asthma, and facial edema while receiving prazosin. Anaphylaxis developed after subsequent rechallenge with subcutaneous prazosin.

D. Tamsulosin (Flomax)
   1. Contraindications: hypersensitivity to quinazolines
   2. Allergic reactions: rash (7%) (R), pruritis (R), urticaria (R); angioedema of face, lips, and tongue (R)
   3. Adverse drug effects: dizziness (C), rhinitis (13% to 18%) (C), headache (C), arthralgias (11%) (C), myalgias (5%) (R), arthritis (5%) (R), back pain (7% to 8%) (R), reversible hepatotoxicity (R), cough (3% to 4%) (R), sinusitis (2% to 4%) (R), pharyngitis (5% to 6%) (R), abnormal ejaculation (R), atypical red blood cell and lymphocyte counts (U)
   4. Comments: In a meta-analysis comparing tamsulosin with placebo, terazosin, prazosin, and alfuzosin (alfuzosin is

not available in the United States), adverse effects increased significantly with escalating tamsulosin doses. Any adverse event reported increased from 5% (0.2 mg) to 75% (0.8 mg), and specific adverse events, including dizziness, rhinitis, headache, and abnormal ejaculation, increased as well. Compared to terazosin, adverse events including headache, dizziness, severe hypotension, and asthenia were lower in patients receiving tamsulosin. Specific adverse events were not included in the prazosin studies.

  E. **Terazosin (Hytrin)**
    1. Contraindications: hypersensitivity to other quinazolines
    2. Allergic reactions: anaphylaxis (R), rash (R)
    3. Adverse drug effects: dizziness (26%) (C), asthenia (14%) (C), postural hypotension (8%) (C), nasal congestion (5.9% to 12%) (C), impotence (6%) (R), headache (6%) (R), dyspnea (1.8% to 3.1%) (R), decreased libido (3%) (R), sinusitis (2% to 2.6%) (R), rhinitis (1.9% to 7%) (R), syncope (1%) (R), thrombocytopenia (R); decrease in white blood cell counts, albumin, hematocrit, hemoglobin (R); ejaculatory abnormality (0.3%) (U)
    4. Comments: One case of rash, pruritus, asthenia, fever, scaling erythematous plaques, and inguinal lymphadenopathy was reported after 3 days of terazosin 2 mg PO qd. Treatment included cessation of the drug, and use of an emollient and steroids. Recovery was within 2 weeks.

IV. Stone agents
  A. **Acetohydroxamic acid (Lithostat)**
    1. Contraindications: renal dysfunction (CrCl < 20 mL/ min, SCr ≥2.5 mg/dL), thrombotic disorders, urinary tract infection caused by non–urease-producing organisms treatable with antibiotics, patients who can be treated with surgery
    2. Allergic reactions: rash with concurrent consumption of ethanol (nonpruritic macular rash on face and upper extremities) (C)
    3. Adverse drug effects: hemolytic anemia (R), platelet aggregation (R), thrombosis (R), alopecia (R), anorexia (R), malaise (R), depression (R)
    4. Comments: Lab findings consistent with hemolytic anemia were reported in 15% of patients, sometimes associated with systemic symptoms (lethargy, malaise, GI upset). Improvement was seen after discontinuation of the drug.

  B. **Allopurinol (Zyloprim, Aloprim)**
    1. Contraindications: hypersensitivity to oxypurinol
    2. Allergic reactions: fever (C), rash (C), hypersensitivity syndrome(<0.1%) (R), hypersensitivity reaction (mild/ moderate, 2%; severe, 0.4%) (R), angioedema (R), vasculitis (R), CNS changes associated with hypersensitivity reaction (R), acute tubular necrosis (R), interstitial nephritis (R), hepatotoxicity (R), anaphylaxis (U), agranulocytosis (+/−rash) (U), arteritis (U), cerebral vasculitis (U)
    3. Adverse drug effects: aplastic anemia (R), cystitis (R)
    4. Comments: Hypersensitivity syndrome reported with allopurinol is life threatening, with a mortality rate as high as 30%. The syndrome appears from within 1 to 50 days of

initiation of treatment and is characterized by any combination of the following: renal failure, rash (maculopapular, 53%; toxic epidermal necrolysis, 25%; exfoliative, 21%; erythema multiforme, 9%), hepatomegaly (16%), fever (95%), eosinophilia, leukocytosis (40%). Hypersensitivity reactions may occur with or without pulmonary symptoms such as bronchospasm, wheezing, and rhinitis. Several types of rash have been reported, including maculopapular, pruritic, erythema multiforme, toxic epidermal necrolysis, Stevens–Johnson syndrome, lichenoid reactions, exfoliative dermatitis, toxic pustuloderma, and granuloma anulare.

C. **Hydrochlorothiazide (multiple brands, including Esidrix, HydroDIURIL, Microzide, Oretic)**

   1. **Contraindications:** hypersensitivity to sulfonamides, anuria

   2. **Allergic reactions:** rash (C), photosensitivity (C), anaphylaxis (R), SLE (R), necrotizing vasculitis (may or may not be immune related) (R), Stevens–Johnson syndrome (R), hemolytic anemia in combination with methyldopa (R), hypersensitivity reaction (R), thrombocytopenia (may or may not be immune related) (<1%) (R), interstitial nephritis (R), cholestatic jaundice (R), fever (U), rigors (U)

   3. **Adverse drug effects:** electrolyte changes (C), porphyria (R), pulmonary edema (R), pancreatitis (R), myalgias (U)

D. **Potassium citrate (Polycitra-K, Cytra-K)**

   1. **Contraindications:** severe renal dysfunction, anuria, oliguria, azotemia, Addison disease, severe cardiovascular disease, hyperkalemia, peptic ulcer disease

   2. **Adverse drug effects:** hyperkalemia/electrocardiographic changes (high doses) (C)

E. **Trichlormethiazide (Aquacot, Diurese, Metahydrin, Naqua, Niazide, Trichlorex)**

   1. **Contraindications:** hypersensitivity to sulfonamides, anuria

   2. **Allergic reactions:** rash (C), photosensitivity (C), SLE (R), necrotizing vasculitis (may or may not be immune related) (R), hypersensitivity reaction (R), thrombocytopenia (may or may not be immune related) (<1%) (R), urticaria (R)

   3. **Adverse drug effects:** electrolyte changes (C), agranulocytosis (R), leukopenia (R), aplastic anemia (R)

V. **Anticarcinogenic agents**

A. **Aminoglutethimide (Cytadren)**

   1. **Contraindications:** hypersensitivity to glutethimide.

   2. **Allergic reactions:** morbilliform rash (18%) (C), pruritis (C), myalgias (C), fever (C), SLE (R), cholestatic jaundice (R), severe mucocutaneous eruption (R), purpura simplex (capillaritis) (U)

   3. **Adverse drug effects:** lethargy/drowsiness (C), anorexia (C), myalgia (R), porphyria (R), leukopenia (R), pancytopenia (R), agranulocytosis (R), thrombocytopenia (R), renal failure (R), somnolence syndrome (R), hypothyroidism (R), adrenal suppression (R), acute renal failure (R), hypercholesterolemia (R), alveolar damage (U), enhanced skin reaction with radiotherapy (U)

4. Comments: Rash associated with aminoglutethimide therapy is commonly transient and subsides with extended treatment. The drug should be stopped if the rash is severe or lasts more than 5 days. Two cases of mucocutaneous reactions were seen as superficial oral ulceration periorbital edema, pustular psoriasis, and stomatitis. The reactions were accompanied with rash, somnolence, fever, CNS depression, and resolved after prednisone was increased to 30 mg qd, and aminoglutethimide was discontinued.

B. Ketoconazole (Nizoral, Nizoral A-D)

1. Contraindications: hypersensitivity to azole antifungals; concurrent use with astemizole, cisapride, terfenadine, or triazolam

2. Allergic reactions: erythema multiforme (29%) (C), anaphylaxis (R), pruritic rash (R), exfoliative erythroderma (U), fixed drug eruption (U), photosensitivity (U), immune hemolytic anemia (U), interstitial pneumonitis (U), angioedema of face, hands, and feet (U), fixed drug eruptions (U)

3. Adverse drug effects: hepatitis/hepatotoxicity (C), arthralgias (R), myalgias (R), hypothyroidism (R), alopecia (R), thrombocytopenia (R), hemolytic anemia (R), adrenal suppression (R), gynecomastia (R), hyperuricemia (R), dizziness (R), papilledema (U), tinnitus (U)

C. Mitomycin C (intravesical administration) (Mutamycin)

1. Allergic reactions: delayed hypersensitivity (R), rash (R), eczematous eruption (R), exfoliative dermatitis (R), pruritis (R), photosensitivity (R), eosinophilic cystitis with generalized urticaria (R)

2. Adverse drug effects: myelosuppression (C), moderate cystitis (C), hemolytic anemia (R), thrombocytopenia (R), bladder contracture (R), bladder fibrosis (R), hemolytic uremic syndrome (R), pulmonary toxicity (R), alopecia (R)

3. Comments: Delayed hypersensitivity was reported after 10 months of monthly intravesical treatment with mitomycin, evidenced as exfoliative dermatitis on palms and soles, purpura, or vasculitis, and resolved upon cessation of treatment. Other reports of hypersensitivity reactions appear similar, with eczematous eruption on the palms and soles, and generalized urticaria.

Some investigators believe that many of the skin reactions reported are due to contact dermatitis and can be prevented by carefully cleansing the hands and perineum after administration.

D. Thiotepa (Thioplex)

1. Contraindications: renal dysfunction, hepatic dysfunction, bone marrow suppression

2. Allergic reactions: rash (C, intravenous form), anaphylaxis (R), laryngeal edema (R), wheezing (R), urticaria (R), generalized hypersensitivity reaction (pruritis, diaphoresis, shortness of breath, and chills) (R)

3. Adverse drug effects: myelosuppression (C, even with intravenous administration)

E. BCG vaccine (bacillus Calmette–Guérin; PACIS, TheraCys, TICE BCG)

    1. Contraindications: fever, urinary tract infection, acute illness, immunodeficiency/immunocompromise, inflammatory skin disease, recent smallpox vaccination, active tuberculosis

    2. Allergic reactions: arthritis (R), myalgia (2% to 3% with intravesical administration) (R); anaphylaxis (R), maculopapular rash (R), urticaria (R), eosinophilia (R), eczema exacerbation (R), lupus vulgaris at injection site when administered intradermally (R), Sweet syndrome (flulike symptoms with fever, fatigue, neutrophilic dermatosis) (R), penile edema (intraurethral instillation) (R)

    3. Adverse drug effects: thrombocytopenia (R), polyneuritis (R), acute iritis with arthritic symptoms (U)

    4. Comments: Due to the many dermatologic effects seen when given intradermally, it is recommended that BCG vaccine be administered percutaneously. With percutaneous administration, a normal reaction, consisting of eruption of small red papules at the site of injection, is seen within 10 days of vaccination. Over several weeks, the papules grow to about 3 mm, scale, and recede.

VI. Hormone/antiandrogen agents

  A. Bicalutamide (Casodex)

    1. Contraindications: women/pregnancy

    2. Allergic reactions: rash (9%) (C), pruruitis (<6%) (R), interstitial pneumonitis (U), eosinophilic lung disease (U)

    3. Adverse drug effects: back pain (25%) (C), pelvic pain (21%) (C), asthenia (22%) (C), bone pain (9%) (C), anemia (11%) (C), concurrent use with luteinizing hormone–releasing hormone analogs: dyspnea (13%) (C), cough (8%) (C), hot flashes (C), gynecomastia/breast tenderness (C), pharyngitis (8%) (C), elevated liver enzymes (≤2%) (R), hepatitis (R), sweating (R), myasthenia (7%) (R), arthritis (5%) (R), impotence (R), hepatic failure (U), pulmonary fibrosis (U)

  B. Flutamide (Eulexin)

    1. Contraindications: severe hepatic dysfunction, women/pregnancy

    2. Allergic reactions: papulovesicular rash (R), pruritis (R), ecchymoses (R), photosensitivity (R)

    3. Adverse drug effects: gynecomastia (C), galactorrhea (C), diarrhea (C), anemia (6%) (R), leukopenia (3%) (R), thrombocytopenia (1%) (R), methemoglobinemia (R), elevated liver enzymes (R), jaundice (R), cholestatic hepatitis (R), hepatic failure (R), blurred vision (R), hepatic necrosis (U), systemic lupus erythmetosis (SLE) (R), hepatic failure with death (U), interstitial pneumonitis (U), pseudoporphyria (U)

  C. Goserelin (Zoladex)

    1. Contraindications: Hypersensitivity to leutonizing hormone receptors (LHRH) or LHRH agonists women of child-bearing potential/pregnancy, breast-feeding

    2. Allergic reactions: rash (R), urticaria (R), hypersensitivity (U)

    3. Adverse drug effects: bone pain (R), hot flashes (R), gynecomastia (R), decreased libido/impotence (R), exacerbation of polychondritis with cutaneous manifestations (U)

    4. Comments: One case report of rash was pruritic and maculopapular rash, resulting in cessation of therapy. Another case of hypersensitivity reaction between the third and sixth injection of 3.6 mg included generalized urticaria, facial and extremity angioedema, and dyspnea.

  D. Leuprolide (Lupron, Eligard, Viadur)
    1. Contraindications: hypersensitivity to gonadotropin-releasing hormone or its analogs, women of child-bearing potential/pregnancy
    2. Allergic reactions: injection site reaction (37.5%) (C), hypersensitivity reaction (generalized hives, shortness of breath, respiratory distress) (U), anaphylaxis (U)
    3. Adverse drug effects: general pain (32.7%) (C), edema (20.8%) (C), hot flashes (C), gynecomastia (R), thrombosis (R), anemia (2.3%) (R), peripheral edema (R), elevated liver enzymes (R), asthenia (7.6%) (R), extremity pain (3.1%) (R), joint disorders (7% to 8%) (R), paresthesias (7% to 8%) (R), neuromuscular disorders (7% to 8%) (R), sweating (5.3%) (R), alopecia (2.3%) (R), sterile abscess (R), acne (R), red cell aplasia (U), leukopenia (U), interstitial pneumonitis (U)

  E. Nilutamide (Nilandron)
    1. Contraindications: severe hepatic dysfunction, severe respiratory disease
    2. Allergic reactions: pruritis (<2%) (R)
    3. Adverse drug effects: interstitial pneumonitis (1% to 2%, but has been reported as high as 17%) (R/C), aplastic anemia (R), elevated liver enzymes (R), hepatitis (R), blurred vision/impaired dark adaptation (R), hypertension (R), impotence (R), dizziness (R), drowsiness (R), malaise (R), hot flashes (R), neutropenia (U)
    4. Comments: A positive relationship between nilutamide and interstitial pneumonitis has been seen in small studies and case reports. Symptoms appear within 2 months of therapy and may be seen with fever, dyspnea, pulmonary fibrosis, or lymphocytosis. Chest x-ray should be obtained before treatment.

  F. Testosterone (multiple brands including Andro, AndroGel, DepoAndro, Depo-Testosterone, Androderm, Testoderm, Testopel)
    1. Contraindications: prostate cancer, breast cancer in men, women/pregnancy, severe liver dysfunction, severe renal dysfunction, severe cardiac disease
    2. Allergic reactions: allergic skin reactions with topical administration (C)
    3. Adverse drug effects: elevated liver enzymes and bilirubin (R), peliosis hepatis (R), hepatic carcinogen (R), alopecia (R), acne (R), flushing (R), gynecomastia (R), edema (R), hypercalcemia (R), change in libido (R), psoriasis exacerbation (U), jaundice (U)

VII. Erectile dysfunction agents
  A. Prostaglandin E$_1$ (Alprostadil, Caverject, Muse, Prostin R Pediatric)
    1. Contraindications: women/children/newborns, history of priapism, multiple myeloma, sickle cell anemia, leukemia,

penile angulation or deformation, Peyronie disease, penile implants, neonates with respiratory distress syndrome
  2. Allergic reactions: erythema (topical) (C), urticaria (U), penile pruritis (topical) (U)
  3. Adverse drug effects: urogenital pain (12%, transurethral) (C), apnea in neonates (C), severe burning (topical) (C), flushing (C), nausea (C), tachycardia (R), malaise (R), edema (R), hyperbilirubinemia (<1%) (R), upper respiratory tract infection (5%) (R), respiratory depression (R), wheezing (R), bradypnea (R), tachypnea (R), hypercapnia (R), dizziness (R), hypotension (U), penile fibrosis (U), Peyronie disease (U)
B. Sildenafil (Viagra)
  1. Contraindications: use with nitroglycerin/nitrates, use in breast-feeding women or in children
  2. Allergic reactions: rash (2%) (R), lichenoid eruption (U)
  3. Adverse drug effects: nasal congestion (C), headache (C), flushing (C), dyspepsia (C), diarrhea (R), dizziness (R), pelvic musculoskeletal pain (R), blurred vision (R), angina (R), heart failure (R), cardiac arrest (R), tachycardia (R), hypertension (R), hypotension (R), stroke (U)
C. Tadalafil (Cialis) *investigational*
  1. Adverse drug effects: myalgias, headache, back pain, dyspepsia
  2. Comments: not yet FDA approved
D. Vardenafil *investigational*
  1. Adverse drug effects (reported in phase I): flushing, sinus congestion, headache

SELECTED READINGS

Arregui MA, Aguirre A, Gil N, et al. Dermatitis due to mitomycin C bladder instillations: study of 2 cases. *Contact Dermatitis* 1991;24:368-370.

Bharija SC, Belhaj MS. Ketoconazole-induced fixed drug eruption. *Int J Dermatol* 1988;27:278.

Bohle A, Kausch I, Jocham D. Treatment of recurrent penile condylomata acuminate with external application and intraurethral instillation of bacillus Calmette–Guerin. *J Urol* 1998;160(2):394–396.

Borroni G, Brazzelli V, Baldini F, et al. Flutamide-induced pseudoporphyria. *Br J Dermatol* 1998;138:711–712.

Carlson DH, Healy J. Pulmonary hypersensitivity to imipramine. *S Med J* 1982;75:514.

Carruthers SG. Adverse effects of alpha1-adrenergic blocking drugs. *Drug Safety* 1994;11:12–20.

Coltart RS. Severe mucocutaneous reaction to aminoglutethamide. *Br J Radiol* 1984;57:531–532.

Colver GB, Inglis JA, McVittie E, et al. Dermatitis due to intravesical mitomycin C: a delayed-type hypersensitivity reaction? *Br J Dermatol* 1990;122:217–224.

Echechipia S, Alvarez MJ, Garcia BE, et al. Generalized dermatitis due to mitomycin C patch test. *Contact Dermatitis* 1995;33:432.

Emtage LA, Trethowan C, Hilton C, et al. Interim report of a randomized trial comparing Zoladex 3.6 mg depot with diethylstilbestrol 3 mg/day in advanced prostate cancer. *Am J Clin Oncol* 1988;11(Suppl 2):S173–S175.

Enomoto U, Ohnishi Y, Kimura M, et al. Drug eruption due to flavoxate hydrochloride. *Contact Dermatitis* 1999;40:337–338.

Evora PRB, Roselino CH, Schiaveto PM. Methylene blue in anaphylactic shock. *Ann Emerg Med* 1997;30:240.

Evora PRB. Should methylene blue be the drug of choice to treat vasoplegias caused by cardiopulmonary bypass and anaphylactic shock? *J Thorac Cardiovasc Surg* 2000;119:632–633.

Goldfinger SE, Marx S. Hypersensitivity hepatitis due to phenazopyridine hydrochloride. *N Engl J Med* 1972;286:1090–1091.

Gonzalez-Delgado P, Florido-Lopez F, De San Pedo BS, et al. Hypersensitivity to ketoconazole. *Ann Allergy* 1994;73:326–328.

Hernandez-Cano N, Herranz P, Lazaro TE, et al. Severe cutaneous reaction due to terazosin. *Lancet* 1998;352:202–203.

Inglis JA, Tolley DA, Grigor KM. Allergy to mitomycin C complicating topical administration for urothelial cancer. *Br J Urol* 1987;59:547–549.

Kahana M, Levy A, Yaron-Shiffer O. Drug eruption following ketoconazole therapy. *Arch Dermatol* 1984;120:837.

Kunkeler L, Nieboer C, Bruynzeel DP. Type III and type IV hypersensitivity reactions due to mitomycin C. *Contact Dermatitis* 2000;42:74–76.

Labarthe MP, Bayle-Lebey P, Bazex J. Cutaneous manifestations of relapsing polychondritis in a patient receiving goserelin for carcinoma of the prostate. *Dermatology* 1997;195:391–394.

Lee M, Sharifi R. Generalized hypersensitivity reaction to intravesical thiotepa and doxorubicin. *J Urol* 1987;138:143–144.

Lepor H, Williford WO, Barry MJ, et al. The efficacy of terazosin, finasteride, or both in benign prostatic hyperplasia. *N Engl J Med* 1996;335:533–539.

Letterie GS, Stevenson D, Shah A. Recurrent anaphylaxis to a depot form of GnRH analogue. *Obstet Gynecol* 1991;78:943–946.

McVary, KT, Polepalle S, Riggi S, et al. Topical prostaglandin E_1 SEPA gel for the treatment of erectile dysfunction. *J Urol* 1999;162:726–730.

Morrow PL, Hardin NJ, Bonadies J. Hypersensitivity myocarditis and hepatitis associated with imipramine and its metabolite, desipramine. *J Forens Sci* 1989;34:1016–1020.

Nissenkorn I, Herrod H, Soloway MS. Side effects associated with intravesical mitomycin C. *J Urol* 1981;126:596–597.

Pohl R, Balon R, Berchou R, et al. Allergy to tartrazine in antidepressants. *Am J Psychiatry* 1987;144:237–238.

Rag SG, Karadsheh AJ, Guillot RJ, et al. Case report: systemic hypersensitivity reaction to goserelin acetate. *Am J Med Sci* 1996;312:187–190.

Raimer SS, Quevedo EM, Johnston RV. Dye rashes. *Cutis* 1999;63:103–106.

Rand R, Sober AJ, Olmstead PM. Ketoconazole therapy and exfoliative erythroderma. *Arch Dermatol* 1983;119:97–98.

Shokeir AA, Alserafi MA, Mutabagani H. Intracavernosal versus intraurethral alprostadil: a prospective randomized study. *Br J Urol Int* 1999;83:812–815.

Stratakis CA, Chrousos GP. Capillaritis (purpura simplex) associated with use of aminoglutethimide in Cushing's syndrome. *Am J Hosp Pharm* 1994;51:2589–2591.

Sweeney JD, Hoernig LA, Behrens AN, et al. Von Willebrand's variant (type II buffalo): thrombocytopenia after desmopressin but absence of in vitro hypersensitivity to ristocetin. *AJCP* 1990;93:522–525.

Taylor JD. Anaphylactic reaction to LHRH analogue, leuprorelin. *Med J Aust* 1994;161:455.

Van Kijke CPH, Veerman FR, Haverkamp HCH. Anaphylactic reactions to ketoconazole. *Br Med J* 1983;287:1673.

Vanek N, Hortobagyi GN, Buzdar AU. Radiotherapy enhances the toxicity of aminoglutethimide. *Med Pediatr Oncol* 1990;18:162–164.

Vilaplana J, Romaguera C, Azon A, et al. Flutamide photosensitivity—residual vitiliginous lesions. *Contact Dermatitis* 1998;36:68–70.

Walter-Ryan WG, Kern EE III, Shirriff JR, et al. Persistent photoaggravated cutaneous eruption induced by imipramine. *JAMA* 1985;254:357–358.

Williams DS, Leslie MD. Skin reaction following aminoglutethimide and radiotherapy. *Br J Radiol* 1987;60:1226–1227.

Williams G, Abbou CC, Amar, ET, et al. Efficacy and safety of transurethral alprostadil therapy in men with erectile dysfunction. *Br J Urol* 1998;81:889–894.

Wilt TJ, Howe W, MacDonald R. Terazosin for treating symptomatic benign prostatic obstruction: a systematic review of efficacy and adverse effects. *Br J Urol Int* 2002;89:214–225.

Wilt TJ, MacDonald R, Nelson D. Tamsulosin for treating lower urinary tract symptoms compatible with benign prostatic obstruction: a systematic review of efficacy and adverse effects. *J Urol* 2002;167:177–183.

Wilton L, Pearce G, Edet E, et al. The safety of finasteride used in benign prostatic hypertrophy: a non-interventional observational cohort study in 14,772 patients. *Br J Urol* 1996;78:379–384.

Yokota M, Matsukura S, Kaji J, et al. Allergic reaction to DDAVP in diabetes insipidus: successful treatment with its graded doses. *Endocrinol Jpn* 1982;29:475–477.

23

Antibody Products and Vaccines

John M. Kelso

23.1 ANTIBODY PRODUCTS (IMMUNE GLOBULINS, ANTITOXINS, ANTIVENINS, AND MONOCLONAL ANTIBODIES)

Passive immunization can be accomplished by the administration of preformed antibody. There are many such "immune globulin" preparations. These products contain antibodies directed against a broad range of pathogens or selectively concentrated to contain a particular antibody. The antibodies can be raised in immunized animals such as horses or sheep, harvested from human beings previously infected or immunized, or be murine, "humanized" murine, or recombitant human monoclonal antibodies. The latter category of monoclonal antibodies can also be used for desired biological outcomes other than neutralizing microbes, toxins, or venoms. Finally, the products are formulated for administration intramuscularly, intravenously, or subcutaneously.

I. **Antibody products.** See Table 23.1.
   A. **Immune-mediated reactions**
      1. **Immediate-type IgE-mediated allergic reactions**
         a. **Antibodies of animal origin.** Nonhuman antibodies clearly have a greater likelihood of causing IgE-mediated allergic reactions because these are foreign proteins. As with any such reaction, prior sensitization is required, by exposure either to the product itself or to cross-reacting animal proteins. Thus, persons who have previously received animal serum of the same origin as well as those with allergy to the animal in which the antibodies were raised may be at increased risk. Products consisting of complete animal antibodies (equine botulism and diphtheria antitoxins, equine spider and snake antivenins, and murine monoclonal antibodies) pose the greatest risk for anaphylaxis. The ovine snake antivenin- and digoxin-binding products have a lower rate of acute allergic reactions, presumably because they consist of only the Fab portions of the ovine antibodies; however, anaphylaxis can still occur. Furthermore, since the enzymatic digestion of the ovine antibodies is by papaya-derived papain, allergy to sheep or papaya might pose special risks. The "humanized" murine and recombitant human antibodies have the least amount of nonhuman protein and pose the lowest risk for anaphylaxis.
            (1) **Skin testing.** The various package inserts for these products describe whether skin testing is recommended and how it should be performed; however, some basic principles apply to any immediate-type skin testing.
               (a) The testing itself can cause a systemic allergic reaction.

Table 23.1. Immune globulins [brand name(s)]

Broad-spectrum immune globulins
Human origin:
IM administration:
Immune globulin (IG) [BayGam]
IV administration:
Intravenous immune globulin (IVIG) [Gamimune, Gammagard, Gammar, Iveegam, Sandoglobulin]

Specific "immune" globulins
Human origin:
IM administration:
Hepatitis B immune globulin (HBIG) [BayHep B, Nabi-HB]
Rabies immune globulin (RIG) [BayRab, Imogam]
Rh o (D) immune globulin [Rhogam, MicRhogam, BayRho-D]
Tetanus immune globulin (TIG) [BayTet]
Vaccinia immune globulin (VIG)
Varicella zoster immune globulin (VZIG)
IV administration:
Botulism immune globulin (BIG)
Cytomegalovirus intravenous immune globulin (CMV-IVIG) [CytoGam]
Respiratory syncytial virus immune globulin (RSV-IGIV) [RespiGam]
Rh o (D) immune globulin [WinRho]

Animal origin (animal):
IM or IV administration:
Black widow spider antivenin (equine)
Botulism antitoxin (equine)
Diphtheria antitoxin (equine)
IV administration:
Crotalidae snake polyvalent antivenin (equine)
Crotalidae snake polyvalent immune Fab (ovine) [CroFab]
Digoxin immune Fab (ovine) [Digibind]
Muromonab-CD3 (anti-CD3) (murine monoclonal) [Orthoclone OKT3]

"Humanized" murine monoclonal antibody
IM administration:
Palivizumab (anti-RSV) [Synagis]
IV administration:
Abciximab (anti-GP IIb/IIIa receptor/anti-vitronectin receptor) [Reopro]
Alemtuzumab (anti-CD52) [Campath]
Basiliximab (anti-IL-2R) [Simulect]
Daclizumab (anti-IL-2R) [Zenapax]
Gemtuzumab ozogamicin (anti-CD33 + calicheamicin) [Mylotarg]
Infliximab (anti-TNF alpha) [Remicade]
Rituximab (anti-CD20) [Rituxan]
Trastuzumab (anti-HER2) [Herceptin]

Recombinant human antibody
SC subcutaneous administration:
Adalimumab (anti-TNF alpha) [Humira]

(b)   Prick tests should be performed prior to intradermal tests and intradermal tests are performed only if the prick tests are negative.

(c)   Positive (histamine) and negative (saline) controls should be placed.

(d)   Prick tests can generally be performed with undiluted serum, but consideration should be given to using a 1:10 or even 1:100 dilution if the history is suggestive of risk for severe reaction.

(e)   Intradermal tests can generally be performed with serum diluted 1:100, but consideration should be given to using a 1:1,000 dilution if the history is suggestive of risk for severe reaction.

(2)   Importantly, **anaphylaxis** has been described with many of these products even after negative skin testing, and they should be administered only under conditions where anaphylaxis can be promptly recognized and treated. Epinephrine must be immediately available for intramuscular subcutaneous administration.

(3)   Desensitization. Again, the various package inserts for these products describe how desensitization should be performed. However, some basic principles apply.

(a)   The procedure can cause anaphylaxis and should be performed only under conditions where anaphylaxis can be promptly recognized and treated. Epinephrine must be immediately available for subcutaneous administration.

(b)   The starting dose is typically 0.1 mL of a 1:100 dilution [more dilute if the skin tests were strongly positive (i.e., reaction to a prick test or higher dilution)].

(c)   The dose is roughly doubled every 15 minutes until a therapeutic dose has been given. This is often accomplished by giving 0.1 mL, followed by 0.2 mL, followed by 0.5 mL of a given concentration before going on to the same volumes of the next higher concentration.

(d)   The intravenous doses must be flushed sufficiently to allow the material to reach the patient.

(e)   In some circumstances the desensitization protocol is too lengthy to allow sufficiently rapid treatment of the patient and consideration may be given to slow intravenous administration after pretreatment with antihistamines and corticosteroids

(4)   Allergic reactions to Immune globulin (human) and intravenous immune globulin (IVIG). "Broad spectrum" immune globulin products for intramuscular or intravenous administration are more than 95% IgG and contain only trace amounts of IgA and IgM. In extremely rare circumstances, some patients with undetectable serum IgA levels have IgE antibodies against IgA. The infusion of any product containing even trace amounts of IgA can cause anaphylaxis in these patients. This complication can be overcome with subsequent infusions by choosing a particular product with especially low IgA, slowing the infusion rate, and perhaps pretreating with antihistamines and/or corticosteroids.

2. Immune complex–mediated reactions. The term "serum sickness" was coined to describe an adverse reaction occurring days after the injection of equine serum diphtheria antitoxin and is a common complication of therapy with any animal serum. The reaction typically occurs 7 to 10 days after the injection or infusion, but may occur much earlier in those previously sensitized. Manifestations include fever, maculopapular or urticarial rash, and arthralgia. Antihistamines, nonsteroidal anti-inflammatory drugs, and corticosteroids are helpful in management. Since serum sickness is due to IgG, not IgE, antibodies, immediate-type skin testing is not predictive.

B. Adverse drug reactions

1. IVIG is associated with several more or less common adverse reactions, the mechanisms of which are largely speculative.

a. "Flulike" symptoms. These include fever, chills, nausea, vomiting, headache, and backache. They are more common with the first infusion and may be related to the interaction of the antibodies with a significant bacterial "load" in the patient leading to release of bacterial products and cytokines. Such symptoms may also be infusion rate related and may respond to slowing the intravenous rate. If the symptoms are recurrent, pretreatment with antihistamines and/or nonsteroidal anti-inflammatory drugs may be helpful.

b. Aseptic meningitis has been reported in up to 11% of those receiving high-dose (2 g/kg) IVIG therapy. Note that this dose exceeds that normally used for antibody replacement (400 mg/kg).

c. Renal failure has been reported within 7 days of IVIG infusions. Most such cases were among the elderly or diabetic, and some had prior renal insufficiency. Ninety percent of the cases have involved sucrose-containing IVIG products, and it is thought that the cause of renal failure might be osmotic damage. In those at risk, consideration should be given to using a non–sucrose-containing product. When infusing sucrose-containing products the rate of infusion should not exceed 3 mg of sucrose per kilogram body weight per minute.

23.2. VACCINES

Vaccines represent perhaps the greatest public health achievement ever, having dramatically reduced the morbidity from infectious diseases. Serious adverse reactions to vaccines overall are quite rare. All such reactions should be reported to the Vaccine Adverse Event Reporting System (VAERS) at http://www.vaers.org/default.htm. Adverse reactions may be due to vaccine constituents other than the immunizing agent or, less often, to the immunizing agent itself.

I. Vaccine generic names and trade names. See Table 23.2.

A. Immune-related reactions

1. **Immediate-type allergic reactions.** When a person who has preformed IgE antibody to a vaccine constituent is given a vaccine containing that constituent, a systemic allergic reaction, including life-threatening anaphylaxis, is possible. Anaphylactic reactions to vaccines are rare but potentially life threatening.

   a. **IgE-mediated reactions to vaccine constituents**

      (1) **Gelatin.** Gelatin is added to many vaccines (see Table 23.3) as a stabilizer and has been shown to be responsible for many anaphylactic reactions to measles–mumps–rubella (MMR), varicella, and Japanese encephalitis vaccines. A history of allergy to the ingestion of gelatin (e.g., Jell-O) should be sought prior to the administration of any gelatin-containing vaccine. However, a negative history may not exclude an allergic reaction to gelatin injected with the vaccine.

      (2) **Egg.** Chicken egg protein is present in yellow fever and influenza vaccines and may cause reactions in egg-allergic recipients. Safe administration of influenza vaccine containing 1.2 μg egg protein/mL to egg-allergic recipients has been reported but the vaccine can contain more than this amount and the egg protein content is not stated on the label. Also, vaccine recipients can be allergic to heat-labile egg proteins in raw egg and thus may not think of themselves as "egg allergic." There is no relationship between anaphylactic reactions to MMR vaccine and egg allergy.

      (3) **Chicken.** Chicken proteins other than egg may be present in yellow fever vaccine and may be responsible for reactions in chicken-allergic recipients.

      (4) **Latex.** Latex is used in rubber stoppers to vials and in other packaging. There is one report of an anaphylactic reaction after hepatitis B vaccine attributed to rubber in the stopper injected into a latex-allergic patient; however, most vaccine vial stoppers are made of synthetic rubber (as opposed to natural rubber latex) and pose no risk to the latex-allergic individual. The U.S. Food and Drug Administration requests that all products that contain natural rubber latex be labeled.

   b. **IgE-mediated reactions to specific vaccines**

      (1) **Diphtheria.** There is only one report of generalized hives attributed to IgE for the diphtheria component of "Di-Te-Pol" (diphtheria–tetanus–polio) vaccine. Also reported was one case of anaphylaxis after *Haemophilus* influenza type B (Hib) conjugate vaccine demonstrated to be due to the diphtheria-conjugating protein.

      (2) **Hepatitis B vaccine.** There are a few reports consistent with anaphylaxis, but none have been confirmed with in vivo or in vitro IgE antibody tests. Hepatitis B vaccines contain up to 5% yeast protein, but no adverse reactions have been attributed to this component per se.

      (3) ***Haemophilus* influenza type b.** There are a few reports consistent with anaphylaxis, but none confirmed with in vivo or in vitro IgE antibody tests. (See also "Diphtheria" above regarding conjugate vaccines.)

Table 23.2.   Vaccines

Adenovirus (no longer made)
Anthrax
  Biothrax (Bioport)
Cholera
  **Cholera vaccine
  (Wyeth-Ayerst) (no longer
  made)**
Diphtheria (*see also* Tetanus)

Diphtheria and tetanus toxoids
  and acellular pertussis
  (DTaP)
  Acel-Immune (Lederle)

  **Infanrix
  (GlaxoSmithKline)**
  Tripedia (Aventis Pasteur)
Haemophilus influenzae type b
  (conjugating protein)
  ActHIB (Aventis Pasteur)
  (tetanus toxoid)
  PedvaxHIB (Merck) (OMPC
  of *Neisseria meningitidis*)
  HibTITER (Lederle)
  (diphtheria CRM 197)
Haemophilus influenzae type b
  (conjugating protein OMPC of
  Neisseria meningitidis) + Hep
  B
  Comvax (Merck)
Hepatitis A
  Havrix (GlaxoSmithKline)

  **Adult formula
  Pediatric/adolescent
  formula**
  Vaqta (Merck)
  **Adult formula
  Pediatric/adolescent
  formula**
Hepatitis B

  **Engerix-B
  (GlaxoSmithKline)
  Adult formula
  Pediatric/adolescent
  formula
  Recombivax HB (Merck)
  Adult formula
  Pediatric/adolescent
  formula
  Dialysis formula**

Measles
  Attenuvax (Merck)
Measles, mumps, and rubella
  MMR II (Merck)
Measles and rubella

  **MRVAX II (Merck) (no
  longer made)**
Meningococcal meningitis

  **Menomune-A/C/Y/W-135
  (Aventis Pasteur)**
Mumps

  Mumpsvax (Merck)
Mumps and rubella

  **Biavax II (Merck) (no
  longer made)**
Pertussis (*see* DTaP)

Plague (no longer made)

Pneumococcal pneumonia
  23-valent
  **Pneumovax 23 (Merck)
  Pnu-Immune 23
  (Lederle)**
  7-valent (conjugate protein)
  Prevnar (Lederle)
  (diphtheria CRM 197)
Poliomyelitis
  IPOL (Aventis Pasteur)
Rabies

  **Imovax rabies vaccine
  (Aventis Pasteur)
  RabAvert (Chiron)**

Rotavirus (no longer made)
Rubella

  Meruvax II (Merck)
Smallpox (Vaccinia)
  Dryvax (Wyeth) (available
  only from CDC)
Tetanus (see also DTaP)

Table 23.2. *(Continued)*

Hepatitis A + hepatitis B	**TD (pediatric) (Aventis Pasteur, Lederle)**
TWINRIX	**Td (adult) (Aventis**
(GlaxoSmithKline)	**Pasteur, Lederle)**
Influenza	**Tetanus Toxoid (Lederle)**
Fluzone (Aventis Pasteur)	Typhoid
FluShield (Wyeth-Ayerst)	**Typhim Vi (Aventis Pasteur)**
Japanese encephalitis	**Typhoid Vaccine (Wyeth-Ayerst) (no longer made)**
JE-VAX (Aventis Pasteur)	**Vivotif Berna (Berna)** (oral)
Lyme disease	Varicella
LYMErix	**Varivax (Merck)**
(GlaxoSmithKline)	Yellow fever
(no longer made)	**YF-VAX (Aventis Pasteur)**

   (4)   Influenza. There are many vague references to anaphylaxis in the literature but no specific reports of cases. As above, vaccine with ≤ 1.2 μg/mL of egg protein was safely administered to egg-allergic children.
   (5)   Japanese encephalitis. Some immediate-type anaphylactic reactions have been reported, including some with IgE antibodies to gelatin. With this vaccine in particular, there have been many reports of late-onset anaphylaxis (many hours to 2 weeks after vaccination).
   (6)   Lyme disease. Although initial clinical trials did not report immediate-type allergic reactions to Lyme vaccine, a postlicensure study of VAERS reports revealed

Table 23.3.   Gelatin content of vaccines 2003

Vaccine	Gelatin Content (μg/dose)
DTaP (Acel-Imune, Lederle)	15 μg per 0.5-mL dose[a]
DTaP (Tripedia, Aventis Pasteur)	28 μg per 0.5-mL dose[a]
Influenza (Fluzone, Aventis Pasteur)	250 μg per 0.5-mL dose[b]
Japanese encephalitis (JE-VAX, Aventis Pasteur)	500 μg per 1.0-mL dose[b]
Measles, mumps, rubella (Attenuvax, BiavaxII, MeruvaxII, MMRII, MRVAXII, Mumpsvax, Merck)	14,500 μg per 0.5-mL dose[b]
Rabies (RabAvert, Chiron)	12,000 μg per 1.0-mL dose[b]
Varicella (Varivax, Merck)	12,500 μg per 0.5-mL dose[b]
Yellow fever (YF-VAX, Aventis Pasteur)	7,500 μg per 0.5-mL dose[a]

[a]Vaccine manufacturers, personal communication.
[b]Package inserts.

22 cases of urticaria. Only seven of these occurred within 24 hours of vaccination and only two were associated with dyspnea. None were confirmed with specific tests for IgE antibody.

(7) MMR. Most anaphylactic reactions are due to gelatin allergy as above. There is no relation to egg allergy because the vaccine contains no, or a miniscule amount of, egg protein.

(8) Pertussis. There are no reports of allergic reactions attributed to pertussis vaccine.

(9) Pneumococcal infection. There is a single report of anaphylaxis in a child who received 23-valent pneumococcal vaccine. IgE antibody to the vaccine was demonstrated by skin testing and in vitro assay.

(10) Rabies. There are a few reports consistent with anaphylaxis, but none confirmed with in vivo or in vitro IgE antibody tests. Some late-onset (several days after vaccination) serum-sickness-like reactions and urticaria associated with IgE antibodies to β-propiolactone-altered human serum albumin in the vaccine have also been reported.

(11) Tetanus. There are a few reports consistent with anaphylaxis (including fatalities), one confirmed with a positive skin test.

(12) Typhoid. There are several reports of severe reactions within one hour of vaccination but the reports are not consistent with anaphylaxis but rather involve high fever, vomiting, and headache.

(13) Varicella. Most anaphylactic reactions are due to gelatin allergy.

(14) Yellow fever. There are many reports consistent with anaphylaxis. The constituent responsible for these apparently IgE-mediated reactions has not been investigated, but the vaccine contains both gelatin and egg protein.

2. **Immune complex–mediated reactions**
   a. **Tetanus.** Local reactions to tetanus toxoid are quite common and are probably related to the level of anti-tetanus toxoid antibodies generated by previous doses of the vaccine via an Arthus reaction.

3. **Autoimmune reactions**
   a. **Lyme Disease.** Persistent arthritis can be a sequela of naturally occurring Lyme disease, and may be an autoimmune phenomenon where self antigen cross-reacts with the spirochetal antigen OspA. Because the vaccine is recombinant OspA, theoretically it could cause persistent arthritis. However, neither the initial clinical trials nor postlicensure monitoring supports such a causal relationship.

4. **Delayed-type hypersensitivity reactions to vaccine constituents**
   a. **Aluminum.** Aluminum-containing vaccines may cause persistent nodules palpable at the injection site, probably due to a delayed-type hypersensitivity to aluminum.

b. Neomycin and thimerosal. Neomycin and thimerosal are present in several vaccines. They have not been reported to cause immediate-type allergic reactions. They can cause delayed-type hypersensitivity reactions when applied topically to the skin, but this has not been associated with adverse reactions to the vaccines and is not a contraindication to receive vaccines.

B. Adverse drug reactions: Virtually all vaccines can cause minor, self-limited side effects. These include local injection site reactions, such as pain, warmth, tenderness, swelling, and erythema, as well as systemic reactions, such as fever. Such reactions are not contraindications to further doses of any vaccine.

1. Anthrax. With the threat of exposure to inhalational anthrax as a biological weapon in the Gulf War, anthrax vaccine was administered. Although studies are ongoing, there is no evidence of an association between anthrax vaccine and "Gulf War illness." Although a small number of serious events have been reported, "analysis of VAERS data documented no pattern of serious adverse events clearly associated with the vaccine, except injection site reactions." Studies are currently underway to determine whether intramuscular administration of anthrax vaccine would result in fewer local reactions than the current subcutaneous route, which often results in the development of persistent subcutaneous nodules.

2. MMR. Transient rashes occur in 5% of measles vaccine recipients, which may represent vaccine-induced modified measles. Measles or MMR vaccine causes a late-onset fever 5 to 12 days after vaccination in as many as 15% of recipients with an increased risk of febrile seizures without long-term sequelae. Measles, rubella, or MMR vaccine can cause thrombocytopenia within 2 months of vaccination, usually without serious consequence, but hemorrhage may rarely occur. This may not preclude a subsequent dose because the rate of thrombocytopenia with natural infection with rubella or measles is tenfold higher than the risk with the vaccine. Determining immunity by antibody titers generated to previous doses of the vaccine may inform this decision. Rubella vaccine causes transient acute arthritis in up to 15% of adult female vaccine recipients due to direct infection of the joints. Experts have differed over whether or not rubella vaccine can lead to chronic arthritis.

3. Pertussis. Pertussis vaccine has generated by far the greatest concern in terms of adverse reactions, including febrile seizures, inconsolable crying, and hypotonic-hyporesponsive episodes. Fortunately, the incidence of these reactions has decreased dramatically with conversion from whole-cell (DTP) to acellular (DTaP) pertussis vaccines. Because these events are not known to have permanent sequelae, they are not absolute contraindications to subsequent pertussis vaccination. More severe neurologic adverse events termed "encephalopathy" are described as "an acute severe CNS disorder occurring within seven days following vaccination and generally consisting of major alterations in consciousness, unresponsiveness, generalized or focal seizures, that persist for more than a few hours with failure to resolve within 24 hours." Such reactions have an incidence estimated at 0 to 10.5 per million doses of DTP, may have permanent sequelae, and are an absolute contraindication to further pertussis vaccination.

4. Smallpox. The expected response to the vaccine is a papule at the site of vaccination within 2 to 5 days, which subsequently becomes vesicular and then pustular. A scab forms subsequently and then separates within 2 to 3 weeks, leaving a scar. Fever is common, especially among children, and lymphadenopathy can occur. The most common complication of vaccinia (smallpox) vaccination is autoinoculation to other sites (1 in 2,000 vaccinees). Most such lesions heal spontaneously. "Generalized vaccinia" (1 in 5,000 vaccinees) describes a blood-borne spread of the vaccine virus causing lesions distant to the site of inoculation. This condition is also usually self-limited. "Eczema vaccinatum" may occur in vaccine recipients who have eczema or other chronic skin conditions or even a history of such in the past (1 in 26,000 vaccinees). Lesions develop at the site of current or former skin conditions. Although this complication is also usually mild, it can be severe or even fatal. "Progressive vaccinia" occurs in persons with underlying immune deficiency. Rather than the usual healing at the site of vaccination, progressive enlargement of the lesion and ultimate necrosis occurs. Secondary lesions with necrosis may develop as well. This condition can also result in fatality. Postvaccination encephalitis may occur about 1 or 2 weeks after vaccination (1 in 300,000 vaccinees). The fatality rate for this complication is 25%, and another 25% of patients are left with permanent neurologic sequelae. Relative contraindications for vaccinia (smallpox) vaccination include the presence or history of eczema or other chronic skin condition, immunosuppression, pregnancy, and known allergy to a component of the vaccine. With a known face-to-face exposure to smallpox, the risk of the disease and its complications are thought to outweigh the risk of vaccine complications, even in those with relative contraindications. Household contacts with the presence or history of eczema or other chronic skin condition and immunosuppression should be housed separately from the vaccinee until the vaccination site has healed. Vaccinia immune globulin (VIG) may be of help in ameliorating eczema vaccinatum, progressive vaccinia, or severe generalized vaccinia. It may also be used for autoinoculation to the eye or eyelid, but it is specifically contraindicated in vaccinia keratitis, where it may promote scarring. VIG is not effective in postvaccination encephalitis or in the management of smallpox itself. The Centers for Disease Control and Prevention (CDC) is the only civilian source for the limited remaining quantities of vaccinia vaccine or VIG.

5. Tetanus. Tetanus toxoid with or without diphtheria toxoid may cause Guillain–BarrÉ syndrome. However, the administration of subsequent doses to persons who have had Guillain–Barré syndrome may be justified to complete a primary immunizing series but perhaps not for routine booster doses. Brachial neuritis is a chronic, deep, steady, aching pain in the shoulder and upper arm, has rarely been associated with TT, Td, and TD administration and may preclude further doses.

6.   Typhoid. Severe systemic reactions, including a fatality, after killed whole-cell typhoid vaccine have been reported. These reactions consist of fever, chills, myalgias, and emesis. No severe reactions have been reported to the newer Typhoid Vi polysaccharide vaccine.

7.   Varicella. A few varicella-like lesions appear at the injection site in about 3% of varicella vaccine recipients. Generalized varicella-like rashes appear in as many as another 3%. These rashes can either result from wild-type virus, representing natural infection, or from the vaccine strain virus, representing attenuated disease caused by the live attenuated vaccine virus. Those caused by vaccine strain virus appear from 5 to 42 days (median 21 days) after vaccination and consist of 1 to 500 (median, 51 lesions). Similarly, a typical dermatomal herpes zoster rash may rarely appear after varicella vaccination and may contain either wild-type or vaccine strain virus.

8.   Yellow fever. Vaccine-associated encephalitis can occur in recipients of yellow fever vaccine. This risk appears greatest for infants, in whom the rate may be as high as 4 per 1,000, and the vaccine should not be given to any infant younger than 4 months and to those 4 to 9 months of age only if the risk of exposure is high. There are reports of fatalities from severe multisystem disease within days of yellow fever vaccination. Some patients had disease strikingly similar to natural yellow fever infection and vaccine strain virus was recovered.

C.   Suggested approach to a suspected IgE-mediated reaction to a vaccine (Fig. 23.1).

1.   Are nature and timing of reaction consistent with anaphylaxis? The first step is to determine if the nature and timing of the reaction are consistent with anaphylaxis (Note 1 to Fig. 23.1). Pertinent too is a history of similar reactions to the same or other vaccines, or to vaccine constituents. The various elements that make up a vaccine are very clearly labeled in manufacturer package inserts. If the reaction occurred with the first dose of a vaccine, the chance that the immunizing agent itself is the allergen is greatly diminished. One should also inquire about allergic reactions to food because influenza and yellow fever vaccines contain egg protein; yellow fever vaccine may also contain chicken proteins, and many vaccines contain gelatin (Table 23.3).

2.   Is there a need for future doses of this vaccine or other vaccines with common components? Once a history has been obtained of a vaccine reaction occurring shortly after administration that is consistent with mast cell degranulation, determine if future doses of the suspect vaccine, or other vaccines with common components, are required. Given the potential for cross-reaction with common components in other vaccines and with foods, a thorough evaluation, even if no further doses are required, is appropriate. Many vaccines are given as a series, however, some recipients may

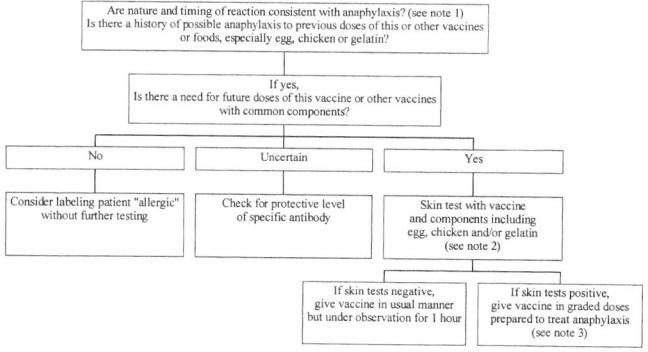

Fig. 23-1. Suggested approach to suspected immediate-type allergic reactions to vaccines.

Note 1: Are nature and timing of reaction consistent with anaphylaxis?

Probable anaphylactic reaction

Reaction occurring within 4 hours of vaccine administration, to include signs and/or symptoms from more than one system as below: 1) dermatologic signs and/or symptoms: pruritus, urticaria, angioedema, flushing; 2) Respiratory signs and/or symptoms: dyspnea, bronchospasm, glossal/pharyngeal edema, hoarseness; 3) nose/eye symptoms: nasal congestion, rhinorrhea, sneezing, red, itchy, watery eyes; 4) Cardiovascular symptoms: hypotension, tachycardia, palpitations, light headedness, loss of consciousness; 5) Gastrointestinal symptoms: nausea, vomiting, diarrhea.

Possible anaphylactic reaction

Signs and/or symptoms from only one system as above
Signs and/or symptoms from more than one system as above, but happened more than 4 hours after vaccination

Note 2: Skin tests with vaccine and components including egg, chicken, and/or gelatin

Vaccine skin tests

Prick test with full-strength vaccine (consider dilution if history of life-threatening reaction)

If prick test with full-strength vaccine negative, intradermal test with 0.02 m^3 vaccine 1:100

Vaccine component/food skin tests

Prick tests with commercial extracts of egg (influenza and yellow fever vaccines) and chicken (yellow fever vaccine)

Prick test with sugared gelatin (e.g., Jell-O: dissolve 1 level teaspoon of gelatin powder in 5 mL normal saline). Vaccines that contain gelatin: DTaP (some brands), influenza (some brands), Japanese encephalitis, measles, mumps, rabies (some brands), rubella, typhoid (oral, in the capsule), varicella, yellow fever

Note 3: Vaccine administration in graded doses

For a vaccine where usual dose is 0.5 mL, administer graded doses of vaccine at 15-minute intervals: 0.05 mL of 1:100 dilution, 0.05 mL of 1:10 dilution, 0.05 mL of full strength, 0.10 mL of full strength, 0.15 mL of full strength, and 0.20 mL of full strength.

generate an adequate response to fewer than the usual number of doses. Thus, it is reasonable to determine the antibody level achieved by the doses already received. Protective levels of specific antibody have been determined for many vaccines and some are routinely available in commercial reference laboratories. If a patient has already mounted a sufficient antibody response, consideration can be given to not giving additional doses of the vaccine. However, the level of protective antibody may not persist as long in persons vaccinated with fewer than the usual number of doses.

3. Skin testing with vaccines and vaccine components. If the patient must receive additional doses of a vaccine, skin testing with the vaccine should proceed. The vaccine should first be tested by the prick method. Full-strength vaccine can be used, unless the history of reaction was truly life-threatening, in which case beginning even the prick test with dilute vaccine is appropriate. If the full-strength prick test is negative, with appropriate positive and negative controls, an intradermal test with the vaccine diluted 1:100 should be performed, again with appropriate controls.

Caution should be exercised in interpreting skin tests to vaccines since, as with all skin testing, clinically irrelevant positive skin test results are possible. For example, among children with egg allergy (but no history of reaction to vaccines), some with positive prick skin tests to influenza vaccine or MMR vaccine have been given the vaccines uneventfully. Also, some healthy adults with positive intradermal skin tests to influenza vaccine diluted 1:100 have been given vaccine uneventfully. Thus, if a patient with a suspected IgE-mediated reaction to a vaccine is skin test positive, the same material should also be placed on persons who have received the vaccine uneventfully. If these controls also have positive skin tests, consider that the patient's positive skin test result may or may not be clinically relevant. Vaccines can induce acute IgE antibody production in a significant number of subjects, the clinical significance of which is unknown. This has been specifically demonstrated with tetanus–diphtheria and tetanus vaccines.

If the suspect vaccine contains egg (influenza and yellow fever), chicken (yellow fever), or gelatin proteins (Table 23.3), the patient should also be skin tested to these. Egg and chicken extracts for skin testing are commercially available. Gelatin can be prepared by simply dissolving one teaspoon of sugared gelatin powder (e.g., Jell-O) in 5 m^3 of normal saline to create a skin prick test solution.

4. Administration of vaccine. If the intradermal skin test is negative, the chance that the patient has IgE antibody to any vaccine constituent is negligible, and the vaccine can be administered in the usual manner. It is prudent nonetheless, in a patient with a history suggestive of an anaphylactic reaction, to administer the vaccine under observation with epinephrine and other treatment available. If vaccine or vaccine component skin tests are positive, the vaccine may still be administered, if necessary, via a graded-dose protocol. Administration of a vaccine to an allergic person even by such a graded-dose protocol would still carry the risk of an anaphylactic reaction and should be undertaken only after obtaining written informed consent and with immediate preparation to treat anaphylaxis.

SPECIFIC VACCINES (SEE ABOVE FOR DETAILS)

1. Anthrax
   a. Allergic reactions (U)
   b. Adverse drug effects: local reactions often result in persistent subcutaneous nodules (C).
2. Diphtheria
   a. Allergic reactions: anaphylaxis (R)
3. *Haemophilus* influenza type b
   a. Allergic reactions: anaphylaxis (U)
4. Hepatitis B
   a. Allergic reactions: anaphylaxis (U), see diphtheria for conjugate vaccine
5. Influenza
   a. Allergic reactions: anaphylaxis (U). See egg constituent above.
6. Japanese encephalitis
   a. Allergic reactions: anaphylaxis, both immediate and delayed (C). See gelatin constituent above.
7. Lyme disease
   a. Allergic reactions: urticaria (R)
   b. Allergic reactions: autoimmune arthritis (U)
8. MMR
   a. Allergic reactions: anaphylaxis (R). See gelatin constituent above.
   b. Adverse drug effect: Transient rash (C), transient acute arthritis (C)
9. Pertussis
   a. Allergic reactions: (U) No reports of allergic reactions.
   b. Adverse drug effect: febrile seizures, inconsolable crying, and hypotonic-hyporesponsive episodes (rare since acellular DtaP vaccine release). Encephalopathy (U)
10. *Pneumococcus*
    a. Allergic reactions: anaphylaxis (U)
11. Rabies
    a. Allergic reactions: anaphylaxis, urticaria, serum sickness (R)
12. Smallpox
    a. Precautions: Do not administer to patients with eczema, other chronic skin condition, immunosuppression, pregnancy; or to someone who will have contact with such patient.
    b. Allergic reactions (U)
    c. Adverse drug effect: fever, autoinoculation (C), progressive vaccinia (R)
13. Tetanus
    a. Allergic reactions: anaphylaxis (R)
    b. Allergic reactions: Arthus-type delayed local reaction (C)
    c. Adverse drug effect: Guillain–Barré syndrome (U), brachial neuritis (U)

   14. Typhoid
      a. Allergic reactions: anaphylaxis (U)
      b. Adverse drug effect: fever, vomiting, headache (R). No severe reactions to the newer Vi polysaccharide vaccine.
   15. Varicella
      a. Allergic reactions: anaphylaxis (R). See gelatin constituent above.
      b. Adverse drug effect: varicella-like lesions, varicella rash (C), herpes zoster (R)
   16. Yellow fever
      a. Precaution: Do not give to infant younger than 4 months. Only give to infants age 4 to 9 months if risk of exposure is high.
      b. Allergic reactions: anaphylaxis (C). See gelatin and egg constituents above.
      c. Adverse drug effect: encephalitis (R), multisystem disease (U)

SELECTED READINGS

Centers for Disease Control and Prevention at http://www.cdc.gov/default.htm.

Centers for Disease Control and Prevention. Update: vaccine side effects, adverse reactions, contraindications, and precautions. Recommendations of the Advisory Committee on Immunization Practices (ACIP), MMWR 45(RR-12):1, 1996. Available online at http://www.cdc.gov/mmwr/preview/mmwrhtml/00046738.htm.

Centers for Disease Control and Prevention. Epidemiology and prevention of vaccine-preventable diseases. The pink book, 7th ed. Atlanta, 2002. Available online at www.cdc.gov/nip/publications/pink.

Pickering LK, ed. 2000 Red book. Report of the Committee on Infectious Diseases, 26th ed. Elk Grove Village, IL: American Academy of Pediatrics, 2003.

24

Herbal and Natural Therapy

Leonard Bielory

I. Overview. Traditional use of herbal medicines refers to the long history of these medicines in the prevention and management of a variety of self-limited to life-threatening illnesses and have been recognized to be the most commonly consumed health care products. Scientific evaluation of herbal products has been limited; however, due to the known potential for adverse effects or intoxications from most herbal remedies, resulting from their inherent toxicity and the fact that nearly all herbal remedies contain multiple, biologically active constituents, interaction with conventional drugs is a concern. It is becoming apparent that clinicians need to know which herbs can cause intoxication and to be cognizant of potential herb–drug interactions.

In many countries the herbal medicines are poorly regulated, may not be registered or controlled, and are rarely monitored by national surveillance systems for adverse events. However, the increasing popularity of herbal medicines has led to concerns over their safety, quality, and efficacy on the part of health authorities and the general public. In response to these concerns, the World Health Organization (WHO) has published formal monographs on selected medicinal plants to establish quality standards of herbal products and outline the parameters for their safe and effective use. These monographs have a high correlation with publications of the special expert committee of the German Federal Institute for Drugs and Medical Devices known as the Commission E monographs and the European Scientific Cooperative on Phytotherapy (ESCOP).

The agents listed below are provided by their English name, Latin name, and pharmacopoeial names followed by their common uses (not necessarily approved by any health authorities), contraindications, drug interactions, and associated reactions (allergic and idiosyncratic) (C = common; R = rare; U = unlikely).

II. Herbal Medicines
 A. Garlic (*Allium sativum*), Bulbus Allii Sativi
  1. Contraindicated in patients undergoing surgery because it can prolong bleeding.
  2. Drug interactions include an increase in the anticoagulant effects of warfarin (C); bleeding times have been noted to be double in patients on warfarin and garlic supplements. Changes pharmacokinetic variables of paracetamol (U), produces hypoglycemia when taken with chlorpropamide (U). May cause large increases in the minimal inhibitory concentration of ampicillin over baseline values (R).
  3. Allergic reactions (R).
  4. Adverse drug effects include gastrointestinal disturbances, change in body odor through sweat and breath.

5. Commonly used for cardiovascular health (hypertension, cholesterol and lipid lowering, atherosclerosis), relief of cough, colds, rhinitis.

B.   Angelica (*Angelica archangelica*), Radix Angelicae Sinensis. Commonly used as an expectorant for bronchial illnesses, colds and coughs; treatment for mild spasms of gastrointestinal tract, loss of appetite (anorexia nervosa), flatulence, feeling of fullness; used in liqueurs such as Benedictine, Boonekamp, and Chartreuse.

   1. Drug interactions (U).

   2. Allergic reactions (U).

   3. Adverse drug effects include skin sensitization to sunlight due to the furanocoumarins (C). Prolonged sunbathing and exposure to intense UV radiation to be avoided.

C.   Chamomile flower, German (*Chamomilla recutita, Matricaria recutita*), Flos Chamomillae. Name originates from the low-lying (*chamos*, "ground") flower that has an apple scent (*melos*, "apple"). Commonly used for gastrointestinal inflammatory disorders, peptic ulcers, and spasms, topical cutaneous inflammation and bacterial infections, oral throat and mouth mucosal irritation, inhalations for the respiratory tract, baths for anogenital inflammation.

   1. Allergic reactions include exacerbation of allergic symptoms in ragweed-sensitive patients who have cross-reactivity with hazelnut, kiwi, birch, several Compositae (ambrosia, chrysanthemum, matricaria, solidago) and grass allergens, primarily the oral allergy syndrome (C), contact dermatitis (U), and anaphylaxis (R).

D.   Echinacea herb and root (*Echinacea augustifolia/ pallida/purpurea*), Herba/Radix Echinacea Augustifolia/Pallida/Purpurea.

   1. Precautions. Although no interactions were found for Echinacea (*E. angustifolia, E. purpurea, E. pallida*), there is a possible risk of hepatotoxicity (R). Therefore, it should not be used with other known hepatotoxic drugs, such as anabolic steroids, amiodarone, methotrexate, and ketoconazole.

   2. Contraindications. Based on theoretical considerations, it is not recommended for use in patients with chronic systemic disease such as acquired immune deficiency syndrome, tuberculosis, and other autoimmune disorders.

   3. Adverse drug effects. Echinacea may cause increases in the minimal inhibitory concentration of ampicillin over baseline values.

   4. Allergic reactions. Urticaria, anaphylaxis to death has been reported (R).

E.   Ephedra (*Ephedra sinica*), Herba Ephedrae. Commonly known as ma huang. Often used in the management of asthma and bronchitis, nasal congestion, diet aids for weight loss, enhancement of athletic performance, stimulation of the central nervous system due to its high content of ephedrine.

   1. Drug interactions include cardiac glycosides and halothane leading to arrhythmias (C), guanethidine enhancement of sympathomimetic effect, monoamine oxidase inhibitors increasing the sympathomimetic effects of ephedrine.

2. Allergic reactions (U).
3. Adverse drug effects include hypertension (U), insomnia (C), tremor (C), heart palpitations (C), headache (C), nausea (C), loss of appetite (C), prostatism (C), cardiac arrhythmias (U), and even fatalities (R).

F. Gingko (*Gingko biloba*), Folium Ginkgo. Commonly used for cerebral insufficiency, memory loss, difficulties in concentration, fatigue, anxiety, headaches, depressed mood, peripheral arterial insufficiency, vertigo, and tinnitus.

1. Contraindications Bleeding when combined with warfarin (U), raised blood pressure when combined with a thiazide diuretic (U), and coma when combined with trazodone (R). Long-term use has been associated with increased bleeding time (R) and spontaneous hemorrhage (R). To be used with caution in patients receiving aspirin, nonsteroidal antiinflammatory drugs, anticoagulants or other platelet inhibitors.

2. Adverse drug effects include stomach or intestinal upsets (C), headaches (U).

3. Allergic reactions. Morbilliform (R) and other allergic skin reactions (R) due to sensitization to the gingkolic acid.

G. Licorice root (*Glycyrrhiza glabra*), Radix Glycyrrhizae. Latin name derived from its common use as a sweetener (*glukos*, "sweet"; *rhiza*, "root") containing glycyrrhizin (or glycyrrhizinic acid) that is 50 times sweeter than sucrose. Commonly used for treatment of gastric and duodenal ulcers, rhinoconjunctivitis, bronchitis, impaired digestion, bloating and flatulence, demulcent for sore throats, anti-inflammatory in managing allergies, adrenocortical insufficiency.

1. Contraindications. Patients with cholestatic liver disorders, cirrhosis, hypokalemia, renal insufficiency.

2. Drug interactions include agents that cause potassium loss, such as thiazide diuretics; offsets the pharmacologic effect of spironolactone; interferes with cardiac glycosides, such as digoxin, pharmacodynamically.

3. Allergic reactions (U).

4. Adverse drug effects noted due to excessive ingestion (>20 g/day) produces excessive levels of aldosterone (pseudoaldosteronism) (U) resulting in headache (C), lethargy (C), sodium and water retention (C), hypertension (C), potassium loss (C), and myoglobinuria (R).

H. St. John's wort (*Hypericum perforatum*), Herba Hyperici. Available in United States as an alcoholic tincture, oral aqueous infusion, topical oil infusion, and dry capsules and tablets; in Germany as a tea (Hyperforat), coated tablet (Jarsin), juice (Kneipp), tincture (Psychotonin), and in combination with valerian (Sedariston). In general use for neuralgia, anxiety, neurosis, micturition (Incontinuria), and depression.

1. Contraindications. Lowers blood concentrations (C) of cyclosporine, amitriptyline, digoxin, indinavir, warfarin, phenprocoumon, and theophylline.

2. Allergic reactions. Photosensitization (R) requires 30 to 50 times the 900-mg recommended dose.

3. **Adverse drug effects.** Intermenstrual bleeding (U) when used concomitantly with oral contraceptives (ethinylestradiol/desogestrel), delirium when used with loperamide, or mild serotonin syndrome (C) when used with monoamine oxidase or selective serotonin reuptake inhibitors (sertaline, paroxetine, nefazodone).

I. **Peppermint oil and leaf (*Mentha piperitae*), Aetheroleum Menthae Piperitae and Folium Menthae Piperitae.** Available as an oral and topical oil, inhalant, liniment, ointment, and tincture. Commonly used for complaints of indigestion, flatulence, irritable colon, and other gastrointestinal tract (spasmolytic) dysfunction, including that of gallbladder and bile ducts. Also used for colds, rheumatic complaints, allergies, pruritus, urticaria, and pain in irritable skin conditions.

1. **Contraindications.** Patients with obstructed bile ducts, gallstones, gallbladder inflammation (U). Contraindicated in infants and children for use on the face due to risk of respiratory spasms (U).
2. **Drug interactions** (U).
3. **Allergic reactions** (R).

J. **Ginseng root (*Panax ginseng*), Radix Ginseng.** Commonly used as an aphrodisiac and a stimulant.

1. Contraindicated in patients with diabetes.
2. **Drug interactions** include interference with digoxin pharmacodynamically, hypoglycemic agents; lowers blood concentrations of alcohol and warfarin (U), and induces mania (R) if used concomitantly with phenelzine; possible additive effect on estrogens or corticosteroids (U).
3. **Allergic reactions (U).**
4. **Adverse drug effects** include headache (U), tremulousness (U), and manic episodes (R) in patients treated with phenelzine sulfate. Long-term use associated with vaginal bleeding (R), mastalgia (R), mental status changes (R), and Stevens–Johnson syndrome (R).

K. **Kava kava rhizome (root) (*Piper methysticum*), Piperis methystici rhizoma.** Used for the short-term management of anxiety.

1. **Drug interactions** include potentiation of the sedative effect of anesthetics inducing a semicomatose state when given concomitantly with alprazolam (R); increasing "off" periods in Parkinson patients taking levodopa (R).
2. **Allergic reactions (U).**

L. **Stinging nettle root, herb, and leaf (*Urtica dioica*), Radix Urticae, herba/folium.** The Latin genus name comes from the term "burn" due to the urticate (stinging) nature of its hairs. Available as a freeze-dried powder, extract, juice, or in combination with saw palmetto. Used homeopathically for the management of allergies such as allergic rhinitis; naturopathically for benign prostatic hypertrophy; and generally for its anti-inflammatory effects in acute arthritis and as a diuretic.

1. **Contraindications** (U).
2. **Drug interactions** (U).
3. **Allergic reactions** (U).

4. **Allergic reactions.** Collection of fresh leaves causes allergic-type reactions, such as urticaria (C), burning, and itching upon application to mucosal surfaces (C); is known to cause mild gastrointestinal disturbances, such as diarrhea (R).

M. **Valerian root (*Valeriana officinalis*), Radix Valerianae.** Commonly used for insomnia, restlessness, anxiety, and poor appetite.

1. **Drug interactions** may occur with concomitant barbiturate use resulting in excessive sedation.

2. **Allergic reactions** (U).

3. **Adverse drug effects** include nephrotoxicity (R), headache (R), chest tightness (R), mydriasis (R), abdominal pain (U), and tremor of the hands and feet (R).

III. **Natural Therapies**

A. **Ayurvedic remedies**

1. **Allergic reactions** (U).

2. **Adverse drug effects.** Contain arsenic or mercury that can produce typical skin lesions (U).

B. **Aromatherapy**

1. Phototoxic dermatitis from 5-methoxypsoralen; photocontact dermatitis, immediate contact reactions, and pigmentary changes (U).

2. Fragrance allergy (C) affects approximately 1% of the general population with axillary dermatitis, dermatitis of the face (including the eyelids) and neck, well-circumscribed patches in areas of "dabbing-on" perfumes (wrists, behind the ears), and (aggravation of) hand eczema.

3. Increasing incidence of lavender oil–associated contact dermatitis (C).

C. **Moxibustion**

1. **Allergic reactions** (U).

2. **Adverse drug effects.** Burns are directly related to burning of various materials (C).

D. **Acupuncture**

1. **Contraindications** include an unstable spine, severe clotting disorder, valvular heart disease, neutropenia, and lymphedema (U).

2. **Allergic reactions.** Contact dermatitis may result from the nickel-based acupuncture needles (C).

SELECTED READINGS

Bielory L, Lupoli K. Herbal interventions in asthma and allergy. *J Asthma* 1999;36:1–65.

Blumental M, Goldberg A, Brinchmann J, et al., eds. *Herbal medicine.* Expanded Commission E Monographs. Newton, MA: Integrative Medicine Communications, 2000.

World Health Organization. *WHO Monographs on Selected Medicinal Plants.* Geneva, 1999.

Latex

Kevin J. Kelly

Allergic reactions to natural rubber latex (referred to as "latex") were documented in modern medicine starting in 1979, although some reports in the German medical literature describe urticaria reactions in the 1920s and contact allergy in the 1930s. The latex used in finished consumer and medical products is a white cytosol secreted by lactifer cells that underlie the bark of the tree *Hevea brasiliensis*. Latex actively circulates throughout lactifer plants, of which there are more than 2,000 species in the world. Because latex is rich in *cis*-1,4-polyisoprene, manufacturers have harvested latex from the *Hevea* circulatory system to create and market more than 40,000 consumer and medical products. Despite the demonstrable lack of immune response to polyisoprene, retained proteins in finished latex products have resulted in IgE-mediated immune responses causing urticaria (C), flushing (C), angioedema (U), rhinoconjunctivitis (U), asthma (U), and the most serious problem of all, anaphylaxis (U) (potentially fatal). Latex allergy is considered in this textbook because of the ubiquitous nature of latex products, the potential contamination of medications, and the fact that latex-allergic reactions in some situations could be mistakenly interpreted as medication allergies or allergic reactions to general anesthesia. Thus, the clinician must have a high index of suspicion when confronted with allergic reactions to medications where latex may be an undetected cause. The picture of latex allergy was further confused by the use of products made of latex that were claimed to be "hypoallergenic." Although this labeling is no longer allowed by the U.S. Food and Drug Administration (FDA), it referred to chemicals used in the manufacturing process that were retained in the finished rubber products in small amounts. These retained chemicals may cause type IV hypersensitivity cellular immune responses of contact dermatitis (C) but rarely are confused with drug hypersensitivity.

Allergic reactions have been characterized by whether the component of latex causes adverse reactions and the nature of the usual clinical manifestation of such reactions: (C) common, (R) rare, or (U) unlikely.

I. Device classification

    A. Latex is not considered a drug and is not classified as such. Although the FDA does not currently regulate the use of latex in consumer products, medical devices such as gloves are regulated as class I medical devices that must meet general controls.

    B. Allergic reactions to latex must always be considered in the clinical setting of immunoglobulin E (IgE)–mediated reactions where contact with skin, mucous membrane, or aeroallergen may occur.

    1. Natural rubber latex (latex) content

        a. *cis*-1,4-Polyisoprene (R) is an inert substance that is rarely reported to cause adverse reactions.

b. Proteins (C). The major components of finished rubber products that cause IgE-mediated allergic reactions. More than 250 polypeptides identified with 13 well-characterized allergens have been identified (*Hev b 1–13*).
c. Rubber accelerator and oxidant chemicals (C). Thiuram and thiazole chemicals used in the manufacture of and retained in latex finished products may cause type IV cell-mediated hypersensitivity reactions manifested as contact dermatitis (C). Urticaria (R) has been described as a result of reactions to these chemicals but the mechanism is unknown.
d. Other components (e.g., magnesium, sodium) are not known to cause allergic or adverse reactions (U).
e. Corn starch powder (C). Many latex products made by a dipping method are coated with a donning powder of highly cross-linked starch. This powder can cause an irritant or nonimmunologically mediated dermatitis (C). It easily carries protein allergen (non-covalent binding), which leads to airborne contamination, subsequent inhalation, allergen dispersion onto other devices (phones, carpet, food), and results in IgE-mediated reactions to the proteins being carried (C).

2. Populations at higher risk of developing latex allergy
   a. Spina bifida (C). Multiple factors, including early and multiple surgeries, frequent bladder and rectal contact with latex, atopy, and neural immune mechanisms, have all been implicated as risk factors for the development of latex allergy in this group. As many as 70% of spina bifida patients were demonstrated in the early 1990s to be allergic to latex. Operating room anaphylaxis (C) was the most severe and important of these reactions. Reactions from intravascular contact from intravenous solutions that flowed through tubing containing latex check valves were implicated as a major cause. This setting is easily confused with **medication administration, barium enema,** or **general anesthesia** as a cause of the allergic response.
   b. Health care workers (C). Latex-allergic reactions are more common in this group because of contact inhalation of latex in latex powder with latex gloves in their daily activities. These workers are at risk of reaction when they become patients.
   c. Occupations in which latex products are worn or produced (C). Housekeepers, food handlers, hair dressers, rubber tire workers, latex doll manufacturers, and others have been reported with allergic reactions to latex. In the future, postal workers and airline security workers may be at risk because of the use of latex gloves.
   d. Atopic (U). Subjects with an atopic genetic predisposition appear to develop latex allergy more frequently than nonatopic subjects
   e. Multiple surgeries (U). It has been found that patients who have had multiple surgeries have a higher risk of IgE-mediated allergy.

f.   Patients with frequent contact with latex gloves (U). premature neonates, chronic mechanical ventilation patients, and persons with bladder extrophy may be at higher risk.

g.   General population (R). Clinical latex allergy in this group is rare despite findings of IgE antibody when screening blood donors. This problem manifested itself initially as allergic reactions to barium enema catheter balloon tips.

h.   Patients allergic to fruit. Cross-reacting proteins to latex proteins that are contained in many fruits (especially banana, kiwi, avocado) have caused clinical reactions. This history raises the suspicion that an allergic reaction attributed to medications may be due to latex.

SELECTED READINGS

Bernardini R, Novembre E, Inhargiola A, et al. Prevalence and risk factors of latex sensitization in an unselected pediatric population. *J Allergy Clin Immunol* 1998;101:621–625.

Kelly KJ, Banerjee B. Latex hypersensitivity. In: Grammer LC, Greenberger PA, eds. *Patterson's allergic diseases,* 6th ed. 2002;653–671.

Kelly KJ, Walsh-Kelly CM. Latex allergy: a patient and health care system emergency. *Ann Emerg Med* 1998;32:723–729.

Natural rubber latex sensitivity. *J Allergy Clin Immunol (Suppl)* 2002;110:S1–S140.

Slater J. Rubber anaphylaxis. *N Engl J Med* 1989;17:1126–1130.

Sussman G, Tarlo S, Dolovich J. The spectrum of IgE-mediated responses to latex. *JAMA* 1991;265:2844–2847.

26

Commonly Used Agents in the Management of HIV-1 Infection

Andrew W. Urban and Frank M. Graziano

I. Principles of HIV therapy. State of the art management of human immunodeficiency virus (HIV) infection has evolved into a complex and highly specialized field of medicine. Highly active antiretroviral therapy (HAART) refers to the use of combination antiretroviral therapy in the management of HIV infection. The decision to initiate HAART is individualized and based on several factors, including level of viral replication (plasma HIV-RNA) and level of immune system deterioration (plasma CD4 T-lymphocyte count), presence of symptoms attributable to HIV or opportunistic complications, ability to adhere to complex multidrug regimens, and patient desire for therapy. When HAART is used, the goals of therapy include (a) reducing HIV-associated morbidity and mortality and improving quality of life; (b) achieving maximal and durable viral suppression; and (c) preserving or enhancing immune system function by immune reconstitution. HAART regimens derive from four major classes of antiretrovirals: nucleoside and nucleotide reverse transcriptase inhibitors (NRTIs), nonnucleoside reverse transcriptase inhibitors (NNRTIs), protease inhibitors (PIs) and fusion inhibitors (FI). In addition to antiretroviral agents, individuals infected with HIV may also receive a variety of other medications including antimicrobials to prevent or treat opportunistic infections [e.g., trimethoprim–sulfamethoxazole (TMP-SMX)], agents to manage metabolic complications (e.g., lipid-lowering agents), or agents to manage other HIV associated complications (e.g., erythropoietin therapy for anemia).

II. Risks of hypersensitivity reactions in HIV therapy. The risk of adverse drug reactions (ADR) is clearly higher for individuals with HIV infection than for those without HIV infection or those with other immunosuppressive conditions. ADRs include drug hypersensitivity reactions and nonhypersensitivity reactions, such as side effects and drug–drug interactions. Drug hypersensitivity reactions include both allergic and pseudoallergic reactions. Because most agents used in the management of HIV infection have been in clinical practice a very short time, little information has been put forth regarding specific hypersensitivity mechanisms for individual drugs or classes of agents. It therefore becomes difficult to categorize hypersensitivity reactions. All reported cases of HIV antiretroviral hypersensitivity reactions fall into the pseudoallergic category, meaning that the timing or clinical features of the reaction resemble an allergic reaction, but immune mechanisms have not been found to be causative for the process.

With the use of HAART and increasingly complex daily medication regimens for managing HIV, the ability to isolate a particular agent as the cause of a drug hypersensitivity reaction can be quite challenging. Although case reports of hypersensitivity reactions can be found for most antiretroviral agents, in general these reactions are rare. The most commonly reported agents associated with hypersensitivity reactions in HIV-infected individuals are sulfonamides and other antimicrobials used in the management of opportunistic infections. With all agents, a history of a severe initial hypersensitivity reaction is a contraindication to the subsequent use of that agent. For some agents (e.g., TMP-SMX), rechallenge (in the absence of a severe or life-threatening initial hypersensitivity reaction) can be useful in trying to confirm the association between an individual drug and hypersensitivity reaction. However, for other agents (e.g., abacavir), rechallenge is contraindicated (even in the absence of a severe initial reaction) as subsequent hypersensitivity reactions can be life threatening. Gender differences, comorbidities, degree of immune suppression, genetic predisposition, and cross-hypersensitivity among agents can influence the risk of a hypersensitivity reaction.

III. Antiretroviral agents
A. Nucleotide Reverse Transcriptase Inhibitors (NRTI)
1. **Allergic reactions** to NRTIs are rare, and a history of severe hypersensitivity to any agent is a contraindication to the future use of that agent. Abacavir has a unique hypersensitivity syndrome that is discussed in detail below.

2. **Class-related adverse drug effects.** The most important NRTI class adverse effect is mitochondrial toxicity (with or without lactic acidosis) secondary to the inhibition of mitochondrial DNA-polymerase-γ by the NRTI agents. Although all NRTIs have been implicated, individual agents vary in their ability to inhibit DNA-polymerase-γ and in their association with this syndrome in clinical studies. Clinical findings are along a spectrum ranging from asymptomatic hyperlactatemia to nonspecific symptoms including fatigue, nausea, abdominal pain, and dyspnea to severe illness with acidosis and in some cases death. Laboratory findings can include elevation of liver function test results, pancreatic enzymes, anion gap, and lactate levels. Hepatomegaly and steatosis are often present. Management consists of supportive care plus discontinuation of NRTIs.

   a. **Zidovudine (AZT, Retrovir)**

      (1) Contraindications. Concurrent use of stavudine (d4T, Zerit)

      (2) Allergic reactions. Rash and fever are rare. Anaphylactoid reaction, urticaria, and leukocytoclastic vasculitis have been reported. While the mechanism of hypersensitivity is unknown, successful zidovudine desensitization protocols have been reported.

      (3) Adverse drug effects. Myelosuppression (anemia, neutropenia), macrocytosis, hepatitis, myopathy, gastrointestinal (GI) intolerance, headaches, malaise, nail pigmentation changes, hypertrichosis.

   b. **Didanosine (ddI, Videx-Ec)**

      (1) Contraindications: History of ddI-induced pancreatitis.

(2) Allergic reactions. Rash and fever (R), Leukocytoclastic vasculitis (R), Stevens–Johnson syndrome (R), Ofuji papuloerythroderma (R). The mechanism of hypersensitivity is unknown.

(3) Adverse drug effects. Pancreatitis, peripheral neuropathy, hepatitis, GI intolerance (more with buffered tablets and powder than enteric-coated Videx-EC formulation), hyperuricemia, optic neuritis, and retinal depigmentation (R).

c. Zalcitabine (ddC, Hivid)

(1) Allergic reactions. Rash (erythematous, macular) may occur in approximately 2% to 3% within the first 2 weeks of therapy and is usually self-limited (R). The mechanism of hypersensitivity is unknown.

(2) Adverse drug effects. Peripheral neuropathy is the major treatment-limiting adverse effect. Stomatitis and esophageal ulcerations can occur in up to 4% of cases and are usually self-limited. In some cases, discontinuation of ddC may be necessary.

d. Lamivudine (3TC, Epivir)

(1) Allergic reactions. Anaphylactoid reaction, angioedema, and urticaria are rare. The mechanism of hypersensitivity is unknown. Contact dermatitis (R).

(2) Adverse drug effects. Minimal toxicity, pancreatitis rarely reported in pediatric clinical trials.

e. Stavudine (d4T, Zerit)

(1) Contraindications. Concurrent use of zidovudine.

(2) Allergic reactions. No published reports, but cases have been reported to the manufacturer. (U).

(3) Adverse drug effects. Peripheral neuropathy, motor weakness in association with lactic acidosis, hepatitis, GI intolerance.

f. Abacavir (Ziagen, also a component of the triformulation Trizivir)

(1) Contraindications. History of prior abacavir hypersensitivity reaction is an absolute contraindication to the use of abacavir.

(2) Allergic reactions. Abacavir hypersensitivity syndrome is a multisystem disorder that occurs in approximately 5% of individuals treated with abacavir. The mechanism of hypersensitivity is unknown. Symptoms usually begin within a few days to 6 weeks after initiation of abacavir therapy, with the median time to onset being 11 days. Genetic factors may influence the risk of a hypersensitivity reaction to abacavir, with a decreased risk reported in individuals of African descent and an increased risk found for those with certain human leukocyte antigen (HLA) haplotypes (HLA-B*5701, HLA-DR7, and HLA-DQ3). The most common initial symptoms include fever, rash, malaise, and GI symptoms such as nausea (with or without emesis), diarrhea, and abdominal pain. The rash may be maculopapular or urticarial, and can begin several days after the onset of constitutional symptoms. Less commonly, respiratory symptoms including sore throat, dyspnea, cough, and bronchospasm can occur, as well as musculoskeletal symptoms such as arthralgia and myalgia. Headache, paresthesia, and edema are rare but have been reported. Initial symptoms may be mild but escalate in severity with continued dosing, and life-threatening reactions can occur if the drug is continued during an ongoing severe reaction. Some individuals note an exacerbation of symptoms soon after taking subsequent doses of abacavir. Laboratory abnormalities most commonly reported include elevated hepatic transaminases, lymphopenia, and elevated creatine phosphokinase. Liver and renal failure are rare but have been reported. Improvement in symptoms is generally noted within 24 to 48 hours following abacavir discontinuation, with resolution of the hypersensitivity reaction within several days in most cases. When abacavir hypersensitivity syndrome is diagnosed, abacavir must be permanently discontinued. An individual with a history of abacavir hypersensitivity should never be rechallenged with abacavir as severe symptoms can develop quickly (within hours), leading to life-threatening reactions and death. One case of Stevens–Johnson syndrome has been reported (R).

    (3) **Adverse drug effects.** GI intolerance, headache, malaise are rarely reported.

  g. **Tenofovir (Viread)**

    (1) **Allergic reactions.** Rash (R).

    (2) **Adverse drug effects.** GI intolerance rarely reported. Case reports describe Fanconi syndrome and renal impairment.

  h. **Emtricitabine (Emtriva)**

    (1) **Allergic reactions.** Rash has been reported with similar frequency to control groups in clinical studies (U).

    (2) **Adverse drug effects.** Skin discoloration including hyperpigmentation involving the palms and/or soles. Headache, diarrhea, nausea are rare. Exacerbations of hepatitis B have been reported after discontinuation of emtricitabine.

B. **Non Nucleotide Reverse Transcriptase Inhibitors (NNRTI)**

  1. Although **Allergic reactions** are quite rare, a history of a severe hypersensitivity reaction to any NNRTI is a contraindication to future use of that agent.

  2. **Class-related adverse drug effects.** Rash and hepatotoxicity are the most common class-related adverse effects and will be described below for each individual agent. Although most NNRTI-associated rashes are mild and do not lead to drug discontinuation, an important minority of cases do represent severe reactions, and life-threatening eruptions, including Stevens–Johnson syndrome, have been reported. All NNRTIs are metabolized by the cytochrome P450 pathways, and the agents differ in their ability to inhibit or induce various CYP450 isoenzyme subsets. Potential drug–drug interactions between NNRTIs, PIs, and a wide variety of commonly used medications must always be carefully considered.

a. **Nevirapine (Viramune)**

  (1) **Contraindications.** History of severe hypersensitivity reaction to nevirapine.

  (2) **Allergic reactions**

    (a) Cutaneous reactions to nevirapine are the most common treatment-limiting side effects (C). These reactions occur in up to 17% of individuals started on nevirapine and lead to drug discontinuation in 7%. Dose escalation (200 mg once daily for 14 days, followed by 200 mg twice daily thereafter) reduces the incidence of rash for individuals beginning nevirapine therapy. One study found that women had a 7-fold increase in risk for severe rash and a 3.5-fold increase in discontinuation rates compared to men. Most cutaneous reactions occur within the first 6 weeks of therapy. Severity ranges from mild self-limited maculopapular rashes to life-threatening eruptions, including Stevens–Johnson syndrome. Systemic features of a hypersensitivity syndrome, including fever, arthralgias, and myalgias, may be present. Drug rash with eosinophilia and systemic symptoms (DRESS) syndrome has been reported. Nevirapine should be discontinued for severe rash, or rash plus fever, blistering, mucosal membrane involvement, or significant systemic features. If rash occurs during the initial 14 day lead-in dosing period, the dose should not be increased until the rash has resolved. Corticosteroid prophylaxis given for the first 14 days of nevirapine administration has been found in a clinical trial to increase the incidence and severity of rash during the first 6 weeks of therapy.

    (3) **Adverse drug effects** Hepatotoxicity can occur with or without signs of systemic hypersensitivity. Most cases present within the first 12 weeks of therapy; however, up to one third of cases have occurred after this period. Clinical presentations range from mild symptoms of hepatitis to life-threatening hepatic failure. Preexisting elevation in transaminases or a history of chronic hepatitis B or C confers an increased risk for nevirapine-associated hepatotoxicity. Clinical and liver function test monitoring should be intensive over the first 12 weeks of nevirapine administration, as well as in the setting of clinically suspected hepatitis or hypersensitivity. If nevirapine is discontinued because of hepatitis, it should not be restarted.

b. **Efavirenz (Sustiva)**

  (1) **Allergic reactions**

    (a) Rash occurs in up to 26% of those initiating efavirenz therapy, with a median time to onset of 11 days (C). Children experience rash more commonly (up to 40% incidence), with greater severity and earlier onset (median time to onset 8 days) than adults. The most common presentation is a diffuse morbilliform rash, with blistering and desquamation in 1% to 2%, and Stevens–Johnson syndrome occurring quite rarely (0.1%). DRESS syndrome has been reported. In adult clinical trials the drug discontinuation rate was 1.7% because of rash, and the vast majority of individuals are successfully treated through a rash without needing to stop or modify the drug administration. While the mechanism of rash is unknown, a successful 14-day desensitization protocol has been reported.

(b) Leukocytoclastic vasculitis (R).

(c) Pulmonary hypersensitivity (R).

(2) Adverse drug effects.

(a) Central nervous system (CNS) side effects are the most common adverse effect, occurring in up to 50% of those initiating therapy with efavirenz and leading to drug discontinuation in approximately 5%. The incidence of CNS side effects is greatest during the first 2 to 4 weeks of therapy, and such effects usually resolve with time and continued drug administration. Giving efavirenz with food may increase the severity of CNS side effects due to increased blood levels. Typical symptoms include impaired concentration, dizziness, confusion, vivid dreams, hallucinations, insomnia or increased somnolence. Serious psychiatric adverse events are rare, but individuals with preexisting mental health disorders are at higher risk for serious psychiatric adverse events. The drug is usually initially administered at bedtime to improve the tolerability of CNS side effects and to minimize the impact of CNS symptoms on daily activities.

(b) Hepatotoxicity occurs less often than with nevirapine, and severe hepatotoxicity leading to efavirenz discontinuation is rare.

(c) Hyperlipidemia, drug interactions.

(d) Teratogenicity. Efavirenz should be avoided during pregnancy, and women of childbearing age receiving efavirenz need to be counseled about this risk.

c. Delavirdine (Rescriptor)

(1) Allergic reactions

(a) Rash is the most common adverse effect, occurring in up to 44%, and usually within the first 7 to 21 days of treatment. Individuals with lower CD4 counts are at greater risk of developing a rash, although the severity is not related to immune status. Typical rashes are diffuse, erythematous maculopapular eruptions, usually pruritic, and last for approximately 2 weeks during which time the drug may be continued without dose adjustment or discontinuation in the absence of severe symptoms. Erythema multiforme and Stevens–Johnson reactions have been rarely reported.

(2) Adverse drug effects. Hepatotoxicity is less common than with other NNRTIs.

C. Protease Inhibitors (PI)

1. Class-related allergic reactions. Hypersensitivity reactions to the PIs are quite rare (R).

2. Class-related adverse drug effects. More common adverse effects with PIs (seen to varying degrees with individual agents) include diarrhea, nausea, anorexia, GI intolerance, and hepatotoxicity. Severe drug-induced liver injury has been reported but is rare. As a class, fat redistribution syndromes, insulin resistance, and hyperlipidemia can be seen with currently available PI agents. The most recently approved PI, atazanavir, has fewer lipid abnormalities associated with its use. All PIs are metabolized by the cytochrome P450 pathways, and the agents differ in their ability to inhibit or induce various CYP450 isoenzyme subsets. Potential drug–drug interactions between PIs, NNRTIs, and a wide variety of commonly used medications should always be carefully considered.

a. **Saquinavir (Invirase, Fortovase)**
(1) **Allergic reactions.** Fixed drug eruption (R).
(2) **Adverse drug effects.** GI intolerance.

b. **Ritonavir (Norvir)**
(1) **Allergic reactions.** Fixed drug eruptions are rare.
(2) **Adverse drug effects.** GI intolerance (can be severe and treatment limiting at full dose), circumoral paresthesias, peripheral paresthesias, fatigue. Lipid elevations may be more severe in comparison to those associated with other PIs.

c. **Indinavir (Crixivan)**
(1) **Allergic reactions.** Maculopapular rashes (R), leukocytoclastic vasculitis (R).
(2) **Adverse drug effects.** GI intolerance, nephrolithiasis, indirect hyperbilirubinemia, nail changes.

d. **Nelfinavir (Viracept)**
(1) **Allergic reactions.** Urticaria (R). While the mechanism of hypersensitivity is unknown, a successful nelfinavir desensitization protocol has been reported.
(2) **Adverse drug effects.** Diarrhea (reported in up to 30%), GI intolerance, tablet formulation can quickly dissolve in mouth.

e. **Amprenavir (Agenerase)**
(1) **Contraindications.** The oral solution has a relatively high amount of propylene glycol and should not be used in the presence of liver failure, renal failure, pregnancy, alcohol ingestion, and coadministration of disulfiram or metronidazole.
(2) **Allergic reactions**
(a) Rash occurs in up to 22% and can lead to drug discontinuation in 3%. (C) Severe or life-threatening rashes (including Stevens–Johnson syndrome) occur in 1%. Most rashes are maculopapular and appear a median of 11 days after beginning amprenavir therapy. Amprenavir is a sulfonamide; however. the potential for cross-hypersensitivity between sulfonamide agents and amprenavir is not known. Amprenavir should be used with caution in patients with known sulfonamide allergy. Amprenavir should be discontinued in the setting of a severe rash or cutaneous reactions in conjunction with systemic symptoms.

(3) Adverse drug effects. GI intolerance, oral paresthesias. Acute hemolytic anemia (R).
f. Atazanavir (Zrivada)
   (1) Allergic reactions. None reported.
   (2) Adverse drug effects. Indirect hyperbilirubinemia, jaundice.
g. Lipinavir/ritonavir (Kaletra)
   (1) Allergic reactions. Rash is rare overall, but is slightly more common in children than in adults (R).
   (2) Adverse drug effects. Diarrhea (C), GI intolerance (C), asthenia (C), pancreatitis (R), thrombocytopenia (R).

D. Fusion Inhibitors
   Introduction. Enfuvirtide is the first FDA-approved agent of a new class of antiretrovirals called fusion inhibitors.
   1. This drug acts by blocking the fusion of the HIV envelope to its target cell membrane. It is given by twice-daily subcutaneous injection. As with other antiretrovirals, it is used as part of combination drug therapy to construct a HAART regimen.
   a. Enfuvirtide (Fuzeon, T. 20)
      (1) Contraindication. Enfuvirtide is contraindicated in patients with known hypersensitivity to the drug or its components.
      (2) Allergic reactions. Systemic hypersensitivity reactions have been reported; however, the mechanism is unclear. Clinical findings have included fever, rash, nausea and vomiting, rigors, hypotension, and transaminitis. Enfuvirtide should be discontinued if a systemic hypersensitivity reaction occurs, and individuals who have experienced a systemic hypersensitivity reaction should not be rechallenged as symptoms may recur. According to the manufacturer's package insert, other adverse events that may be immune mediated include primary immune complex reaction, respiratory distress, Guillain–Barré syndrome, and glomerulonephritis.
      (3) Adverse drug effects. Local injection site reactions are common (seen in 98% of individuals receiving enfuvirtide), and in clinical studies led to drug discontinuation in 3% and local site infections in 1%. The mechanism and risk factors for injection site reactions are unknown. Clinical features include local pain, induration, erythema, pruritus, nodules, cysts, and ecchymosis. Increased rates of bacterial pneumonia were seen in individuals receiving enfuvirtide in clinical trials. Other adverse events noted in clinical trials include diarrhea, nausea, fatigue, anorexia, myalgia, weight loss, appetite loss, influenza-like illness, sinusitis, herpes simplex, skin papilloma, taste disturbance, cough, peripheral neuropathy, insomnia, anxiety, depression, eosinophilia, transaminitis, pancreatitis, constipation, abdominal pain, conjunctivitis, and lymphadenopathy.

IV. Miscellaneous agents used in the management of HIV-1

**Table 26.1. Protocol for oral desensitization
to trimethoprim–sulfamethoxazole**

Hour	Dose of TMP-SMX
0	0.004/0.02 mg[a]
1	0.04/0.2 mg[a]
2	0.4/2 mg[a]
3	4/20 mg[a]
4	40/200 mg[a]
5	160/800 mg[b]

[a]Dilution of TMP-SMX oral suspension (40 mg TMP and
200 mg SMX per 5 mL).
[b]TMP-SMX (160/800 mg) tablet.
TMP, trimethoprim; SMX, sulfamethoxazole.
Adapted with permission from Gluckstein D, Ruskin J. Rapid
oral desensitization to trimethoprim–sulfamethoxazole
(TMP-SMZ): use in prophylaxis for *Pneumocystis carinii*
pneumonia in patients with AIDS who were previously intolerant to TMP-SMZ. *Clin Infect Dis* 1995;20:849–853.

**A. Trimethoprim–sulfamethoxazole (TMP-SMX; Bac-
trim, Septra, Cotrimoxazole)** is used against a variety of
opportunistic pathogens encountered in the management of
HIV, including *Pneumocystis carinii, Toxoplasma gondii, No-
cardia* spp, and some enteric pathogens. Sulfonamides, including TMP-SMX, are associated with the highest rates of
hypersensitivity reactions in HIV-infected individuals (C).
Prior to the HAART era, it was recognized that up to 65% of
persons treated with high-dose TMP-SMX for *P. carinii* pneumonia would develop a hypersensitivity reaction, versus approximately 3% for those with other immunosuppressive conditions. Hypersensitivity to TMP-SMX is dose dependent (more
common with higher dosages used for treatment versus lower
dosages used for prophylaxis) and time dependent (earlier onset with higher dosages). The degree of immune suppression at
the time of TMP-SMX initiation may influence the risk of hypersensitivity. The cause of TMP-SMX hypersensitivity is unclear, but potential mechanisms include the formation of toxic
metabolites (e.g., hydroxylamines) in combination with genetic
(e.g., slow acetylation) or acquired defects (e.g., glutathione deficiency) in drug metabolism. Cross-hypersensitivity between
TMP-SMX and other sulfonamides as well as dapsone has been
reported.
   1. Contraindication. History of severe hypersensitivity
   reaction to sulfonamides.
   2. Allergic reactions
      a. Hypersensitivity reactions commonly include fever
      and rash (typically morbilliform or maculopapular, dif-
      fuse and pruritic), and less commonly severe reactions,
      including serum sickness, erythema multiforme, and
      Stevens–Johnson syndrome, can occur. Gradual initiation

of TMP-SMX is associated with fewer ADRs when used as prophylaxis. Individuals who experience mild to moderate initial reactions can be rechallenged successfully, either by dose escalation or direct rechallenge. Gradual dose escalation using desensitization protocols can be utilized and may increase the likelihood of a successful rechallenge. One published desensitization protocol is outlined below in Table 26.1.

b. Adverse drug effects. GI intolerance, myelosuppression, hyperkalemia, renal impairment, hepatitis, tremor, ataxia, clonus.

SELECTED READINGS

Carr A, Cooper DA. Adverse effects of antiretroviral therapy. *Lancet* 2000;356:1423–1430.

Carr A, Garsia R. How HIV leads to hypersensitivity reactions. *Med J Aust* 1996;164:227–229.

Carr A, Penny R, Cooper DA. Allergy and desensitization to zidovudine in patients with acquired immunodeficiency syndrome (AIDS). *J Allergy Clin Immunol* 1993;91(2):683–685.

Demoly P, Messaad D, Trylesinski A, et al. Nelfinavir-induced urticaria and successful desensitization. *J Allergy Clin Immunol* 1998;102:875–876.

Gluckstein D, Ruskin J. Rapid oral desensitization to trimethoprim–sulfamethoxazole (TMP-SMZ): use in prophylaxis for *Pneumocystis carinii* pneumonia in patients with AIDS who were previously intolerant to TMP-SMZ. *Clin Infect Dis* 1995;20:849–853.

Immunology/urban.handbook.hiv drug

Mallal S, Nolan D, Witt C, et al. Association between presence of HLA-B*5701, HLA-DR7, and HLA-DQ3 and hypersensitivity to HIV-1 reverse-transcriptase inhibitor abacavir. *Lancet* 2002;359: 727–732.

Para MF, Finkelstein D, Becker S, et al. Reduced toxicity with gradual initiation of trimethoprim-sulfamethoxazole as primary prophylaxis for *Pneumocystis carinii* pneumonia: AIDS clinical trials group 268. *J AIDS* 2000;24:337–343.

Phillips EJ, Kuriakose B, Knowles SR. Efavirenz-induced skin eruption and successful desensitization. *Ann Pharmacother* 2002;36: 430–432.

Ryan C, Madalon M, Wortham DW, et al. Sulfa hypersensitivity in patients with HIV infection: onset, treatment, critical review of the literature. *WMJ* 1998;97(5):23–27.

27

Genetically Engineered Medications

Burton Zweiman

This is a recent and rapidly developing field with new products undergoing clinical evaluation all the time. Therefore, the evidence in selected agents summarized below must understandably be limited and preliminary.

I. **Genetically engineered drugs**
   A. **Infliximab (Remicade).** Chimeric monoclonal antibody against tumor necrosis factor-α (TNF-α).
      1. **Contraindications.** Anaphylactic reaction to previous infliximab infusion, active tuberculosis.
      2. **Allergic reactions.** Pruritus, urticaria, anaphylaxis ($<1\%$) (R).
      3. **Nonallergic reactions.**
         a. **Infusion reactions.** Within 1 to 2 hours: fever, chills, chest pain, hypotension, dyspnea (up to 20%) (C).
         b. Rash (various types) (C).
         c. Activation of underlying tuberculosis.
   B. **Etanercept (Enbrel).** Soluble TNF receptor Fc fusion protein (competes with TNF-α for binding to its receptor).
      1. **Contraindications.** None known.
      2. **Allergic reactions.** Urticaria (R).
      3. **Nonallergic reactions.** Injection site reactions: generally mild (C).
   C. **Rituximab (Rituxan).** Chimeric monoclonal anti-CD20 antibody: depletes circulating B cells.
      1. **Contraindications.** Anaphylactic reactivity to murine proteins.
      2. **Allergic reactions.** Cough, dyspnea, bronchospasm, serum sickness (C).
      3. **Nonallergic reactions.** Central nervous system, rash, dyspepsia (R).
   D. **Recombinant tissue plasminogen activator (t-PA, TNKase)**
      1. **Contraindications.** Bleeding (active or diathesis), history of cerebrovascular accident, aneurysm.
      2. **Allergic reactions.** Anaphylaxis, angioedema are rare, but angioedema likely more common in individuals receiving concomitant angiotensin-converting enzyme inhibitor therapy.
      3. **Nonallergic reactions.** Bleeding, cardiogenic (U).
   E. **Alemtuzumab (Campth–1H).** Monoclonal antibody against CD52 epitope present on almost all B lymphocytes in chronic lymphocytic leukemia.
      1. **Contraindications.** Anaphylactic reaction to prior Campth–1H infusion.

   2. Allergic reactions (R).

   3. Non-allergic reactions. Fever, rigor, nausea, vomiting, hypotension [thought due to excess release of TNF-α and interleukin-6 (IL-6); generally responsive to corticosteroid treatment]. These manifestations are usually less severe with subsequent infusions.

  F. Daclizumab (Zenapax). Humanized monoclonal antibody against the CD25 epitope in the receptor for IL-2.

   1. Tolerability reported similar to that of placebo.

  G. Trastuzumab (Herceptin). Humanized monoclonal antibody against the epidermal growth factor receptor (HER2) on breast cancer cells in 25% of cases.

   1. Contraindications. None yet (no known way of screening for risk for cardiotoxicity adverse effects described below).

   2. Allergic reactions. Anaphylaxis, infusion reactions (R).

   3. Nonallergic reactions. Cardiotoxicity (ventricular dysfunction, CHF) (C). Sequential monitoring required.

  H. Palivizamab (Synagis). Humanized monoclonal antibody against the respiratory syncytial virus.

   1. Contraindications. None.

   2. Allergic reactions (R).

   3. Non-allergic reactions. Fever, irritability, injection site reactions common (10% but more common than in controls).

  I. Sargramostim (Leukine). Recombinant human granulocyte-macrophage colony-stimulating factor cytokine.

   1. Contraindications. Hemopoietic malignancy, concomitant chemotherapy, radiotherapy. Sensitivity to yeast-derived products.

   2. Allergic reactions. Rash at injection site (C).

   3. Nonallergic reactions. Fever, myalgia (C).

  J. Omalizumab (Xolair). See page 61.

  II. Concluding remarks. Immediate reactions (local and systemic) during infusion of a number of genetically engineered agents are not unusual, as described above. However, it is not clear whether these manifestations are due to true immune responses or to other mechanisms, such as the release of proinflammatory mediators.

SELECTED READING

Huston JS, George AJ. Engineered antibodies take center stage. *Hum Antibodies* 2001;10:127–142.

28

Approach to the Patient with Multiple Drug Allergies

James H. Sussman

I. Overview.
  A. History is most important.
  B. Classify adverse drug reaction.
  C. Assess risk for multiple drug allergy syndrome.
  D. Diagnostic testing.
  E. Treatment of the patient with multiple drug allergies.
  F. Other considerations.
II. History.
  A. List all recent and current drugs.
    1. Prescriptions.
    2. Over the counter.
    3. Alternative or homeopathic.
    4. Herbals.
  B. History of exposure to drug or cross-reacting drugs.
  C. Timing between drug administration and onset of symptoms.
    1. If no prior exposure, interval usually 1 to 4 weeks.
    2. If prior exposure, reaction occurs within minutes to hours.
    3. Construct a graph denoting start and stop days of drugs and symptoms.
  D. Drug dosing.
    1. Small doses may trigger severe allergic reactions.
    2. Larger doses more likely trigger drug toxicity.
  E. Symptoms.
    1. Compatibility with immunopathogenic response.
    2. Characteristics of skin lesions.
    3. Vasovagal symptoms.
    4. Hysterical symptoms.
  F. Reported propensity for drug to cause observed reaction.
  G. Drugs most frequently involved in allergic drug reactions (80% of reactions occur from drugs belonging to classes 1 to 3 below).
    1. Aspirin and Nonsteroidal anti-inflammatory drugs (NSAIDs).
    2. β-Lactam antibiotics.
    3. Sulfonamides (antibacterial, hypoglycemics, diuretics, some cyclooxygenase-2 inhibitors).
    4. Antituberculous drugs (isoniazid, rifampin).
    5. Nitrofurans.
    6. Anticonvulsants (hydantoin, carbamazepine).
    7. Anesthetics (muscle relaxants, thiopental).
    8. Allopurinol.
    9. Antipsychotics.

    10. Radiocontrast media.
    11. Antihypertensives (angiotensin-converting enzyme inhibitors, methyldopa).
    12. Antiarrhythmics (procainamide, quinidine).
    13. Heavy metals (gold salts).
    14. Biologics (insulin, other hormones).
    15. Antisera (antitoxins, monoclonal antibodies).
    16. Enzymes (L-asparaginase, streptokinase, chymopapain).
    17. Vaccines.
    18. Latex.
  H. Drugs least likely to cause allergic reactions.
    1. Estrogens.
    2. Thyroid preparations.
    3. Vitamins.
    4. Minerals.
III. Classification of adverse drug reactions.
  A. Type A reactions (80% of all reactions).
    1. Features: Predictable, dose-dependent, related to known drug action.
    2. Toxic reactions.
    3. Side effects.
    4. Secondary effects.
    5. Drug interactions.
  B. Type B reactions (20% of reactions).
    1. Features: Unpredictable, not related to known pharmacologic actions.
    2. Drug intolerance.
    3. Idiosyncratic reactions.
    4. Allergic.
    5. Pseudoallergic.
  C. Allergic reactions.
    1. Require period of sensitization (prior exposure with no reaction).
    2. Appears after minimum of several days of treatment if no prior exposure.
    3. Restricted to a limited number of syndromes associated with immunopathologic responses (anaphylaxis, asthma, urticaria, angioedema, skin eruption).
    4. Occur in a small percentage of the population.
    5. Triggered by small, subtherapeutic doses.
    6. Resolve after withdrawal of offending drug (although some reactions may persist for days to months).
    7. Often difficult to classify by Gell and Coombs mechanisms.
    8. Not prevented by pretreatment with corticosteroids and antihistamines.
  D. Pseudoallergic reactions.
    1. Refers to immediate generalized reaction not caused by immunoglobulin E (IgE). Independent mast cell mediator release.
    2. Mimics anaphylaxis without involving drug-specific IgE antibodies.
    3. May occur in patients without a prior exposure to the offending agent.

    4. Caused by agents that directly stimulate mast cell mediator release such as opiates, vancomycin, polymyxin B, and D-tubocurare.

    5. Can be prevented by pretreatment with corticosteroids and antihistamines or by slowing infusion rate (e.g., "red man syndrome" with vancomycin).

  E. Multiple drug allergy syndrome.

    1. Penicillin-allergic patients have a tenfold risk of having an allergic reaction to non–β-lactam antimicrobials (57% of allergic reactions are to sulfonamides).

    2. Reactions include rash, urticaria, angioedema, anaphylaxis, Stevens–Johnson syndrome, serum sickness, and immune cytopenias.

    3. Likely related to a propensity for the individual to make immune responses to haptens expressing variable immunopathology.

    4. Risk factors: genetic factors, family history, prior drug reaction, concurrent medical illness.

IV. Diagnostic tests for drug hypersensitivity.

  A. Limitations.

    1. Limited by incomplete understanding of clinically relevant drug metabolites and immunopathologic mechanisms.

  B. Immediate hypersensitivity.

    1. Skin testing for immediate hypersensitivity reactions is limited to penicillin, streptokinase, antilymphocyte globulin, and other high molecular weight polypeptides.

    2. Skin testing to nonirritative concentrations of other antibiotics might be useful but false negatives are problematic.

    3. In vitro IgE tests limited (radioallergosorbent test, enzyme-linked immunosorbent assay).

    4. Assays for IgM and IgG unlikely to have clinical relevance.

  C. T-cell-mediated reactions.

    1. Patch testing may predict T-lymphocyte-mediated reactions such as drug-induced morbilliform eruptions, fixed drug eruptions, bullous reactions, erythroderma, and erythema multiforme.

    2. General laboratory tests such as liver function tests, metabolic profile, complete blood count, total hemolytic complement, and antinuclear antibodies to assess for hepatic or renal involvement or drug-induced lupus.

    3. Lymphocyte blast transformation, leukocyte toxicity assays, and mast cell–and basophil-derived mediator assays await standardization before they will be clinically useful.

  D. Summary.

    1. No single diagnostic tool is the "gold standard" in evaluating drug allergy.

V. Treatment of the patient with multiple drug allergies.

  A. Establish connection between the drug and the reaction.

  B. Seek alternative therapy.

  C. If particular agent is absolutely essential and mechanism is thought to be pseudoallergic, may administer after pretreatment with corticosteroids and antihistamines (see Chapter 20 for pretreatment protocol for radiocontrast media).

D.   If mechanism is allergic (IgE mediated), consider desensitization in an intensive care unit setting (see Chapters 1 and 2 for antibiotic protocols).

E.   Desensitization should not be performed if patient has had a prior severe drug-induced cutaneous skin reaction such as Steven–Johnson syndrome, erythroderma, exfoliative dermatitis, or toxic epidermal necrolysis.

F.   In non-IgE-mediated immunologic reactions, consider graded drug challenge.

VI.   Other considerations.

A.   Employ aggressive measures to prevent infections in patients with multiple antibiotic sensitivity, including vaccination and avoidance of exposures.

B.   Use antibiotics only for well-documented infections.

C.   Reassure fearful patient that if other alternative medications cannot be found, premedication, desensitization, and graded drug challenge are available.

D.   Provide detailed feedback to the patient's other health care providers.

SELECTED READINGS

Bonner JR. Drug allergy. In: Goldman L, Bennett JC, eds. Cecil textbook of medicine. Philadelphia: W. B. Saunders, 2000:1463–66.

Demoly P, Bousquet J. Drug allergy diagnosis work up. *Allergy* 2002;57:37–40.

Gruchalla RS. Approach to the patient with multiple antibiotic sensitivities. *Allergy Asthma Proc* 2002;21(1):39–44.

Gruchalla RS. Drug allergy. *J Allergy Clin Immunol* 2003;111:S548–59.

Sullivan TJ. Drug Allergy. In: Middleton E, Reed CE, Ellis EF, Adkinson NF, Yunginger JW, Busse WW, eds. Allergy principles and practice, 4th Ed. New York: Mosby Book Publishing, 1993:1726–46.

29

When to Refer Patients with Adverse Drug Reactions to a Specialist

George R. Green

I. When to refer. The diagnosis and management of adverse drug reactions is an integral part of the practice of all physicians. In many cases, when an adverse drug reaction is suspected, it is common practice to have them discontinue the medication, advise the patient of the reaction, and document same in medical record. When a medication is necessary for treatment, a substitute will be made preferably using a medication that is sufficiently chemically and structurally different that it will not likely cross-react.

However, there are situations in which the problem becomes more complex either because the diagnosis is uncertain or because it is not easy to identify the offending agent, particularly in patients who are on multiple medications. These instances may precipitate a referral to a specialist to help manage the problem of the adverse drug reaction.

II. To Whom to Refer. Often the most appropriate referral would be to a specialist who manages the condition for which the medications are being prescribed. He or she will have a great deal more familiarity with the adverse drug reaction profile of the suspect medication, as well as alternative ways to manage the problem without using a cross-reacting drug. A majority of the chapters of this book are written by specialists in various fields because they have the most familiarity with the adverse drug reaction profile of the medications that they use most frequently.

The β-lactam antibiotics present a unique instance in which referral to an allergist can be very useful. This is the only widely used group of medications where studies have shown a close correlation of skin test results and true sensitivity to these medications. The introduction and licensing of the peniclloyl polylysine in the 1970s provided a unique opportunity whereby the physician could clarify if there is a reasonable likelihood that the patient was indeed allergically sensitive to β-lactam antibiotics. It is unfortunate that the minor determinate mixture has yet to be approved for commercial use, but nevertheless multiple studies have shown that testing with peniclloyl polylysine as well as penicillin gives highly useful information in the management of patients with reputed sensitivity to the β-lactam antibiotics. This information not only allows us to frequently treat patients with serious infections with the appropriate β-lactam antibiotic despite a history of reputed sensitivity to the drugs, but also allows us to reduce the cost and toxicity of alternative medications such as vancomycin for these common infections.

The allergist may also be useful in consultation to help sort out and treat the patient with what appears to be an adverse drug reaction, except that the agent is unconfirmed or the patient is sensitive to multiple drugs, creating a serious therapeutic dilemma in management.

Skin testing is also useful for a limited array of other drugs, primarily those that are proteins, such as insulin. There are instances in which the allergist can also use this skill in developing a desensitization protocol when it is absolutely necessary to use a drug to which the patient is sensitive.

III. Summary. Physicians who prescribe a medication are generally able to manage the issue of adverse drug reactions in their patients. However, some situations are complicated by a patient history in which the nature of the offending agent is unclear, especially if the patient was or is on multiple medications, or it appears necessary to continue the same or similar agents for the care of the patient. In these instances, referral to a specialist whose primary practice involves the use of the suspect class of medication may be warranted. In some instances, a physician with training in allergy and immunology may be consulted, particularly if clinical management can be affected by specific testing, the problem involves multiple drugs where there is marked uncertainty as to the likely offending agent, or a desensitization protocol may be required for clinical management. Dermatologists may be of help when the skin manifestations are unusual or severe, and a physician in this specific specialty who commonly uses the suspect drugs may be of greatest assistance when decisions regarding alternative therapy are complex.

30

Drug Reporting

Richard W. Honsinger

I. Before a drug is released to the public, it is tested on average on only 2,500 to 3,000 patients. These patients are highly selected for treatment and thus cannot represent a wider population. Consequently, adverse drug reactions often become apparent in the period of postmarketing surveillance. Anaphylaxis to a drug is often not apparent until a patient has been exposed several times. Angioedema from angiotensin-converting inhibitors was rare enough that it was not apparent until the drug had been marketed.

Patient reports often occur before physicians are aware of the problem. However, the U.S. Food and Drug Administration (FDA) has found that patient reports are incomplete and thus encourages patients to report through their physicians.

II. In the United States the FDA offers the program MedWatch. This program offers safety information and compiles safety information before release to the public. The MedWatch voluntary reporting forms are easily accessed on the internet at www.fda.gov/ or found in publications such as the *Physicians' Desk Reference (PDR)*. You may also report to the FDA by telephone at 1-800-FDA-1088. A form can be faxed to the FDA at 1-800-FDA-0178.

Other countries likewise are installing programs to report adverse drug reactions. The United Kingdom Medicines Control Agency has extended reporting to nurses as well as physicians and pharmacists. In 2003 the United Kingdom National Health Service will have a direct phone line for reporting adverse drug reactions by patients.

III. A severe adverse drug reaction that is unsuspected at the time of release may lead to a drug's being withdrawn. Only one half of drug withdrawals occur in the first 2 years after release. Health care providers are morally obligated to participate in this volunteer reporting system. User facilities such as hospitals and nursing homes are legally required to report suspected medical device–related deaths to both the FDA and the manufacturer. Serious injuries must be reported to the manufacturer or, if the manufacturer is unknown, they must be reported to the FDA.

IV. The FDA's MedWatch site does not include vaccines. There is a vaccine adverse event reporting system web site at www.vaers.org.

V. The administration of a drug to a patient who has a known allergy to the drug is a preventable error. When paper charts are being used, there should be a system in place that labels the front of the chart and any medication lists. As our hospitals and outpatient practices convert to computerized medical records, prescriptions, and medication orders, systems must be in place that will alert the practitioner when a drug allergy exists. Such actions should prevent the prescribing of drugs that can cause serious reactions in patients who have a known drug allergy.

The Institute of Medicine report in 1999 focused on the morbidity, mortality, and expense of medical errors. The economic impact of drug allergy is addressed in Chapter 31.

SELECTED READINGS

Kohn LT, Corrigan JM, Donaldson MS, eds. *To err is human: building a safer health system.* Washington, DC: National Academy Press, 1999. Also available on line at Institute of Medicine: www.iom.edu.

Lasser DE, Allen PD, Woolhander SJ, et al., eds. *Timing of new black box warnings and withdrawals for prescription medications* JAMA 2002;287:2215–2220.

U.S. Food and Drug Administration. MedWatch Reporting System: www.fda.gov/.

Vaccine Adverse Event Reporting System: www.vaers.org.

31

Economic Impact of Adverse Drug Reactions

David B. Nash, Adam Stuart Evans, and
Stephen J. Tai

I. **Definition of adverse drug events (ADEs), adverse drug reactions (ADRs), and medication errors**
  A. **Adverse drug events (ADE)**
    1. Any injury caused by a drug-related medical intervention.
    2. Consists of both ADRs and medication errors.
  B. **Adverse drug reaction (ADR)**
    1. The World Health Organization defines an ADR as any response to a drug "which is noxious and unintended and which occurs at doses used in man for prophylaxis, diagnosis, or therapy."
  C. **Medication errors**
    1. Errors that occur in ordering, dispensing, and administering medications.
II. **Incidence of ADRs**
  A. ADRs occur in about 5% of all hospitalized patients.
  B. ADRs occur in 5% to 10% of all outpatients.
    1. Less than 1% of all outpatients are sent to the hospital because of ADRs.
    2. ADRs represent approximately 5% of all hospital admissions.
  C. ADRs result in more than 100,000 deaths annually.
III. **Overall costs**
  A. Costs can be broken down as direct and indirect.
    1. **Direct costs.** Caused by hospitalization, laboratory tests, invasive procedures, etc.
    2. **Indirect costs.** Caused by mortality, loss of productivity and unemployment, disability.
  B. **Estimates**
    1. Annual direct costs estimated at 76.6 billion dollars with majority (47 billion dollars) being related to hospital admissions.
    2. Compared to annual medical spending on:
      a. Obesity: 45.8 billion dollars
      b. Diabetes: 45.2 billion dollars
      c. Cardiovascular disease: 117 billion to 154 billion dollars
IV. **Direct costs**
  A. **Hospitalization**
    1. Occurrence of ADRs significantly prolongs hospital length of stay, increases costs as well as mortality.
    2. ADRs found to increase length of stay from 2 to 3 days at a cost of approximately 2,000 to 3,000 dollars.
  B. **Additional diagnosis, treatment, and physician fees**

    1. Examples of ADRs are rash, nausea, itching, fever, vomiting, and diarrhea.

    2. Estimated costs per patient due to:

        a. Fever: 9,022 dollars [including average length of stay (LOS) increase 5.5 days]

        b. Itching: 677 dollars (LOS increase by 0.7 day)

        c. Rash: 1,868 dollars (LOS increase by 1.4 days)

        d. Diarrhea: 4,631 dollars (LOS increase by 4.4 days)

        e. Vomiting: 712 dollars (LOS increase by 1.4 days)

    3. One hospital found that the cost of additional outcomes from ADEs was 1.5 million dollars per year.

        a. Noninvasive procedures 2.8%

        b. Additional laboratory tests 3.5%

        c. Additional treatment 9.8%

        d. Invasive monitoring or procedures 16.8%

        e. Increased LOS 19.9%

        f. Transfer to ICU 47.2%

V. **Indirect costs**

  A. **There are no studies that have estimated the indirect costs of ADRs.**

    1. Difficult to quantify costs

  B. **Types of indirect costs**

    1. Mortality. Estimated that patients who experience an ADE face twice the risk of death.

    2. Loss of productivity and unemployment

    3. Disability. Estimated that approximately 10% of ADEs cause permanent disability.

VI. **Limitations of economic analysis**

  A. Difficult to attribute the adverse reaction directly to the drug. Could be due to an underlying disease or interactions with other medications.

  B. Most of the research has been with hospitalized patients; not much research in other settings.

  C. Difficult to measure indirect costs.

  D. Debate over what exactly constitutes ADEs, ADRs, and medication errors.

  E. Much of the research has been conducted by a few hospitals.

VII. **Preventable ADEs**

  A. Two types of ADE

    1. Type A: Preventable

        a. Approximately one third of ADEs are avoidable.

        b. Related to dosage or pharmacology of drug.

    2. Type B: Unpreventable

  B. Preventable ADEs are approximately twice as costly as average ADEs

    1. Average ADEs–Approximate LOS increase by 2 days: 3,000 dollars

    2. Preventable ADEs–Approximate LOS increase 4 to 5 days: 6,000 dollars

  C. Preventable ADEs accounted for half of all ADE costs in one hospital study, despite constituting fewer than one third of all ADEs

  D. Total cost of preventable drug-related morbidity and mortality in the United States, including both direct and indirect costs, may range from 138 billion dollars to 182 billion dollars annually.

VIII. Possible solutions for reducing ADEs, ADRs, and medication errors

   A. Pharmacy/pharmacist-based solutions

     1. Development of pharmacy-based intravenous and unit dosing systems.

       a. Advantages. System of checks requires multiple-provider approval for medication distribution.

       b. Obstacles

         (1) Lack of understanding on the part of health care professionals about how these systems work.

         (2) Requires significant effort by hospitals and pharmacists to maintain system.

     2. More involvement of pharmacists in clinical areas.

     3. Advantages. Cooperation of pharmacists and providers should reduce incidence of ADEs.

     4. Obstacles. Increased costs of hiring more qualified pharmacists for care and medicine distribution

     5. Make 24-hour pharmacist support available.

   B. Education solutions

     1. Health care providers

       a. Limited training on prevention of ADRs and ADEs to medical students and residents.

       b. ADE training programs do not exist in more than half of all medical schools.

       c. Only about two thirds of internal medicine residencies have official lectures pertaining to ADRs.

     2. Patients

       a. Greater efforts in instruction of proper uses of their medication.

       b. Increased educational efforts should also reduce non-compliance.

   C. Information technology solutions

     1. Computerized surveillance system. Analyzes clinical signs described by nurses, laboratory tests, drug concentrations, and pharmacy orders for possible ADEs.

       a. Advantages

         (1) Reduces medication errors.

         (2) Early feedback to physicians, which results in potential problems being averted.

       b. Obstacles

         (1) Concern of liability for the ADE.

         (2) Insufficient resources for surveillance and reporting.

         (3) Difficult to attribute the ADE directly to the drug.

         (4) No incentive for monitoring and reporting ADEs.

     2. Computerized physician order entry

       a. Advantages

         (1) Prevent prescribing, dispensing, and administration errors.

         (2) Superior accuracy and speed in communicating orders.

         (3) Can gather information for electronic patient medical records.

(4) Can automatically notify providers of medication interactions, allergies, and possible dosage errors.
   b. Obstacles
   (1) Large installation costs.
   (2) Significantly increased time to enter orders.
   (3) Varying levels of comfort with computers among providers.
3. Machine-readable coding in hospitals
   a. Advantages. Increases safety by ensuring match of medication orders, preparation, dispensation, and administration of medication to the proper patient.
   b. Obstacles
   (1) Cost of hardware that produces and reads the coded labels.
   (2) Most drug manufacturers do not code labels down to the unit dose package level.

SELECTED READINGS

Bates DW, Burrows AM, Grossman DG, et al. Top priority actions for preventing adverse drug events in hospitals: recommendations of an expert panel. *Am J Health Syst Pharm* 1996;53:747–751.

Bates DW, Spell N, Cullen DJ, et al. The costs of adverse drug events in hospitalized patients. Adverse Drug Events Prevention Study Group. *JAMA* 1997;277:307–311.

Classen DC, Pestotnik SL, Evans RS, et al. Adverse drug events in hospitalized patients. Excess length of stay, extra costs, and attributable mortality. *JAMA* 1997;277:301–306.

Evans RS, Pestotnik SL, Classen DC, et al. Preventing adverse drug events in hospitalized patients. *Ann Pharmacother* 1994;28:523–527.

Karch FE, Lasagna L. Adverse drug reactions. A critical review. *JAMA* 1975;234:1236–1241.

Moore N, Lecointre D, Noblet C, et al. Frequency and cost of serious adverse drug reactions in a department of general medicine. *Br J Clin Pharmacol* 1998;45:301–308.

Subject Index

Note: Page numbers followed by "f" refer to figures; those followed by "t" refer to tables.